Dear Linh:
I hope you enjoy my
recent book!
Best, Gerardo Chowell.
09/12/16

Mathematical and Statistical Modeling for Emerging and Re-emerging Infectious Diseases

Gerardo Chowell · James M. Hyman
Editors

Mathematical and Statistical Modeling for Emerging and Re-emerging Infectious Diseases

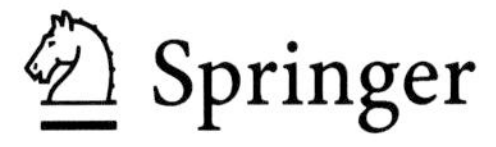

Springer

Editors
Gerardo Chowell
School of Public Health
Georgia State University
Atlanta, GA
USA

James M. Hyman
Department of Mathematics
Tulane University
New Orleans, LA
USA

ISBN 978-3-319-40411-0 ISBN 978-3-319-40413-4 (eBook)
DOI 10.1007/978-3-319-40413-4

Library of Congress Control Number: 2016942897

Printed on acid-free paper

This Springer imprint is published by Springer Nature
The registered company is Springer International Publishing AG Switzerland

Preface

Mathematical modelers are joining with biological, epidemiological, behavioral, and social science studies to produce better projections and better understanding of the transmission dynamics of infectious diseases. They are working with public health workers to create new tools for devising effective strategies to minimize the emergence, impact, and spread of epidemics. For these tools to be useful and used, the decision-makers must fully understand the assumptions, such as any behavior changes of the population during an epidemic, used in defining the model and how sensitive the model predictions, such as the number of people infected, depend upon these assumptions. That is, a clear description of the model formulation and sensitivity analysis of the predictions are both necessary to quantify the uncertainty in the model forecasts.

This collection of articles by epidemic modeling experts describe how these models are created to capture the most important aspects of an emerging epidemic. It provides examples of how these models can help public health workers better understand the spread of infections and reduce the uncertainty of the estimates of disease prevalence. That is, the analysis and model simulations can quantify the relative importance of the complex mechanisms driving the spread of an infection and anticipate the future course of an epidemic. In addition to models focusing on forecasting and controlling infections, the volume contains a discussion on the modern statistical modeling methods to design, conduct, and analyze clinical trials measuring the effectiveness of potential vaccines.

The focus of the volume is on models based on the underlying transmission mechanisms of an infectious agent, rather than statistical forecasting of past trends to predict future incidence. These mechanistic models can help anticipate the emergence and evaluate the potential effectiveness of different approaches for bringing an epidemic under control. Recently, the models have been used to help understand and predict the spread of emerging and re-emerging infectious diseases including Zika, Middle East Respiratory Syndrome, chikungunya, and Ebola. They have been helpful to better understand the impact of increased resistance of well-established diseases such as gonorrhea, tuberculosis, and bronchitis to the antibiotics that once held them in check. The models are being developed to help guide public health workers in controlling infections that have proven difficult to immunize against and to treat once they occur, including influenza, HIV/AIDS, and the common cold. The transmission models are being coupled with cost–benefit analysis to facilitate estimating the relative impact of possible interventions and forecast the requirements that an epidemic will place on the health care system.

In the first chapter, Richard Rothenberg discusses the role of epidemic models to confront public health emergencies including the HIV/AIDS epidemic in the US and the recent 2014 Ebola epidemic in West Africa. This is followed by chapters on how modeling the transmission and control of the Ebola virus disease can capture the behavior changes in the population, the effect of movement restrictions on Ebola control, the impact of early diagnosis and isolation, the performance of ring vaccination strategies, and the use of optimal control theory to guide the number of sickbeds during epidemics.

The volume contains articles on how structured models can be used to address public health policy questions relevant for infectious diseases ranging from waterborne diseases, such as cholera to sexually transmitted infections, such as chlamydia. The articles include an analysis of the role of mass immunization campaigns in controlling measles in Sao Paulo, Brazil in the 1990s in the presence of behavior-dependent vaccination. Other contributions include an evaluation of the impact of including or excluding disease-induced mortality rates on disease dynamics using detailed agent-based model simulations of pandemic influenza and a quantitative framework for modeling household transmission using compartmental models of infectious disease.

We hope the contributions in this volume will incite further research in the field of mathematical epidemiology.

Atlanta, GA, USA Gerardo Chowell
New Orleans, LA, USA James M. Hyman

Contents

A Reality of Its Own

Richard Rothenberg

> *But however small it was, it had, nevertheless, the mysterious property of its kind—put back into the mind, it became at once very exciting, and important; and as it darted and sank, and flashed hither and thither, set up such a wash and tumult of ideas that it was impossible to sit still.*
>
> –Virginia Woolf, A Room of One's Own, 1929

In September 2014, the CDC published a supplement to the MMWR that announced a worst-case estimate of 1.4 million cases of Ebola in Liberia and Sierra Leone [1]. The epidemic was then 6 months old and 8,000 cases had been reported. It was estimated that at least 2.5 times that many had occurred, and the 1.4 million was based on the then estimated incidence of 21,000 cases in 6 months. The method was mathematically simple—based primarily on mean incubation period, contact index, and specific sets of patient circumstances—but the details were complicated. *Ex post facto*, the estimate was roundly criticized in the media [2]. It was defended with the imperative that attention must be paid; that a large number draws that attention; and that being wrong is a lesser sin than ignoring the problem. They might have added that the quantitation was, in essence, a qualitative statement: if we don't do something NOW, this will get very BIG.

From a public health perspective, the NOW…BIG approach has a lot to recommend it. From a modeling perspective, not so much. In fact, modelers shudder at the thought of being so wrong, of ignoring the nuances, of using simplistic methods when subtle ones, taking advantage of the enormous computing power available, are bypassed. The polarization of these positions is perhaps unavoidable, and despite attempts at rapprochement (CDC did make it clear that this was a "quick and dirty" approach that was seeking the worst case scenario), the gulf is difficult to bridge. That may be because, like so many polarizations in our current life, the two sides

R. Rothenberg (✉)
Georgia State University, Atlanta, USA
e-mail: rrothenberg@gsu.edu

G. Chowell and J.M. Hyman (eds.), *Mathematical and Statistical Modeling for Emerging and Re-emerging Infectious Diseases*,
DOI 10.1007/978-3-319-40413-4_1

represent competing world views. CDC is a practical, pragmatic and action oriented organization. Some people at CDC were crunching numbers, but a lot more people were on the ground, exposed, digging in. Modelers rarely use Hazmat suits in their daily lives, and consciously create a reality within which they can pose and answer questions. For them, the immediate stakes are low, but the intermediate and longer term stakes are higher; for CDC, the immediate stakes are paramount (though it would be unfair to accuse them of ignoring the long term). Of course, both world views are justifiable: we have to deal with the here and now, and we must also let the "wash and tumult of ideas" lead us to good answers.

But short or long, the path to good answers is tortuous. Often, the first problem cited is parsimony versus complexity [3]. It is usually a given that the "best" model is the most parsimonious: it is the best description of the data with the fewest variables [4]. To borrow Einstein's famous phrase, a model should be "…as simple as possible, but not simpler." This view is consonant with statistical modeling, wherein the addition of a variable to, say, a regression equation fails to improve its explanatory value (for example, provides little or no increase in R^2). But in modeling transmission dynamics, the comparison may be a distraction. A better contrast may be between simplicity and reality. In this comparison, the tension is between a model that tries to define a few critical elements (a kind of parsimony) and examine an hypothesis about their interaction, and a model that tries to mimic the actual state of things (a kind of reality) and see what happens when something changes. The former has a number of superb exemplars, perhaps the best known of which is the 1998 Watts–Strogatz small world model [5]. The models that strive for reality, on the other hand, often generate more controversy than insight.

Such controversy frequently centers on the role of data, an issue about which modelers have heightened sensitivity (a recent set of articles collectively identified 23 such challenges) [6–9]. The different roles that data play in models are not mutually exclusive, but roughly fall into four categories. Some models are data-free. Most (these days) are data driven (that is, they use parameters derived from empirical studies). Many are data-generating (they create one or multiple data sets that are then analyzed). A few, perhaps the most important ones, are data-seeking. They generate or even test hypotheses based on some combination of actual data, derived parameters, and estimated or presumed properties, but explicitly seek to inform empirical data collection that can verify or refute their suppositions. A heightened sensitivity to the role of data stems, in part, from course corrections for predictions about HIV, both in the United States [10], and globally [11], and possibly from early work in modeling HIV in Africa, wherein the parameters for sexual activity had to be grossly inflated for the model to match actual events [12–15]. But whatever the history, the admonition to connect modeling to data in a meaningful way [8–16] has gained considerable currency, to which the contributions in this volume attest.

But why, it may be asked, should models be restricted by false dichotomies like parsimony versus complexity, or simplicity versus reality, and why be limited to a tight connection with empirical observations. The answer lies in the fact that models create a reality of their own. They are a simulacrum of the perceived world, and occupy a different orbit. They can be argued about, agonized over, vilified or exalted, just as if they were a tangible object. The leap from the reality of models to the reality of reality demands a credible connection. The goldilocks model (not too simple, not too complex, just right) with a firm connection to empirical observations meets that requirement (though it may be one of those things that is hard to define but recognizable when you see it).

An ingenious use of concepts and network connections (Fig. 1) provides a metaphor for the reality compartment in which modelers dwell. The Springer designers have created this network from the concepts in a single article [17], for which one or more congeners were identified in 197 articles. If the viewer presses on a concept, the subset of articles that contain that concept appears in an accompanying text box. The inherent value of a reality compartment, then, is that it provides a space for conversation; the downside is disconnection from the reality we actually live in. For those outside the space, for whom entry is technically restricted, disconnection from the measurable world undermines the usefulness and influence of models.

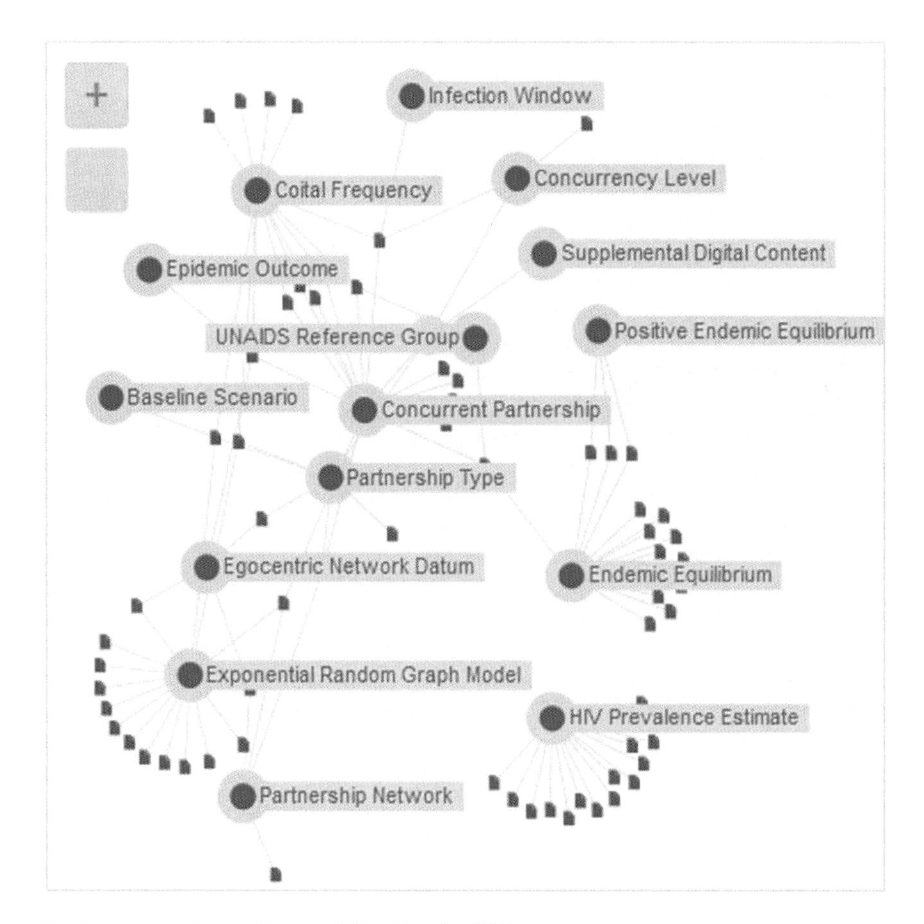

Fig. 1 A concept map of key modeling ideas for HIV

References

1. Meltzer, M.I., Atkins, C.Y., Santibanez, S., et al.: Estimating the future number of cases in the Ebola Epidemic–Liberia and Sierra Leone, 2014–2015. MMWR **63**(3), 1–14 (2014)
2. Stobbe, M.: CDC's overblown estimate of Ebola outbreak draws criticism. The Seattle Times, 1 Aug 2015
3. Regan, D.G., Wilson, D.P.: Modelling sexually transmitted infections: less is usually more for informing public health policy. Trans. R. Soc. Trop. Med. Hyg. **102**, 207–208 (2008)
4. Grassly, N.C., Fraser, C.: Mathematical models of infectious disease transmission. Nat. Rev. Microbiol. **6**, 477–487 (2008)
5. Watts, D.J., Strogatz, S.H.: Collective dynamics of 'small-world' networks. Nature **393**, 440–442 (1998)
6. De Angelis, D., Presanis, A.M., Birrell, P.J., Tomba, G.S., House, T.: Four key challenges in infectious disease modelling using data from multiple sources. Epidemics **10**, 83–87 (2015)
7. Klepac, P., Funk, S., Hollingsworth, T.D., Metcalf, C.J.E., Hampson, K.: Six challenges in the eradication of infectious diseases. Epidemics **10**, 97–101 (2015)
8. Lessler, J., Edmunds, W.J., Halloran, M.E., Hollingsworth, T.D., Lloyd, A.L.: Seven challenges for model-driven data collection in experimental and observational studies. Epidemics **10**, 78–82 (2014)
9. Metcalf, C.J.E., Edmunds, W.J., Lessler, J.: Six challenges in modelling for public health policy. Epidemics **10**, 93–96 (2015)
10. Rothenberg, R.B.: Chronicle of an epidemic foretold. Millbank Q. **71**, 565–574 (1993)
11. UNAIDS: AIDS epidemic update. Geneva: Joint United Nations Programme on HIV/AIDS (UNAIDS) and World Health Organization (WHO), pp. 1–50 (2007)
12. Anderson, R.M., May, R.M., Boily, M.C., Garnett, G.P., Rowley, J.T.: The spread of HIV-1 in Africa: sexual contact patterns and the predicted demographic impact of AIDS. Nature **352**, 581–589 (1991)
13. Auvert, B., Buonamico, G., Lagarde, E., Williams, B.: Sexual behavior, heterosexual transmission, and the spread of HIV in sub-Saharan Africa: a simulation study. Computers and biomedical research, an international journal **33**, 84–96 (2000)
14. Bongaarts, J.: A model of the spread of HIV infection and the demographic impact of AIDS. Stat. Med. **8**, 103–120 (1989)
15. French, K., Riley, S., Garnett, G.: Simulations of the HIV epidemic in sub-Saharan Africa: sexual transmission versus transmission through unsafe medical injections. Sex. Transm. Dis. **33**, 127–134 (2006)
16. Rothenberg, R.B., Costenbader, E.: Empiricism and theorizing in epidemiology and social network analysis. Interdiscip. Perspect. Infect. Dis. **2011**, 1–5 (2011)
17. Goodreau, S., Cassels, S., Kasprzyk, D., Montaño, D., Greek, A., Morris, M.: Concurrent partnerships, acute infection and HIV epidemic dynamics among young adults in Zimbabwe. AIDS Behav. **16**, 312–322 (2012)

Modeling the Impact of Behavior Change on the Spread of Ebola

Jessica R. Conrad, Ling Xue, Jeremy Dewar and James M. Hyman

Abstract We create a compartmental mathematical model to analyze the role of behavior change in slowing the spread of the Ebola virus disease (EVD) in the 2014–2015 Western Africa epidemic. Our model incorporates behavior change, modeled as decreased contact rates between susceptible and infectious individuals, the prevention of traditional funerals, and/or increased access to medical facilities. We derived the basic reproductive number for the model, and approximated the parameter values for the spread of the EVD in Monrovia. We used sensitivity analysis to quantify the relative importance of the timing, and magnitude, of the population reducing their contact rates, avoiding the traditional burial practices, and having access to medical treatment facilities. We found that reducing the number of contacts made by infectious individuals in the general population is the most effective intervention method for mitigating an EVD epidemic. While healthcare interventions delayed the onset of the epidemic, healthcare alone is insufficient to stop the epidemic in the model.

Keywords Ebola virus disease · EVD · Mathematical model · Reproductive number · Behavior changes · Epidemic model · Differential equations · Western Africa

J.R. Conrad · L. Xue · J. Dewar · J.M. Hyman (✉)
Department of Mathematics, Tulane University, New Orleans, LA 70118, USA
e-mail: mhyman@tulane.edu

J.R. Conrad
e-mail: jconrad4@tulane.edu

L. Xue
e-mail: lxue2@tulane.edu

J. Dewar
e-mail: jdewar@tulane.edu

G. Chowell and J.M. Hyman (eds.), *Mathematical and Statistical Modeling for Emerging and Re-emerging Infectious Diseases*,
DOI 10.1007/978-3-319-40413-4_2

1 Introduction

Ebola virus disease (EVD) is a zoonotic tropical disease [36] with an average fatality rate of 50 % and a range of 25–90 % in past outbreaks. It was first identified in 1976 in Yambuku, Zaire and Nzara, South Sudan [34]. While its circulation among humans is rare, around 30 outbreaks occurred since EVD was first identified, causing less than 1,600 deaths before 2014 [36]. However, the current West Africa 2014 outbreak has led to more than 28,600 probable cases and 11,300 deaths [32].

Typical symptoms of the disease include fever, weakness, and diarrhea. Bleeding complications occur in less than half of all infectious people, and heavy bleeding is relatively rare. EVD's incubation period, i.e. the time from infection of the virus to onset of symptoms, is typically between five and seven days, but can range from 2 to 21 days. Humans are not infectious until they develop symptoms [34]. Blood samples usually start to show positive results by PCR one day before the symptoms appear [36], which have been used to confirm 15,216 cases since the onset of the West Africa 2014 EVD epidemic [32]. Early supportive care with rehydration, symptomatic treatment improves survival rate, but no licensed treatments proven to neutralize the virus are available yet, though blood, immunological, and drug therapies are under development [34].

Although the reservoir for EVD is in the animal population, once a human is infectious it can be sustained through person to person transmission until the conditions change. The infection spreads through direct contact with bodily fluids such as blood, vomit, urine, or sweat. Transmission can also occur through contact with objects contaminated by bodily fluids. EVD can persist for several hours after the death of an infectious person and traditional burial practices, which involve bathing the bodies contributes to the spread of infection, thus accelerating the early spread of the infection [36]. The primary transmission routes are through individuals in close contact with the infectious person, such as health workers and family members.

Prior to the current West African 2014 EVD outbreak, the epidemics were in rural areas. These outbreaks were quickly controlled with contact tracing and isolation and quarantine of the patients to break the chain of transmission. The previous epidemics were mitigated by combining the active isolation of people who came in contact with infected individuals, an effective community response, and preventative education programs [36]. The community support is important for identifying and isolating infectious people and stopping traditional funerals where people can come in contact with infectious postmortem bodily fluids.

Early EVD models were developed to quantify transmission in different settings (illness in the community, availability of medical care, and traditional burial) [8, 21]. These models simulated the 1995 EVD outbreak in the Democratic Republic of the Congo, the 2000 outbreak in Uganda, and the current outbreak in Liberia and Sierra Leone. Although the models took into account common places where infection spreads, they failed to consider different specialized medical care and funeral settings, such as EVD Treatment Centers, local EVD Community Centers, and home-based medical care respectively. These subclasses were considered by Lofgren et al. [22]

to identify where healthcare-only interventions would be the most effective. They found that healthcare initiatives can decrease the burden of the disease significantly on a community, making it a key role in mitigating the EVD epidemic.

Recent models forecasted disease progression in Sierra Leone and Liberia during the epidemic to compare the potential impact of some other common interventions, such as contact tracing, medical care access, as well as pharmaceutical intervention [10]. Rivers et al. adapted Legrand et al.'s EVD epidemic model, and determined that increased contact tracing in addition to infection control could have a substantial impact on the number of EVD cases, though they also predicted that this would not be sufficient to halt the progression of the epidemic [10].

Most models for the recent West Africa EVD are based on ordinary differential equation (ODE) compartmental models [5, 8–10, 10, 14, 16, 17, 27, 28, 28], network-models [2, 13, 18, 26, 39], or individual based models (IBMs) [24, 29, 33]. The ODE compartmental models are the easiest to analyze and estimate threshold conditions for an epidemic. The network models can capture the complexity of human contact interactions, but are usually static and don't account for the rapid change in the contact patterns of an infectious person. The large-scale IBMs usually require synthetic population data that is not yet available for this epidemic.

In past EVD epidemics, behavior change has been the primary method to bring epidemics under control [15]. These behavior changes, coupled with community support and prevention education, are key to mitigating ebola outbreaks. Most of the existing models do not directly account for behavior change, and therefore cannot accurately reproduce, or forecast, the transmission pathways. In our model, we account for behavior changes as they affect the contact rates between susceptible and infectious individuals, the prevention of traditional funerals, and/or increased access to medical facilities.

We found that the most effective intervention method for mitigating an EVD epidemic is reducing the number of contacts made by infectious individuals in the general population. While increasing medical care access delayed the onset of the epidemic, this form of intervention failed to prevent or stop the epidemic overall. One way to measure the impact of behavior changes or medical interventions dynamic effects on the transmission rate is to measure the resulting change in the effective reproductive number of how many new infections that add a single new infected person would create.

After describing the mathematical model and the parameters, we derive the basic and effective reproduction numbers and use sensitivity analysis to quantify the relative importance of the behavior changes and availability of medical facilities in stopping the epidemic. We find that the effective reproduction number is most sensitive to the number of contacts that an infected person has with the susceptible population.

2 Mathematical Model

This model in Fig. 1 can be expressed as the system of ordinary differential equations (ODEs):

$$\frac{dS}{dt} = -\lambda S \tag{1a}$$

$$= -\alpha_i I - \alpha_m M - \alpha_f F \tag{1b}$$

$$\frac{dE}{dt} = \lambda S - \gamma_{ei} E \tag{1c}$$

$$= \alpha_i I + \alpha_m M + \alpha_f F - \gamma_{ei} E \tag{1d}$$

$$\frac{dI}{dt} = \gamma_{ei} E - (\gamma_{if} + \gamma_{ib} + \gamma_{ir} + \gamma_{im}) I \tag{1e}$$

$$\frac{dM}{dt} = \gamma_{im} I - (\gamma_{mr} + \gamma_{mb}) M \tag{1f}$$

$$\frac{dF}{dt} = \gamma_{if} I - \gamma_{fb} F \tag{1g}$$

$$\frac{dB}{dt} = \gamma_{ib} I + \gamma_{mb} M + \gamma_{fb} F \tag{1h}$$

$$\frac{dR}{dt} = \gamma_{ir} I + \gamma_{mr} M. \tag{1i}$$

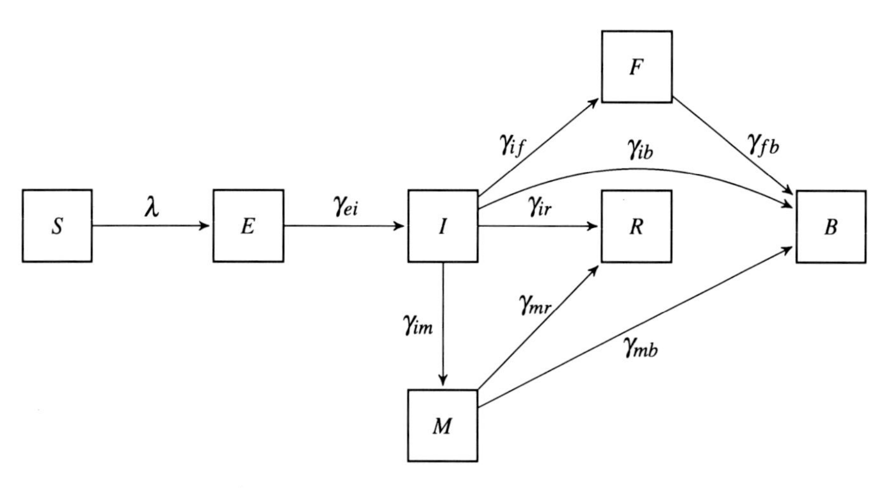

Fig. 1 When susceptible people (S) are infected, they progress to the exposed, but not infectious, state (E). From there, they become infectious (I) to the susceptible population. An infected person either enters a medical facility (M), or does not. If they do not enter a medical facility, they may recover (R) or die. When they die, they may have a traditional funeral (F), where others can be infected, or a 'safe' burial (B). People in a medical facility are more likely to recover and if they die that have a safe burial. The dynamics are described by differential equations (1)

The susceptible population, S, is infected at a rate λ and progresses to an infected, but not infectious, exposed (E) state. Then they advance to an infectious state in the general population, I, (at rate γ_{ei}). An infectious person can recover, R, (at rate γ_{ir}), go to a medical treatment facility (at rate γ_{im}), or, if they die, the person either as a traditional funeral, F, (at rate γ_{if}), or is safely buried, B, (at rate γ_{ib}). The people in a medical facility can recover, R, at an adjusted rate γ_{mr}, or die and be safely buried (at rate γ_{mb}). In this simplified model, because of the short duration of the epidemic, we do not include natural birth, death, or migration into, or out of, our population.

We have included two formulations for rates that people are infected, $\lambda S = \alpha_i I + \alpha_m M + \alpha_f F$. The more traditional formulation is expressed in terms of the susceptible viewpoint where the *force of infection*, λ, represents the rate that the susceptible population is being infected. The other formulation is expressed in terms of the infectious viewpoint where the *force from infectious*, α_*, represents the rate that an infectious person in compartment $* = I,\ M$, or F infects the susceptible population. The mathematical models are equivalent when $\lambda = (\alpha_i I - \alpha_m M - \alpha_f F)/S$. We include the force from infectious viewpoint because it clarifies the mathematical analysis, such as computing the basic reproductive number, and has advantages in estimating the model parameter values when only a small fraction of the population is infected.

The model parameters λ and α_* are nonlinear functions of other variables and time. To simplify the notation, we will not explicitly list all of the parameters unless doing so clarifies the analysis. In particular, the time variable, t, will be listed when we want to emphasize that contact rates or healthcare availability, can change in time. A description of the parameters used and the baseline values are in Table 1. The rate γ_{i*} is the progression from state I to another state $*$, where $*$ is M, F, B, or R. Similarly, the rates γ_{e*} and γ_{m*} are the progressions out of states E and M respectively into other states $*$.

We use the model to investigate the impact of behavior changes and the availability of medical facilities on the spread of the 2014–2015 EVD epidemic in Western Africa. We ignored the natural birth-death cycle in the model because of the short duration of the epidemic. We did not include the migration of people in, and out, of the modeled population, as would need to be included if this local population model is used as the local community in a larger networked model. These effects can be easily added to the model and would not affect the conclusions of our study.

2.1 Rates of Infection

Although both the susceptible and infectious viewpoint models are identical, the model parameters that determine the rates of infection are different. When there are only a few people infectious, as in the EVD epidemic, then there are advantages to estimating the parameters that define the force from infectious, α_*, rather than the traditional force of infection, λ.

2.1.1 Force of Infection

The force of infection, λ, can be decomposed into sum of three terms, $\lambda = \lambda_i + \lambda_m + \lambda_f$, where each term is factored into

$$\lambda_* = c_s \beta_* P_* = \begin{pmatrix} \text{Number of} \\ \text{contacts a} \\ \text{susceptible} \\ \text{has per day} \end{pmatrix} \begin{pmatrix} \text{Probability of} \\ \text{transmission} \\ \text{per contact with} \\ \text{someone in } * \end{pmatrix} \begin{pmatrix} \text{Probability the} \\ \text{contact is with} \\ \text{someone in} \\ \text{state } * \end{pmatrix}$$

Here the subscript $* = i,\ m,\ f$ refers to one of the infectious states, I, M, or F. A susceptible person has c_s contacts per day and the probability of transmission per contact with an infected person is β_*. There are a total of $c_s S$ contacts per day by people in the susceptible population out of $C_{tot}(t) = c_s S + c_e E + c_i I + c_m M + c_f F + c_r R + c_b B$ total contacts in the entire population. The probability that a random contact by a susceptible is with a person in state I is $P_i(t) = c_i I(t)/C_{tot}(t)$ and changes exponentially early in the epidemic. The formulas for the other states are similar.

2.1.2 Force from Infectious

To consider how infection spreads from the perspective of the infectious individuals, we define α as the force of infection *from* the infectious population. This force (α_i, α_m, and α_f) depends upon what state the infectious population is in. Here we assume that the exposed population is not infectious, $\alpha_e = 0$. The rate that the susceptible population is being infected is the sum of the product of each of these forces times the people who are in that state, (1a).

Each force from the infectious states I, M, and F can be decomposed into three factors

$$\alpha_* = c_* \beta_* P_s = \begin{pmatrix} \text{Number of contacts} \\ \text{an infectious} \\ \text{person in state } * \\ \text{has per day} \end{pmatrix} \begin{pmatrix} \text{Probability of} \\ \text{transmission} \\ \text{per contact from} \\ \text{someone in } * \end{pmatrix} \begin{pmatrix} \text{Probability} \\ \text{the contact is} \\ \text{with a} \\ \text{susceptible} \end{pmatrix}$$

The *number of contacts* per day, c_*, a person in state $*$ has depends upon the state. A contact is defined as an interaction between two individuals where the disease transmission could take place. We assume that the infectious populations, I and M, have fewer contacts per day than the susceptible and exposed populations. The contacts for the people in a traditional funeral, F, are averaged over the length of time for the funeral. In this model, we treat every contact as an independent event and do not explicitly account for repeated contacts between the two same individuals.

The *probability that contact by an infectious person is with a susceptible person*, P_s, depends on how the infectious person mixes with the current population. These contacts are not random and, to be accurate, the model should include a mixing matrix between people in each of the states [11, 19]. For simplicity, we assume that the mixing is random and will investigate the importance of this assumption in a later analysis of this model. The probability that a random contact will be with a susceptible person is $P_s(t) = c_s S(t)/C_{tot}(t)$ and $P_s = 1$ early in the epidemic.

The *probability of transmission per contact*, β_*, depends on the state that the infectious person is in. We assume that contacts with an infectious individual, who is not under medical care, are more likely to transmit the disease than contact with a person using protective measures at a medical facility.

In summary, the forces from each of the infectious states are

$$\alpha_i(t) = c_i \beta_i \frac{c_s S(t)}{C_{tot}(t)}, \quad \alpha_m(t) = c_m \beta_m \frac{c_s S(t)}{C_{tot}(t)}, \quad \alpha_f(t) = c_f \beta_f \frac{c_s S(t)}{C_{tot}(t)}. \tag{2}$$

Model forecasts are sensitive to accurately modeling the contacts of an infected person. This is complicated when considering behavior change since an infected person is more likely to change their behavior than the general susceptible population. An advantage of the infectious viewpoint is that it is formulated in terms of these infectious contacts, not the susceptible's contacts. That is, in the susceptible viewpoint, the first factor, c_s, in the force of infection is the average number of contacts that a susceptible person has, while in the infectious viewpoint the first factor, c_i, is the number of contacts that an infectious person has. If disease changes behavior, as it does in EVD, then c_i is likely to change more than c_s, and changes in c_i have a greater impact on the spread of an infection than do changes in c_s. It is especially important when investigating the impact of behavior changes.

Another advantage is that the infected viewpoint is formulated based on estimating the probability that a random contact is with a susceptible person, which is in the early stages of an epidemic $P_s(t) \approx 1$, since nearly every contact is with a susceptible person. In the susceptible viewpoint, the model is based on estimating the probability that a random contact is with an infectious person, which is changing rapidly. That is, from the susceptible viewpoint, we must estimate the probability for a susceptible person that a random contact is with an infectious person, P_*, $* = i,\ m,\ f$. This can be a difficult parameter to estimate when there are few infectious people and the behavior is changing quickly early in the epidemic.

2.2 Progression Rates

The rates that people advance between the model compartments depends upon the disease progression rates and branching probabilities among the next possible compartments where a person could go. We find that using a branching diagram (Fig. 2) greatly simplifies the complexity of having multiple pathways among the model components. The branching probability, p_{jk}, is defined as the fraction of people who progress from state j to state k. The nodes in the diagram for staying at home,

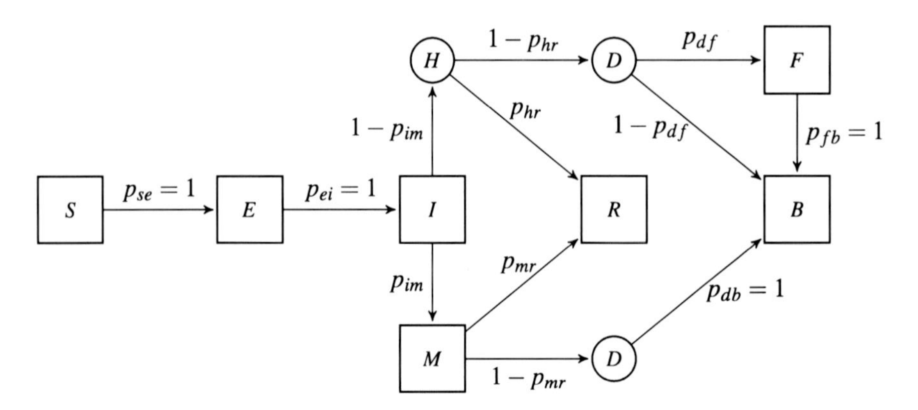

Fig. 2 The probabilities that an individual progresses from one state to the next, denoted as p_{jk}, where j is the state they are leaving and k is the state they are entering. In the branching diagram, the nodes for staying at home, the *circled* H, and dead, the *circled* D, are branching points, and are not compartments of the model

Ⓗ, and dying, Ⓓ, are not compartments in the model. They represent nodes in the branching process that are useful when defining the probabilities of going from one state to another.

In our model, we define four progression rates in terms of the probability of going from one state to another, p_{im}, p_{mr}, p_{hr}, and p_{df} (Table 1). The other branching probabilities are defined in terms of these four probabilities. For example, the probability that an infectious person, I, will have a traditional funeral, F, is $p_{if} = p_{ih}p_{hd}p_{df} = (1 - p_{im})(1 - p_{hr})p_{df}$. Similarly, $p_{ib} = p_{im}p_{md}p_{db} + p_{ih}p_{hd}p_{df}$ and $p_{ir} = p_{ih}p_{hr} + p_{im}p_{mf}$. When describing the meaning of terms that arise in defining the basic reproductive number, we also find it useful to define probabilities that a person will progress through multiple states, such as $p_{ijk} = p_{ij}p_{jk}$ is the probability of going from state i to state j and then to state k.

In addition to the branching probabilities, the transition rates are defined in terms of the average time (in days) spent in a state τ_e, τ_i, and τ_f and the time that entering the medical facility can reduce the time to recovery, t_r days. For example, τ_e is the average time it takes an infected person to become infectious, and τ_i is the time that would be spent in state I for someone not going to the medical facility.

The branching probabilities and average times for the disease progression are then used to define the compartment progression rates, γ_{jk} from compartment j to compartment k. That is, instead of directly defining the progression rates, we define them in terms of parameters that can be directly measured or are easier to interpret.

From these parameters, we define the progression rates as:

$$\gamma_{ei} = p_{ei}/\tau e = 1/\tau_e \qquad \gamma_{ib} = p_{ib}/\tau_f$$

$$\gamma_{if} = p_{if}/\tau_f \qquad \gamma_{ir} = p_{ir}/\tau_i$$

Table 1 The baseline values are chosen selected so that the model is consistent with the Montserrado EVD epidemic incidence data [6, 7, 10, 23, 38]

Symbol	Parameter description	Baseline
c_*^-	Number of contacts per day when $t < t_c$ $c_s^- = 30,\ c_e^- = 30,\ c_i^- = 8.1657,\ c_m^- = 5,\ c_f^- = 20,\ c_r^- = 30$	
c_*^+	Number of contacts per day when $t \geq t_c$ $c_s^+ = 30,\ c_e^+ = 30,\ c_i^+ = 3.0311,\ c_m^+ = 5,\ c_f^+ = 20,\ c_r^+ = 30$	
β_*	Probability of transmission per contact with state $*$ $\beta_i = 0.017,\ \beta_m = 0.0005,\ \beta_f = 0.05$	
τ_e	Average days spent in exposed state	7
τ_i	Average days spent in I	20
τ_f	Average days spent in funeral state	1
p_{hr}	Probability an infectious person recovers (at home)	0.55
p_{mr}	Probability an infectious person recovers (medical care)	0.75
p_{df}^-	Probability a person dying at home has a traditional burial $t < t_f$	0.9
p_{df}^+	Probability a person dying at home has a traditional burial $t \geq t_f$	0.18
p_{im}^-	Probability an infected goes to a medical facility $t < t_m$	0.1
p_{im}^+	Probability an infected goes to a medical facility $t \geq t_m$	0.71
t_c	Date (days) when people change their contact rates	122
t_m	Date (days) when medical facilities become more available	140
t_f	Date (days) when number of traditional funerals drops	84
γ_{jk}	Rate of going from state j to state k (derived from p_* and τ_*)	
P_*	Probability of random contact with state $*$. e.g. $P_s = c_s S/C_{tot}$	

The basic reproductive number for the baseline case is $\mathbb{R}_0 = 2.64$

$$\gamma_{im} = p_{im}/\tau_m \qquad \gamma_{imr} = p_{imr}/\tau_m = p_{im}\,p_{mr}/\tau_m$$

$$\gamma_{imb} = p_{imb}/\tau_m = p_{im}(1 - p_{mr})/\tau_m \qquad \gamma_i = \gamma_{if} + \gamma_{ib} + \gamma_{ir} + \gamma_{im}$$

where γ_i is the total rate that people exit from the I compartment.

2.3 *Behavior Change, Healthcare Availability, and Traditional Funerals*

The number of contacts $c_*(t)$ per day for someone in compartment $*$ can change as the epidemic progresses to avoid being infected or to avoid infecting others. We realize that, in general, $c_*(t)$ is a complex function of time. Our goal is to analyze the relative importance of the behavior changes and we make the simplifying assumption that $c_*(t)$ is a piecewise constant function that changes t_c days after the first (index) case when the epidemic starts. That is,

$$c_*(t) = \begin{cases} c_*^- & \text{if } t < t_c \\ c_*^+ & \text{if } t \geq t_c. \end{cases} \tag{3}$$

This simplified form of the behavior change makes it easy to quantify the importance of the time the behavior change takes place and the magnitude of the change.

As medical treatment units become available and traditional funerals become less frequent, we change the probabilities that an infected person will go to the medical facility p_{im} and the probability that a person dying at home will have a traditional funeral p_{df} as step functions:

$$p_{im}(t) = \begin{cases} p_{im}^- & \text{if } t < t_m \\ p_{im}^+ & \text{if } t \geq t_m \end{cases} \quad \text{and} \quad p_{df}(t) = \begin{cases} p_{df}^- & \text{if } t < t_f \\ p_{df}^+ & \text{if } t \geq t_f. \end{cases} \tag{4}$$

3 Reproduction Numbers

The effective reproductive number, $\mathbb{R}_e(t)$, is the expected number of new infections that a newly infected person will create [12]. Thus, $\mathbb{R}_e(t)$ depends upon the state of the entire system at the time when a susceptible person is infected, $\mathbb{R}_e(t) = \mathbb{R}_e(t, S, E, I, M, F, B, R)$. The basic reproduction number, $\mathbb{R}_0$, measures the average number of secondary cases produced by introducing one infected individual into the disease free equilibrium (DFE).

We will first derive the reproductive numbers from the viewpoint of a stochastic Markov Chain process. It is natural to define the transition probabilities from perspective and to connect relationship between the effective and basic reproductive numbers. We will then use the next generation approach to derive $\mathbb{R}_0$ based on a mathematical analysis of the differential equations.

3.1 Branching Process Derivation of the Reproductive Numbers

We can view the model (1) as a stochastic Markov Chain branching process where the progression rates are defined in terms of a probability per day that a person will progress to another state. This viewpoint has the advantage that each step in the process has a natural epidemiological interpretation.

The reproductive number is derived by estimating the probable number of new infections that would be created by a single individual in each of the infectious states. Since all the new infections must come from one of the three infectious states, we can decompose $\mathbb{R}_e$ into a sum of the compartmental basic reproductive numbers for each state:

$$\mathbb{R}_e = \mathbb{R}_e^i + \mathbb{R}_e^m + \mathbb{R}_e^f,$$

where $\mathbb{R}_e^*$ is the average number of new infections caused by an infectious person, while in state $*$, ($* = i, m$ and f). Each of these reproduction numbers can be factored into three terms:

$$\mathbb{R}_e^* = P_* \tau_* \alpha_*(t) = \begin{pmatrix} \text{Probability an} \\ \text{infected person} \\ \text{enters state } * \end{pmatrix} \begin{pmatrix} \text{Time a} \\ \text{person is} \\ \text{in state } * \end{pmatrix} \begin{pmatrix} \text{Force from infectious} \\ \text{for a person} \\ \text{in state } * \end{pmatrix}.$$

We define P_* as the probability that an infected person ever enters state $*$. In a large infectious population, P_* is also the fraction of the infected people that will eventually enter state $*$. This is determined by the progression rates of all the possible paths someone can enter state $*$.

Since all infected people enter state I, $p_{ei} = 1$. The probability that an infected person goes to a medical facility is $p_{em} = p_{im} = \gamma_{im}/\gamma_i = \gamma_{im}\tau_i$. Similarly, the probability that an infected person will have a traditional funeral can be expressed as $p_{ef} = p_{if} = \gamma_{if}/\gamma_i = \gamma_{if}\tau_i$,

The third term in $\mathbb{R}_e^*$ is the force from infectious for person in state $*$, α_* as defined in (2). Combining these terms, we can express the effective reproductive number as

$$\begin{aligned} \mathbb{R}_e(t) &= \mathbb{R}_e^i(t) + \mathbb{R}_e^m(t) + \mathbb{R}_e^f(t) \\ &= p_{ei}\tau_i\alpha_i(t) + p_{em}\tau_m\alpha_m(t) + p_{ef}\tau_f\alpha_f(t) \\ &= \frac{1}{\gamma_i}c_i\frac{c_sS(t)}{C_{tot}(t)}\beta_i + \frac{\gamma_{im}}{\gamma_i}\frac{1}{\gamma_i}c_m\frac{c_sS(t)}{C_{tot}(t)}\beta_m + \frac{\gamma_{if}}{\gamma_i}\frac{1}{\gamma_{fb}}c_f\frac{c_sS(t)}{C_{tot}(t)}\beta_f. \end{aligned}$$

If at $t = 0$, the population is at the DFE where everyone in the population is susceptible, then the effective reproductive number is also called the basic reproductive number, $\mathbb{R}_0 = \mathbb{R}_e^*(0, S, 0, 0, 0, 0, 0, 0) = \mathbb{R}_e(0)$ and represents the number of new infections that would be caused by a single infected person being introduced into the population. $\mathbb{R}_0 = 2.64$ in this model for the baseline parameter values.

At the DFE, the probability that a contact will be with susceptible person is $P_s(0) = 1$, and the transmission rates simplify to $\alpha_*(0) = c_*\beta_*P_s(0) = c_*\beta_*$. Hence,

$$\begin{aligned} \mathbb{R}_0 &= \mathbb{R}_0^i + \mathbb{R}_0^m + \mathbb{R}_0^f \\ &= p_{ei}\tau_i c_i\beta_i + p_{em}\tau_m c_m\beta_m + p_{ef}\tau_f c_f\beta_f \\ &= \frac{1}{\gamma_i}c_i\beta_i + \frac{\gamma_{im}}{\gamma_i}\frac{1}{\gamma_i}c_m\beta_m + \frac{\gamma_{if}}{\gamma_i}\frac{1}{\gamma_{fb}}c_f\beta_f \end{aligned} \tag{5}$$

3.2 *Next Generation Method Derivation of the Basic Reproductive Number*

The next generation matrix algorithm [12, 37] can be used to explicitly define $\mathbb{R}_0$ by computing the number of new infections that are generated from the infected states. We define the vector $x = [E, I, M, F,]^T$ and write the equations for these variables as $\frac{dx}{dt} = \mathscr{F} - \mathscr{V}$ by defining the vectors $\mathscr{F}$ and $\mathscr{V}$ so that $\mathscr{F}_i$ is the rate new infections are introduced into state i, and $\mathscr{V}_i$ is the rate of transfer out of state i;

$$\mathscr{F} = \begin{bmatrix} \alpha_i I + \alpha_m M + \alpha_f F \\ 0 \\ 0 \\ 0 \end{bmatrix}, \quad \mathscr{V} = \begin{bmatrix} \gamma_{ei} E \\ -\gamma_{ei} E + (\gamma_{if} + \gamma ib + \gamma_{ir} + \gamma_{im}) I \\ -\gamma_{im} I + (\gamma_{mr} + \gamma_{mb}) M \\ -\gamma_{if} I + \gamma_{fb} F. \end{bmatrix} \tag{6}$$

The Jacobian matrices $J_{\mathscr{F}}$ and $J_{\mathscr{V}}$ for this system of differential equations at the DFE have the property that the $(i, j)^{th}$ element of the matrix, $J_{\mathscr{F}}(i, j) = \frac{\partial \mathscr{F}_i}{\partial x_j}$, is the rate at which infected individuals in state j produce new infections in state i. Similarly, $J_{\mathscr{V}}(j, k) = \frac{\partial \mathscr{V}_j}{\partial x_k}$, is the rate at which individuals in compartment k transfer to compartment j.

At the DFE $\alpha_*(0) = c_* \beta_*$ and the Jacobian matrices of $\mathscr{F}$ and $\mathscr{V}$ are:

$$J_{\mathscr{F}} = \begin{bmatrix} 0 & \beta_i c_i & \beta_m c_m & \beta_f c_f \\ 0 & 0 & 0 & 0 \\ 0 & 0 & 0 & 0 \\ 0 & 0 & 0 & 0 \end{bmatrix}, \tag{7}$$

$$J_{\mathscr{V}} = \begin{bmatrix} \tau_e^{-1} & 0 & 0 & 0 \\ -\gamma_{ei} & \tau_i^{-1} & 0 & 0 \\ 0 & -\gamma_{im} & \tau_m^{-1} & 0 \\ 0 & -\gamma_{if} & 0 & \tau_f^{-1} \end{bmatrix} = \begin{bmatrix} \tau_e^{-1} & 0 & 0 & 0 \\ -\tau_e^{-1} & \tau_i^{-1} & 0 & 0 \\ 0 & -p_{im}/\tau_m & \tau_m^{-1} & 0 \\ 0 & -p_{if}/\tau_f & 0 & \tau_f^{-1} \end{bmatrix} \tag{8}$$

We can express the inverse of $J_{\mathscr{V}}$ in terms of the transition probabilities as

$$J_{\mathscr{V}}^{-1} = \begin{bmatrix} \tau_e & 0 & 0 & 0 \\ p_{ei} \tau_i & \tau_i & 0 & 0 \\ p_{im} \tau_m & p_{im} \tau_i & \tau_m & 0 \\ p_{ei} p_{if} \tau_f & p_{if} \tau_i & 0 & \tau_f \end{bmatrix} = \begin{bmatrix} \tau_e & 0 & 0 & 0 \\ p_{ei} \tau_i & \tau_i & 0 & 0 \\ p_{em} \tau_m & p_{im} \tau_i & \tau_m & 0 \\ p_{ef} \tau_f & p_{if} \tau_i & 0 & \tau_f \end{bmatrix}$$

Note that each row of $J_{\mathscr{V}}^{-1}$ is the probability of going from state i to state j scaled by the time in state j.

The next generation matrix is $\mathscr{N} = J_{\mathscr{F}} J_{\mathscr{V}}^{-1} =$

$$\begin{bmatrix} p_{ei} \tau_i c_i \beta_i + p_{em} \tau_m c_m \beta_m + p_{ef} \tau_f c_f \beta_f & \tau_i c_i \beta_i + p_{if} \tau_i c_f \beta_f + p_{im} \tau_i c_m \beta_m & c_m \beta_m \tau_m & c_f \beta_f \tau_f \\ 0 & 0 & 0 & 0 \\ 0 & 0 & 0 & 0 \\ 0 & 0 & 0 & 0 \end{bmatrix}$$

The basic reproduction number can be defined as the spectral radius of $\mathscr{N}$. In this case, the matrix is upper triangular, so the eigenvalues are on the diagonal, and the largest eigenvalue, $\mathcal{N}(1, 1) = p_{ei}\tau_i c_i \beta_i + p_{em}\tau_m c_m \beta_m + p_{ef}\tau_f c_f \beta_f$, which agrees with the previous calculation (5).

4 Parameter Estimation from Montserrado EVD Cases

Most of the model parameters, such as the number of contacts per day, are approximations for the expected value of stochastic events with broad probability distribution. Some model parameters, such as the probability of transmission per contact, independent of the region where the epidemic is taking place. Others, such as the behavior change of the local community in reducing their number of contacts, depend upon the specific region we are studying. Our goal is to define the baseline parameters for our best guess at what actually happened during the epidemic in a specific region. We will then use sensitivity analysis to ask "what if" questions and quantify the relative importance of the mitigation efforts, such as the how sensitive the course of the epidemic will be to the time that the Ebola treatment units are established, or to the time it takes to stop traditional funerals.

To illustrate our approach, we used the EVD incidence from Montserrado, Liberia (Fig. 3). This data can be easily fit with a three, or four parameter spline. It is inappropriate to fit any model using more than the degrees of freedom evident in the data, and therefore we limit our fits to 3 or 4 parameters. In fitting the data, we first defined all the parameters in Table 1 based on our best estimate from the published literature [1, 6, 7, 10, 23, 30, 35, 38]. The dates for the ban of traditional funerals, and increase in medical availability were obtained by press releases [1, 35]. We then identified the parameters that are most likely to vary from region to region and used these to fit the model to the data using the sequential quadratic programming (SQP) MATLAB program *fmincon*.

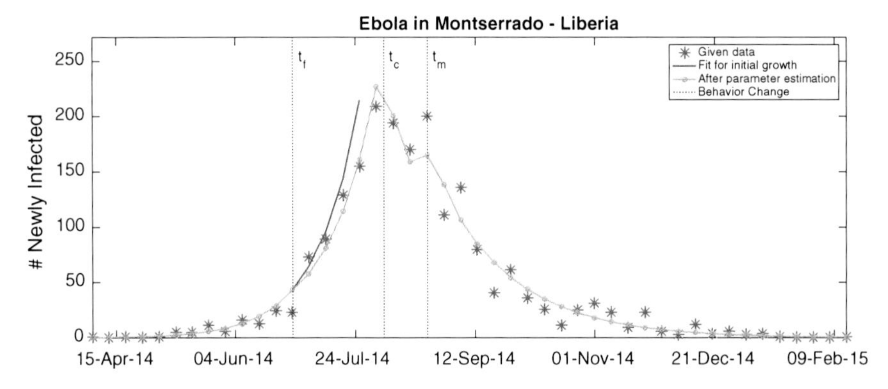

Fig. 3 The weekly EVD cases [31] for Montserrado (∗) are fit with the model (*solid line*) by varying: (1) the behavior change in the infected population, c_i^+; (2) the fraction of infected people who go to a medical facility, p_{im}; and (3) the fraction of people who have a traditional funeral p_{if}

The first step in initializing a multicompartmental model is to create balanced initial conditions for the number of people in each compartment that is consistent with a real epidemic [20]. We achieved this balanced initial state by starting the epidemic with a small (0.001 %) infected population, and letting the epidemic advance until there is one person infected. We then reset the integration time to zero as the time of the first index case.

Starting with the balanced initial conditions, we varied the single parameter c_i to match the early growth of the epidemic based on the difference between the model predictions and the WHO data for the number of weekly cases [31]. That is, we started by fitting the model with a single parameter match to the initial growth of the epidemic in the first four months of the epidemic, before there were significant behavior changes or new medical facilities available. We then verified that our fitted parameter, $c_i^- = 8.2$, was relatively insensitive to the four month window. The fit is shown as the solid red line in Fig. 3 and would continue growing exponentially unless we account for the decreased contact rates, reduced traditional funerals, and availability of medical treatment facilities.

Once we have the model agreeing with the initial growth, we then varied the:

- magnitude, c_i^+, and time, t_c, that the infected population changed behavior,
- increase in the fraction of people receiving medical treatment p_{im}, and
- reduction in the fraction of people having a traditional funeral p_{if}. The fitted values are given in Table 1.

The resulting baseline solution of the model (Fig. 4) is in good agreement with the published incidence data.

5 Sensitivity Analysis

In local sensitivity analysis [3, 4], we perturb our reference (baseline) solution to quantify how quantities of interest (QOIs), such as the reproductive numbers or size of the infected population, change in response to small changes in the parameters of interest (POI), such as the time people change their behavior (t_c) or the probability that an infected person will be treated at a medical facilities (p_{im}). The sensitivity indices tell us the relative importance of each parameter to the QOIs and how sensitive they are to changes in parameters, such as the magnitude of the behavior change. The sign of the index indicates the direction of the response, and its magnitude tells us the relative importance of each parameter in our model predictions. Because the analysis is based on a linearization of the solution with the baseline parameters, the local sensitivity analysis indices are only valid in a small neighborhood of the baseline parameter values.

We define $\hat{q} = q(\hat{p})$ as the value of the QOI when the model is solved with the baseline parameter values $\hat{p}$. If the POI, $\hat{p}$, is perturbed by a small amount, $p = \hat{p}(1 + \theta_p)$, then the QOI will change by $q = q(\hat{p} + \theta_p^q \hat{p})$ where $\theta_q := \theta_p \frac{\hat{p}}{\hat{q}} \frac{\partial q}{\partial p}$. The

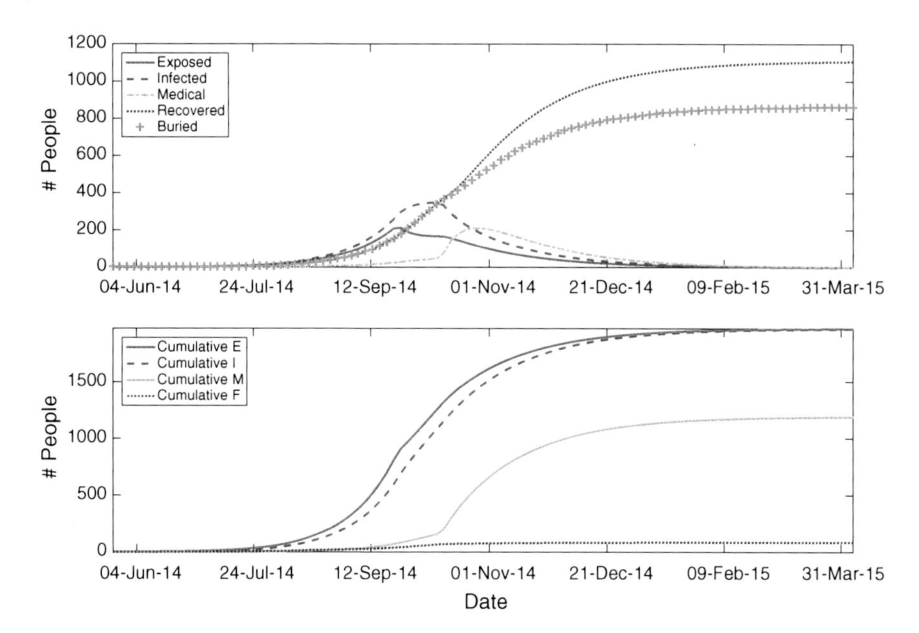

Fig. 4 The baseline solution of the model (1) using the fitted parameters (Table 1) has a noticeable jump in the number of people receiving medical treatment at time $t_m = 22 - Oct - 2014$

ratio of the change in q with respect to a change in p is defined as the dimensionless relative sensitivity index as

$$\mathsf{S}_p^q := \frac{\hat{p}}{\hat{q}} \times \left.\frac{\partial q}{\partial p}\right|_{p=\hat{p}} = \frac{\theta_q}{\theta_p}. \tag{9}$$

That is, this local normalized relative sensitivity index S_p^q is the percent change in the output given the percent change in an input parameter. If the $\hat{p}$ changes by $x\%$, then $\hat{q}$ will change by $\mathsf{S}_p^q x\%$. Note that the sign of the sensitivity index indicates whether the QOI increases (> 0) or decreases (< 0) with the POI.

The sensitivity indices in the Table 2 show that, by far, the most efficient way for slowing the epidemic is to reduce the number of contacts that an infectious person has in state I. The impact of the general susceptible public S reducing their contacts c_s has a much smaller effect since the vast majority of these contacts are with other susceptible people that have little impact on the epidemic. This suggests that the emphasis of mitigation efforts should be focused on urging the infected people to isolate themselves, rather than have everyone reduce all their contacts.

In extended sensitivity analysis [25], we vary the POIs over a wide range of values. In Fig. 4, the total number of people dying increases with the fraction p_{df}^+ of people not in medical care who continued to have a traditional funeral after the funeral restrictions went into effect. Note that the epidemic would have been over three times worse if everyone continued to have a traditional funeral ($p_{df}^+ = 1$) compared to

Table 2 The sensitivity indices of $\mathbb{R}_0$ with respect to the model parameters for the baseline case (Table 1)

Total	c_s	c_e	c_i	c_m	c_f	c_r	p_{df}	$\frac{c_i^+}{c_i^-}$	p_{im}
Exposed	0.0015	–0.00047	9.5	0.048	1	–0.00086	0.12	1.2	–0.4
Dead	0.0014	–0.00045	9.3	0.044	1	–0.00079	0.12	1.1	–0.44

Note that the sensitivity index for the total dead with respect to c_i is 9.3 meaning that if the infected population reduced their contacts by 1 %, then the number of people who died would be reduced by 9.5 %

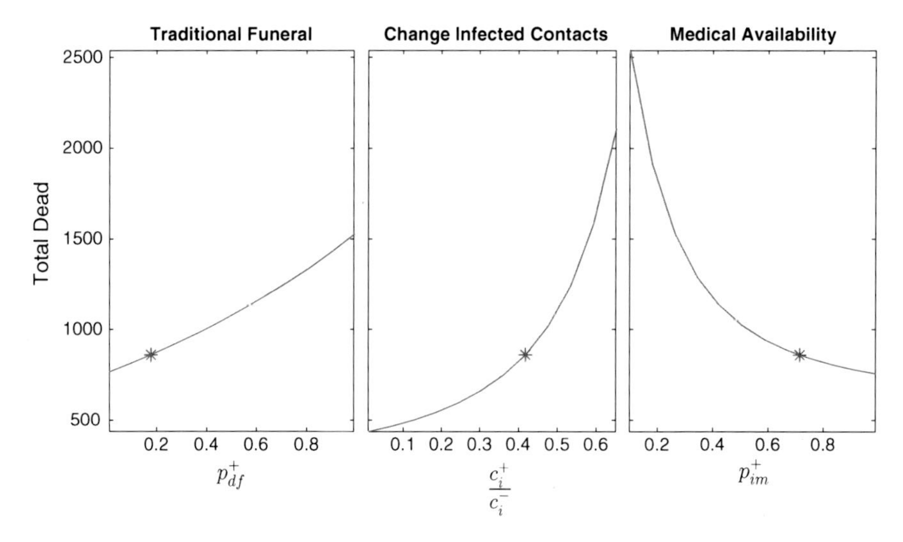

Fig. 5 The baseline case in these extended sensitivity analysis plots is indicated by an $*$. The y-axis for the total number of people dying is plotted as a function of p_{df}^+, c_i^+/c_i^-, and p_{df}^+ over a wide range of possible values. Notice that in the center figure, reducing the number of contacts an infectious person has after the behavior change has begun has the greatest impact on slowing the epidemic

completely stopping the funerals ($p_{df}^+ = 0$). The center plot illustrates the sensitivity of the epidemic growth as a function of the relative reduction (c_i^+/c_i^-) in the number of contacts that an infectious person has after the behavior change begins. The baseline case is that infected people reduce their contacts to 40 % of what they were before time t_c. The model predicts that the death toll would have been cut in half if they they had cut their contacts to 10 % of c_i^-. The plot on the right shows the dramatic effect that increasing the fraction p_{if} of infected people who are admitted to a medical treatment unit can have on reducing the total number of people dying in the epidemic. Without the availability of medical treatment ($p_{if} = 0$) the model predicts that the epidemic would have been far worse (Fig. 5).

6 Summary and Conclusions

Our simulations indicate that reducing the contacts that infectious people have with the general public is the most important mitigation strategy of those considered in the model. These contacts include both the contacts with an infected person at home, under medical care, and in a traditional funeral. Reducing the number of contacts that the general susceptible population has per day by the same factor is a more difficult task to have the same impact on the epidemic. The simulations predict that medical care intervention alone would have been insufficient to stop this epidemic from spreading through a population.

We acknowledge that ordinary differential equations, such as this model, are best used to simulate large epidemics and may not be valid in representing how the infection would spread through small rural communities. Also, our simple model also fails to account for the important role that family structure had in the EVD epidemic where infectious individuals are more likely to infect family members than people in the general community. Even though it would be inappropriate to use a simple model, such as this one, for forecasting an epidemic where so few people are infected, these models can provide insights into the relative importance of mitigation strategies, such as the effectiveness of behavior change and the availability of medical interventions in stopping the epidemic.

Acknowledgments MH, LX, and JD were partially supported by NIH/NIGMS Models of Infectious Disease Agent Study (MIDAS) grants U01-GM097658-01 and U01-GM097661-01. This work was also partially supported by the NSF/DEB RAPID award B53035G and the Louisiana Board of Regents, SURE program.

References

1. All Africa.: Liberia: Ellen Enforces Cremation as Measure Against Ebola (2014). Available from: http://allafrica.com/stories/201408051276.html
2. Arino, J., Van den Driessche, P.: A multi-city epidemic model. Math. Popul. Stud. **10**(3), 175–193 (2003)
3. Arriola, L., Chowell, G., Hyman, J.M., Bettencourt, L.M.A., Castillo-Chavez, C.: Sensitivity Analysis for Quantifying Uncertainty in Mathematical Models (2009)
4. Arriola, L.M., Hyman, J.M.: Being sensitive to uncertainty. Comput. Sci. Eng. **9**(2), 10–20 (2007)
5. Browne, C., Huo, X., Magal, P., Seydi, M., Seydi, O., Webb, G.: A Model of the 2014 Ebola Epidemic in West Africa (2014). arXiv:1410.3817 [q-bio.PE]
6. Bwaka, M.A., Bonnet, M.J., Calain, P., Colebunders, R., De Roo, A., Guimard, Y., Katwiki, K.R., Kibadi, K., Kipasa, M.A., Kuvula, K.J. et al.: Ebola Hemorrhagic Fever in Kikwit, Democratic Republic of the Congo: Clinical Observations in 103 Patients. J. Infect. Dis. **179**(Supplement 1), S1–S7 (1999)
7. Camacho, A., Kucharski, A.J., Funk, S., Breman, J., Piot, P., Edmunds, W.J.: Potential for large outbreaks of ebola virus disease. Epidemics **9**, 70–78 (2014)
8. Chowell, G., Hengartner, N.W., Castillo-Chavez, C., Fenimore, P.W., Hyman, J.M.: The basic reproductive number of ebola and the effects of public health measures: the cases of congo and uganda. J. Theor. Biol. **229**(1), 119–126 (2004)

9. Althaus, C.L.: Estimating the reproduction number of ebola virus (EBOV) during the 2014 outbreak in West Africa. PLOS Curr. Outbreaks (2014)
10. Rivers, C.M., Lofgren, E.T., Marathe, M., Eubank, S., Lewis, B.L.: Modeling the impact of interventions on an epidemic of ebola in sierra leone and liberia. PLOS Curr. Outbreaks (2014)
11. Valle, S.Y.D., Hyman, J.M., Hethcote, H.W., Eubank, S.G.: Mixing patterns between age groups in social networks. Soc. Netw. **29**(4), 539–554 (2007)
12. Diekmann, O., Heesterbeek, J.A.P., Metz, J.A.J.: On the definition and the computation of the basic reproduction ratio r 0 in models for infectious diseases in heterogeneous populations. J. Math. Biol. **28**(4), 365–382 (1990)
13. Eubank, S., Guclu, H., Kumar, V.S.A., Marathe, M.V., Srinivasan, A., Toroczkai, Z., Wang, N.: Modelling disease outbreaks in realistic urban social networks. Nature **429**(6988), 180–184 (2004)
14. Tuite, A., Fisman, D., Khoo, E.: Early epidemic dynamics of the West African 2014 ebola outbreak: Estimates derived with a simple two-parameter model. PLOS Curr. Outbreaks (2014)
15. Garrett, L.: Ebola: Story of an Outbreak. Hachette Books, New York (2014)
16. Gomes, M.F.C., Piontti, A.P., Rossi, L., Chao, D., Longini, I., Halloran, M.E., Vespignani, A.: Assessing the international spreading risk associated with the 2014 West African ebola outbreak. PLOS Curr. Outbreaks (2014)
17. Thomas House. Epidemiological Dynamics of Ebola Outbreaks. eLife (September 2014)
18. Hyman, J.M., LaForce, T.: Modeling the spread of influenza among cities. Bioterrorism Math. Model. Appl. Homel. Secur. 211–236 (2003)
19. Hyman, J.M., Li, J.: Disease transmission models with biased partnership selection. Appl. Numer. Math. **24**(2), 379–392 (1997)
20. Hyman, J.M., Li, J., Stanley, E.A.: The initialization and sensitivity of multigroup models for the transmission of HIV. J. Theor. Biol. **208**(2), 227–249 (2001)
21. Legrand, J., Grais, R.F., Boelle, P.Y., Valleron, A.J., Flahault, A.: Understanding the dynamics of ebola epidemics. Epidemiol. Infect. **135**(04), 610–621 (2007)
22. Lofgren, E.T., Rivers, C.M., Marathe, M.V., Eubank, S.G., Lewis, B.L.: The Potential Impact of Increased Hospital Capacity to Contain and Control Ebola in Liberia (2014). arXiv:1410.8207
23. Maganga, G.D., Kapetshi, J., Berthet, N., Ilunga, B.K., Kabange, F., Kingebeni, P.M., Mondonge, V., Muyembe, J.-J.T., Bertherat, E., Briand, S., et al.: Ebola virus disease in the democratic republic of congo. N. Engl. J. Med. **371**(22), 2083–2091 (2014)
24. Manore, C., McMahon, B., Fair, J., Hyman, J.M., Brown, M., LaBute, M.: Disease properties, geography, and mitigation strategies in a simulation spread of rinderpest across the United States. Vet. Res. **42**(1), 1–12 (2011)
25. Manore, C.A., Hickmann, K.S., Xu, S., Wearing, H.J., Hyman, J.M.: Comparing dengue and chikungunya emergence and endemic transmission in a. aegypti and a. albopictus. J. Theor. Biol. **356**, 174–191 (2014)
26. McMahon, B., Manore, C., Hyman, J., LaBute, M., Fair, J.: Coupling Vector-host Dynamics with Weather, Geography and Mitigation Measures to Model Rift Valley Fever in Africa. Submitted (2014)
27. Martin, I.M., Atkins, C.Y., Santibanez, S., Knust, B., Petersen, B.W., Ervin, E.D., Nichol, S.T., Damon, I.K., Washington, M.L.: Estimating the future number of cases in the ebola epidemicliberia and sierra leone, 2014–2015. MMWR Surveill Summ **63**(suppl 3), 1–14 (2014)
28. Nishiura, H., Chowell, G.: Early transmission dynamics of ebola virus disease (EVD), West Africa, March to August 2014. Eurosurveillance, **19**(36) (2014)
29. University of Pittsburg MIDAS National Center of Excellence. Framework for Reconstructing Epidemiological Dynamics (2012). https://midas.pitt.edu/index.php?option=com_content&view=article&id=78&Itemid=72
30. World Health Organization. Ebola Epidemic Liberia, Marchoctober 2014 (2014). Available from: http://www.cdc.gov/mmwr/preview/mmwrhtml/mm63e1114a4.htm
31. World Health Organization. Who Ebola Data and Statistics (2016). Available from: http://time.com/3478238/ebola-liberia-burials-cremation-burned

32. Parpia, A.S., Ndeffo-Mbah, M.L., Wenzel, N.S., Galvani, A.P.: Effects of response to 2014–2015 ebola outbreak on deaths from malaria, HIV/AIDS, and tuberculosis, West Africa. Emerg. Infect. Dis. **22**(3), 433–441 (2016)
33. Stroud, P., Del Valle, S., Sydoriak, S., Riese, J., Mniszewski, S.: Spatial dynamics of pandemic influenza in a massive artificial society. J. Artif. Soc. Soc. Simul. **10**(4), 9 (2007)
34. WHO Ebola Response Team. Ebola virus disease in west africathe first 9 months of the epidemic and forward projections. N. Engl. J. Med. **371**(16), 1481–1495 (2014)
35. Time. Liberia burns its bodies as ebola fears run rampant (2014). Available from: http://apps.who.int/gho/data/node.ebola-sitrep
36. Troncoso, A.: Ebola outbreak in West Africa: a neglected tropical disease. Asian Pac. J. Tropical Biomed. **5**(4), 255–259 (2015)
37. Van den Driessche, P., Watmough, J.: Reproduction numbers and sub-threshold endemic equilibria for compartmental models of disease transmission. Math. Biosci. **180**(1), 29–48 (2002)
38. Van Kerkhove, M.D., Bento, A.I., Mills, H.L., Ferguson, N.M., Donnelly, C.A.: A review of epidemiological parameters from ebola outbreaks to inform early public health decision-making. Sci. Data, **2** (2015)
39. Xue, L., Scott, H.M., Cohnstaedt, L.W., Scoglio, C.: A network-based meta-population approach to model Rift Valley fever epidemics. J. Theor. Biol. (2012)

A Model for Coupled Outbreaks Contained by Behavior Change

John M. Drake and Andrew W. Park

Abstract Large epidemics such as the recent Ebola crisis in West Africa occur when local efforts to contain outbreaks fail to overcome the probabilistic onward transmission to new locations. As a result, there may be large differences in total epidemic size from similar initial conditions. This work seeks to determine the extent to which the effects of behavior changes and metapopulation coupling on epidemic size can be characterized. While mathematical models have been developed to study local containment by social distancing, intervention and other behavior changes, their connection to larger-scale transmission is relatively underdeveloped. We make use of the assumption that behavior changes limit local transmission before susceptible depletion to develop a time-varying birth-death process capturing the dynamic decrease of the transmission rate associated with behavior changes. We derive an expression for the mean outbreak size of this model and show that the distribution of outbreak sizes is approximately geometric. This allows a probabilistic extension whereby infected individuals may initiate new outbreaks. From this model we characterize the overall epidemic size as a function of the behavior change rate and the probability that an infected individual starts a new outbreak. We find good agreement between the analytical results and stochastic simulations leading to novel findings including critical learning rates that demarcate large and small epidemic sizes.

Keywords Ebola · Epidemic model · Behavior change · Transmission rate · Birth-death process · Metapopulation model

1 Introduction

Many questions arise during outbreaks of emerging infectious diseases. How transmissible is the new pathogen within the initially exposed population? How fast will it spread to other populations? What must be done to achieve containment? How large

J.M. Drake (✉) · A.W. Park
Odum School of Ecology, University of Georgia, Athens, GA 30602-2202, USA
e-mail: jdrake@uga.edu

G. Chowell and J.M. Hyman (eds.), *Mathematical and Statistical Modeling for Emerging and Re-emerging Infectious Diseases*,
DOI 10.1007/978-3-319-40413-4_3

will the final epidemic be? These questions and others are amenable to theoretical analysis using dynamic models [12]. Most models of disease transmission, however, assume time constant parameters and do not account for changing human behavior or other interventions. The 2014–2015 West Africa Ebola epidemic illustrates this point. With an R_0 around 1.7–3.0 [4, 6, 17] and a population of around 20 million persons [16] in the three primarily affected countries, the final size of an outbreak contained by susceptible depletion [13] would be from 11.7 to 18.8 million persons. In contrast, the actual epidemic size of $\approx$30,000 persons is much less than 1 % of this size.

Because standard models admit containment only after the outbreak becomes self-limiting through depletion of susceptible persons, they are inappropriate for making predictions about apparent infections, where self-protective behaviors may be quickly adopted, and in modern societies, where global financial, medical, and logistic resources are rapidly mobilized to contain emerging pathogens like SARS, MERS, and Ebola. But, if behaviors change and resources are quickly mobilized, then why have outbreaks of these emerging pathogens persisted as long as they have? One possible explanation is that behavior change and intervention are *local* events that occur only around transmission clusters and are not completely efficient, so that while behavior change and intervention act to reduce transmission where it is high, a small fraction of infections escape isolation to seed new outbreaks in spatially or socially adjacent populations. According to this idea, the persistence of the pathogen in the population—and the propensity to transition from outbreak to epidemic proportions—is based on a balance between the ability of the pathogen to spark new outbreaks and the capacity of behavior change and intervention to contain these outbreaks before further spread occurs.

Our motivation for this idea comes from the 2014–2015 West Africa Ebola epidemic. For instance, spread among counties in Liberia seems to be consistent with this picture (Fig. 1). Here we see that the epidemic was maintained by a series of outbreaks, each of which recapitulates a common pattern of explosive transmission, followed by a decline in the rate of transmission and eventual containment. Because the transmission process in each county occurs almost independently of the other counties (coupling is primarily important for the initial spark and possibly subsequent reinfections), a single compartmental model cannot accurately represent the associated dynamics. Instead, what is required is a model of coupled epidemics. In the following sections we develop a simple, conceptual model of this process. We imagine an epidemic starting with an *outbreak* originating at a single location. In contrast to most models, we assume that this outbreak is quickly contained by reductions in transmission. The stochastic nature of transmission when only a small number of persons are infected gives rise to a probability distribution in the outbreak size. Although the outbreak is quickly contained, there is a small chance that the infection is spread to an adjacent population before complete containment is achieved. If this occurs, then the process is repeated until finally no further outbreaks occur. It is this outbreak-of-outbreaks that we call an *epidemic*. To model this two-scale process, we first propose a simple model for the stochastic dynamics of an outbreak subject to behavior change, for which we obtain the mean outbreak size, denoted M. M is

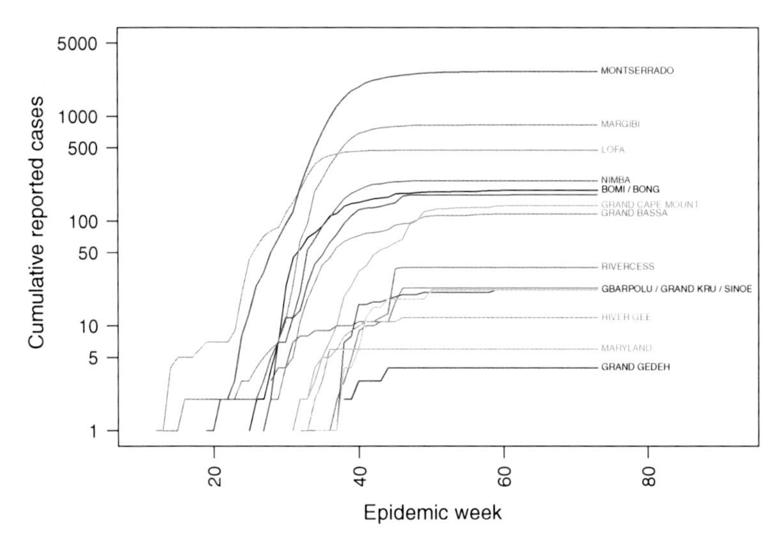

Fig. 1 In the 2014–2015 West Africa Ebola epidemic, the virus spread throughout the administrative units of Liberia during weeks 20 through 40 despite the fact that nation-wide containment measures, including border closure, were put in place beginning in week 30 and the World Health Organization declared the Ebola epidemic to be a Public Health Emergency of International Concern one week later. Here, the cumulative number of cases in each administrative unit is plotted against epidemiological week. These nearly parallel epidemic curves suggest that the same process of outbreak and control was replicated in one county after the next with local interventions and behavior change realized some finite time after cases began accumulating. For instance, approximately the same take-off rate was exhibited by Montserrado as by Grand Cape Mount, despite the fact that their first cases were separated by twelve weeks. Data from the World Health Organization situation reports

important for three reasons. First, it enables calculation of the chance that a secondary outbreak is caused, which may be iterated until no further outbreaks result. Guided by numerical experiments, we propose to approximate the probability distribution of the number of outbreaks by a geometric distribution. The second role played by the mean outbreak size is to parameterize the geometric distribution of outbreak number. Finally, by summing a random number of outbreaks with the mean size M, we obtain an approximation for the *epidemic size*, i.e., the size of all outbreaks added together. The accuracy of this approximation is studied through comparison with simulations.

Models that explicitly take account of within and between household transmission have yielded important understanding of the role of host social structure on epidemic development. Part of their success lies in the relatively simple task of enumerating all possible infection statuses of individuals in small households and of assuming a constant hazard of transmission to uninfected cohabitors [2]. In contrast, when attempting to describe connections between local outbreaks (involving population sizes much bigger than households) and larger-scale epidemics against the backdrop of reduced transmission over time, tracking the local outbreak sizes can be challenging. Previous modeling studies of behavior change to limit transmission have generally assumed that transmission dynamics may additionally be slowed by susceptible depletion, e.g., [3, 5, 15]. By instead assuming that behavior changes act before susceptible depletion, birth-death branching process techniques can be utilized. As well as lending analytical tractability, these models likely capture the rapid social distancing and learned risk-averse behavior associated with deadly diseases such as Ebola. In the recent West African outbreak, outbreak sizes were considerably smaller than population sizes (Fig. 1).

2 Final Size of a Single Outbreak with Behavior Change

We assume that local outbreaks are contained by behavior changes over time that act to reduce transmission (rather than the standard assumption of susceptible depletion). We employ a simple time-varying function for the transmission rate, $\beta_0 e^{-\phi t}$. Parameter β_0 is the intrinsic transmission rate operating in the absence of behavior change, and ϕ is the rate of decay in the transmission rate where large values of ϕ imply that effective behaviors such as social distancing are adopted rapidly. Because the removal rate μ is assumed constant then local transmission dynamics are described by

$$\frac{dI}{dt} = \beta_0 e^{-\phi t} I - \mu I; \qquad \frac{dR}{dt} = \mu I. \tag{1}$$

This is a generalized continuous-time birth-death process with time-varying birth rate, as discussed by Kendall [10]. Following Kendall, the mean final size, $R(\infty)$, is given by

$$M = 1 + \int_0^\infty e^{-\rho(\tau)} \beta(\tau) d\tau \tag{2}$$

where

$$\begin{aligned} \rho(t) &= \int_0^t (\mu - \beta(\tau)) d\tau & (3)\\ &= \mu t - \int_0^t \beta(\tau) d\tau & (4)\\ &= \mu t - \beta_0 \int_0^t e^{-\phi t} d\tau & (5)\\ &= \mu t + \frac{\beta_0}{\phi}[e^{-\phi\tau}]_0^t & (6)\\ &= \mu t + \frac{\beta_0}{\phi}(e^{-\phi t} - 1). & (7) \end{aligned}$$

So consequently, we are seeking to solve

$$\int_0^{\infty} e^{-\mu\tau-\frac{\beta_0}{\phi}(e^{-\phi\tau}-1)}\beta_0 e^{-\phi\tau}\,d\tau \tag{8}$$

$$\beta_0\int_0^{\infty} e^{-(\mu+\phi)\tau-\frac{\beta_0}{\phi}e^{-\phi\tau}}\,d\tau \tag{9}$$

$$\beta_0 e^{\frac{\beta_0}{\phi}}\int_0^{\infty} e^{-(\mu+\phi)\tau}e^{-\frac{\beta_0}{\phi}e^{-\phi\tau}}\,d\tau. \tag{10}$$

Let $z=\frac{\beta_0}{\phi}e^{-\phi\tau}$, then $dz=-\beta_0 e^{-\phi\tau}d\tau$, $d\tau=\frac{-1}{\beta_0}e^{\phi\tau}dz$, $\frac{\phi z}{\beta_0}=e^{-\phi\tau}$, $\ln(\frac{\phi z}{\beta_0})=-\phi\tau$, $\tau=\frac{-1}{\phi}\ln(\frac{\phi z}{\beta_0})$. Now the integral can be written as

$$\frac{-\beta_0}{\beta_0}e^{\frac{\beta_0}{\phi}}\int_{\frac{\beta_0}{\phi}}^{0} e^{\frac{\mu+\phi}{\phi}\ln(\frac{\phi z}{\beta_0})}e^{-z}e^{-\ln(\frac{\phi z}{\beta_0})}dz \tag{11}$$

$$-e^{\frac{\beta_0}{\phi}}\int_{\frac{\beta_0}{\phi}}^{0}\frac{\phi z}{\beta_0}^{\frac{\mu+\phi}{\phi}-1}e^{-z}dz \tag{12}$$

$$-e^{\frac{\beta_0}{\phi}}\frac{\phi}{\beta_0}^{\frac{\mu+\phi}{\phi}-1}\int_{\frac{\beta_0}{\phi}}^{0} z^{\frac{\mu+\phi}{\phi}-1}e^{-z}dz \tag{13}$$

$$e^{\frac{\beta_0}{\phi}}\frac{\phi}{\beta_0}^{\frac{\mu+\phi}{\phi}-1}\gamma\left(\frac{\mu+\phi}{\phi},\frac{\beta_0}{\phi}\right), \tag{14}$$

and the final size is

$$M=1+e^{\frac{\beta_0}{\phi}}\frac{\phi}{\beta_0}^{\frac{\mu+\phi}{\phi}-1}\gamma\left(\frac{\mu+\phi}{\phi},\frac{\beta_0}{\phi}\right), \tag{15}$$

where γ is the lower incomplete gamma function. This expression yields some insights into how underlying processes govern outbreak size. Particularly, the left panel of Fig. 2 shows the expected outbreak size to increase greater than exponentially as β_0 increases. Similarly, the outbreak size initially drops dramatically with learning rate (between 0 and ≈ 0.05 in the right panel of Fig. 2), diminishing as the realized transmission rate becomes small ($\phi > 0.05$). In this figure, the shoulder occurs when ϕ is about one fortieth of β_0.

Stochastic simulations of Eq. 1, obtained using Gillespie's direct method, show that outbreak size is "fat-tailed" with high variance, considerable right skew, and a spike at zero (Fig. 3). This suggests the outbreak size distribution might be approximated by a geometric distribution with mean M (Eq. 15). Figure 3 compares 5,000

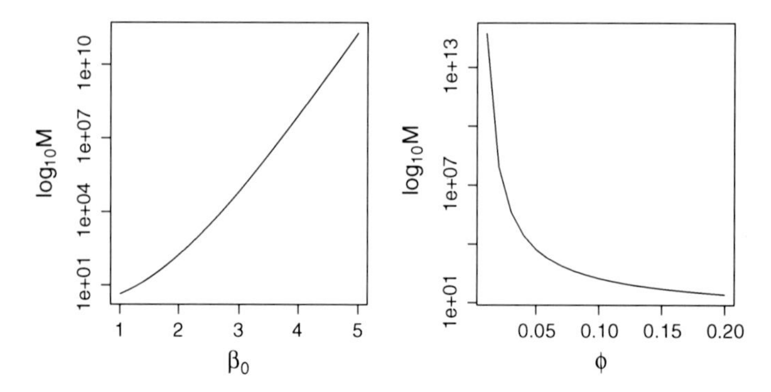

Fig. 2 Mean outbreak size, M, as a function of β_0 and ϕ (with μ held at 1.0, ϕ is fixed at 0.1 in the *left panel*, and β_0 fixed at 2 in the *right panel*). Note the non-linear functions in semi-log space

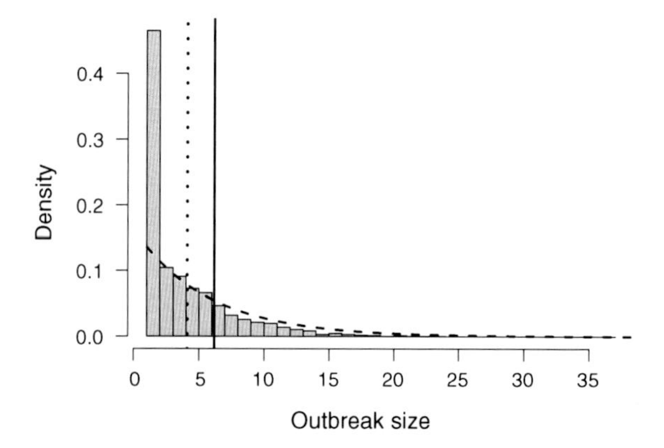

Fig. 3 Histogram of the final outbreak size based on 5000 replicates of the stochastic version of Eq. 1 with $I(0) = 1$, $\beta_0 = 2.0$, $\phi = 0.5$ and $\mu = 1.0$. The *vertical dotted line* shows the sample mean oubreak size from these stochastic simulations. The *solid vertical line* represents the theoretical mean outbreak size (Eq. 15) and the *dashed curve* is the density of the geometric distribution parameterized with the sample mean outbreak size

simulated outbreak sizes with the corresponding approximation (dashed line). The mean of the approximating distribution (solid line) is only slightly larger than the mean of the simulations.

3 Global Epidemic Model

To scale up from local outbreaks to epidemics we adopt a probabilistic model in which local outbreaks are connected by movement of infected individuals among communities. In general, we assume that the number of uninfected communities is large so that the chance that an infected individual sparks an outbreak in another community may be represented by a small constant $0 < \varepsilon \ll 1$. Let p_x be the probability mass function for an outbreak of size x. Since the probability that an individual doesn't spark a secondary outbreak is $1 - \varepsilon$, the probability that an outbreak of size x fails to spark a secondary outbreak will be $(1 - \varepsilon)^x$ by an assumption of independence. The probability that there is an outbreak of size x and that it fails to spark any secondary outbreaks is therefore $p_x(1 - \varepsilon)^x$. By enumeration of all possible outbreak sizes, the probability that an outbreak of unknown size will spark at least one secondary outbreak is

$$\alpha = 1 - \sum_{x=1}^{\infty} p_x(1 - \varepsilon)^x. \tag{16}$$

With $\varepsilon \ll 1$, we assume that each outbreak sparks, at most, only one secondary outbreak.

Let $j = 1, 2, 3, \ldots, N$ index the local outbreaks so that N is the total number of local outbreaks. The probability that the first outbreak is also the last one is just $p(N = 1) = 1 - \alpha$. By contrast, the probability that the first outbreak gives rise to a secondary outbreak (with probability α) and that the second outbreak fails to give rise to a third (with probability $1 - \alpha$) is $p(N = 2) = \alpha(1 - \alpha)$. Proceeding to $j = 3$, the probability that both outbreaks one and two give rise to a secondary outbreak and that the third outbreak is the last yields $p(N = 3) = \alpha^2(1 - \alpha)$. By induction, we see that the general rule is given by

$$f(m) = p(N = m) = \alpha^{m-1}(1 - \alpha). \tag{17}$$

The next challenge is to ascertain the total number of cases in these m outbreaks. Let X_j be the random number of cases in the jth outbreak. The total number of cases in the epidemic will be the sum of cases in the local outbreaks, i.e.,

$$Y_m = \sum_{j=1}^{m} X_j. \tag{18}$$

Since the X_j are independently and identically distributed according to distribution p_x, it follows that the distribution of Y_m is just the m-fold convolution of p_x, denoted p_x^{m*}. The probability that there are exactly m outbreaks and that these give rise to Y cases is

$$p_y = p_x^{m*} f(m). \tag{19}$$

Using the notation of Johnson et al. [8], we have the following re-parameterization for the distribution of outbreak sizes.

$$M = (1 - p)/p \to p = 1/(M + 1), \tag{20}$$

$$P = (1 - p)/p = M, \tag{21}$$

and

$$Q = 1/p = M + 1. \tag{22}$$

If k outbreaks are summed, the result is negative binomially distributed with parameters k and P. Let k be the number of non-primary outbreaks. Applying the same rationale used to arrive at Eq. 17, we obtain $P(k = 0) = 1 - \alpha = a$ and in general $P(k = n) = (1 - a)^n a$. So, the number of non-primary outbreaks is a geometric distribution with parameter $p = a$.

Following Johnson et al. [8], the distribution formed by taking a negative binomial with k drawn from a geometric distribution with parameters Q' and P' is also a geometric distribution with parameter $QQ' - P'$. Identifying parameters in Eq. 17, we have $Q' = 1/(1 - \alpha)$ and $P' = \alpha Q'$ yielding $Q = (M + 1)(\frac{1}{1-\alpha}) - \frac{\alpha}{(1-\alpha)}$. Expanding to obtain the unconditional total epidemic size distribution, we have

$$P(Y = y) = \pi(1 - \pi)^{y-1}, \tag{23}$$

where

$$\pi = \left((M + 1)(\frac{1}{1 - \alpha}) - \frac{\alpha}{(1 - \alpha)}\right)^{-1}. \tag{24}$$

This simplifies to

$$P(Y = y) = \frac{(1 - \alpha)(M/(M + 1 - \alpha))^{y-1}}{M + 1 - \alpha} \tag{25}$$

with expected value

$$1/\pi = (M + 1)\left(\frac{1}{1 - \alpha}\right) - \frac{\alpha}{(1 - \alpha)}. \tag{26}$$

4 Comparison with Numerical Results

This derivation of Eq. 25 relies on approximations for the probability of a secondary outbreak given an outbreak of unknown size (Eq. 16) and the distribution of outbreak sizes (assumed to be approximated by a geometric distribution), as well as the assumption that outbreak number and outbreak sizes are independent. We evaluated these assumptions by comparing Eq. 25 with numerical simulations in which chains of outbreaks were probabilistically generated by linking individual outbreaks simu-

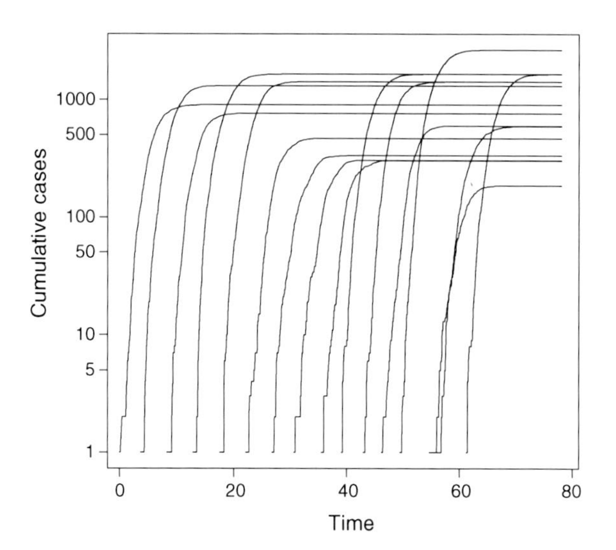

Fig. 4 Example output from model simulating coupled outbreak dynamics initiated by a single individual. The local outbreak dynamic parameters are $\beta_0 = 3.0$, $\mu = 1.0$ and $\phi = 0.1$. The per capita rate of sparking a new outbreak is $\varepsilon = 0.25$. In this example, there are 16 local outbreaks before the process stops

lated as in Sect. 2. Figure 4 shows an example solution that is visually similar to the data on Ebola shown in Fig. 1. Figure 5 compares the mean and 99th percentile of epidemic size for the approximation and simulated results over a range of ε and ϕ. The two solutions are similar to order of magnitude for most combinations of these parameters, failing primarily when ϕ becomes very small.

5 Discussion

The goal of this work has been to develop a relatively simple model that nevertheless provides valid insight into the effects of behavior change and coupling among local populations on the final size of potentially extensive outbreaks. Such processes are invariably at work in outbreaks of novel pathogens that ultimately affect large, distributed populations, notably outbreaks of Ebola [17], SARS [11], and MERS [14]. The model we developed considers *epidemics* to consist of multiple coupled *outbreaks* where outbreak trajectories are contained by local behavior response. Containment is counteracted with the potential of each local outbreak to spark secondary outbreaks through the movement of infected persons so that the final epidemic size reflects the tension between these two processes.

Focusing first on the distribution of outbreak sizes, this work shows that initially supercritical outbreaks that are intrinsically contained through a decline in the transmission rate (assumed to be exponential with time since the outbreak began), give rise to a fat-tailed distribuion of local outbreak sizes. Moreover, the outbreak size distribution changes in a strongly nonlinear fashion with respect to both the initial rate of transmission and the learning rate. Approximating this distribution by a geometric

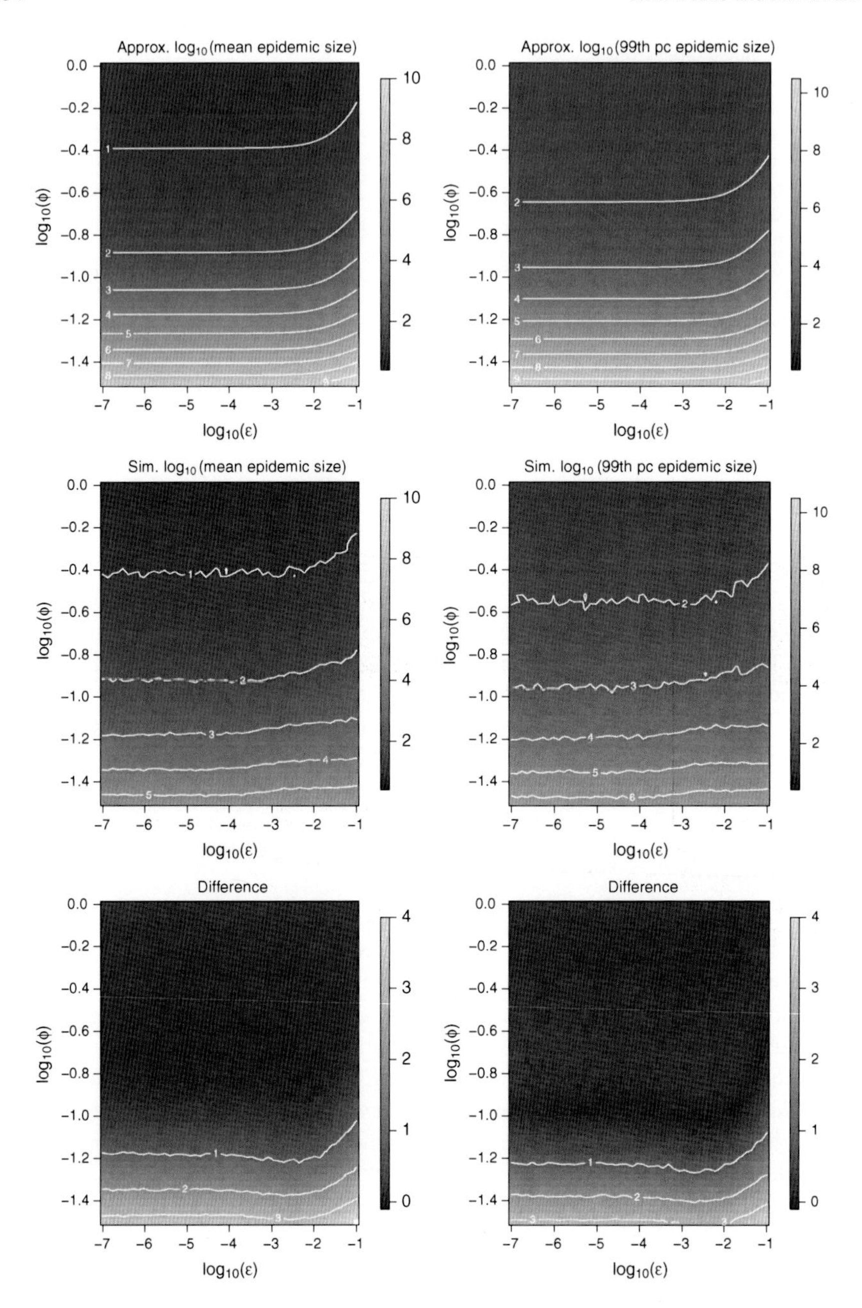

Fig. 5 *Left-hand panels* (*top* to *bottom*) show the predicted mean epidemic size, Eq. 26, the simulated mean epidemic size and the difference between the two as a function of model parameters ε and ϕ. *Right-hand panels* show analogous information for the 99th percentile of epidemic sizes. Constant model parameters are $\beta_0 = 2.0$ and $\mu = 1.0$. Epidemic sizes are simulated from 5000 replications. Contours are indicated by *white lines*

distribution with mean given by Eq. 15 enables one to investigate the tension between containment and expansive spread, i.e., epidemics. Figure 5 shows there to be a large region of the upper left of the $\varepsilon - \phi$ parameter space in which epidemics (i.e., extensive outbreaks with multiple communities affected) are exceedingly unlikely. To the right hand of each panel in Fig. 5, i.e., as $\varepsilon \to 1$, the outbreak size contours turn up rapidly, beyond which movement of infected individuals is so common that the epidemic is effectively well mixed. Outside this range, the outbreak size contours are practically horizontal, illustrating very little dependence on the rate of individual movement so that learning—and the propensity to self-containment—becomes the much more important process. We are unaware of prior results suggesting this transition between epidemics dominated by movement and epidemics dominated by learning.

The super-exponetial scaling of the outbreak size shown in Fig. 2 is recapitulated in the distribution of outbreak sizes. Thus, for instance, as one moves from the top of each panel in Fig. 5 the contours become closer together. Similarly, the fat-tail in the outbreak size distribution (Fig. 3) propagates to the epidemic size distribution. This is perhaps most easily seen by noting that there is an approximately one logarithm displacement between the contours for the average epidemic size and the 99th percentile in Fig. 5. Thus, for an average epidemic size of 1,000, it is not improbable for an epidemic of 10,000 to be realized. Comparison of the approximate analytic results in the first row of Fig. 5 with the exact results from stochastic simulation in the second row shows that although the approximation comes at a small cost in terms of bias, these qualitative conclusions are robust to the range of assumptions required for their solution, particularly the assumption that the zero-inflated distribution of outbreak sizes can be reasonably approximated by a geometric distribution.

Other assumptions we have made include that the probability any local outbreak sparks more than one secondary outbreak is negligible and that there is no effect of susceptible depletion. The first of these assumptions biases downward our expression for the total number of outbreaks (Eq. 17). This bias becomes more severe as $\varepsilon \to 1$, i.e., to the right in each panel of Fig. 5, which would further differentiate our two modes for epidemic expansion. The second issue is of negligible consequence unless the total epidemic size tends to be large relative to the population size (precisely what containment prevents) or where the contacts among susceptible persons are highly structured. While there has been a great deal of theory about this latter condition [9], whether it obtains in generalized epidemics like Ebola remains poorly understood. Additionally, the modeling approach adopted here may admit other assumptions (particularly concerning the underlying distribution of local outbreak sizes) and extensions, including the seeding of multipe new outbreaks from a single outbreak and a time-varying "death" rate in the birth-death process, representing more rapid treatment/isolation with increasing experience.

Multiscale modeling of infectious diseases remains a significant mathematical and computational challenge [7]. The simplifying, plausible assumptions made here have allowed us to relate ultimate epidemic size to the rate at which transmission at a local scale is reduced by behavior change and the probability that a new outbreak is seeded elsewhere before local containment. These analytical results are achieved even though the model does not describe a stationary process and illustrates the value of combining modeling approaches, here the outcome of a potentially large number of branching processes accumulated via convolution. One of the key results is that epidemic size grows faster than exponential with decreasing behavioral learning rate, suggesting that there are critical rates above which behaviors acting to reduce transmission will dramatically reduce the overall number of persons infected during a series of outbreaks. Qualitatively, this phenomenon points to a potential connection between the approach undertaken here and random network modeling [1] where the addition of a few links can lead to explosive percolation suddenly connecting a large proportion of nodes. Practically, it underscores the importance of early response to epidemic containment.

Acknowledgments Research reported here was supported by the National Institute Of General Medical Sciences of the National Institutes of Health under Award Number U01GM110744 and the National Science Foundation under Rapid Award Number 1515194. The content is solely the responsibility of the authors and does not necessarily reflect the official views of the National Institutes of Health or the National Science Foundation.

References

1. Achlioptas, D., D'Souza, R.M., Spencer, J.: Explosive percolation in random networks. Science **323**(5920), 1453–5 (2009)
2. Ball, F., Britton, T., House, T., Isham, V., Mollison, D., Pellis, L., Scalia Tomba, G.: Seven challenges for metapopulation models of epidemics, including households models. Epidemics **10**, 63–67 (2015)
3. Brauer, F.: A simple model for behaviour change in epidemics. BMC Public Health **11 Suppl 1**, S3 (2011)
4. Drake, J.M., Bakach, I., Just, M.R., ORegan, S.M., Gambhir, M., Fung, I.C.H.: Transmission models of historical Ebola outbreaks. Emerging Infect. Dis. **21**, 1447–1450 (2015)
5. Drake, J.M., Chew, S.K., Ma, S.: Societal learning in epidemics: intervention effectiveness during the 2003 SARS outbreak in Singapore. PLOS One **1**, e20 (2006)
6. Drake, J.M., Kaul, R.B., Alexander, L.W., Regan, S.M.O., Kramer, M., Pulliam, J.T., Ferrari, M.J., Park, A.W.: Ebola cases and health system demand in Liberia. PLOS Biol. **13**(1), e1002,056 (2015)
7. Guo, D., Li, K.C., Peters, T.R., Snively, B.M., Poehling, K.A., Zhou, X.: Multi-scale modeling for the transmission of influenza and the evaluation of interventions toward it. Sci. Rep. **5**, 8980 (2015)
8. Johnson, N.L., Kotz, S., Kemp, A.W.: Univariate Discrete Distributions. Wiley, New York (1992)
9. Keeling, M.: The implications of network structure for epidemic dynamics. Theor. Popul. Biol. **67**(1), 1–8 (2005)
10. Kendall, D.G.: On the generalized "birth-and-death" process. Ann. Math. Stat. **19**(1), 1–15 (1948)
11. Lai, P.C., Wong, C.M., Hedley, A.J., Lo, S.V., Leung, P.Y., Kong, J., Leung, G.M.: Understanding the spatial clustering of severe acute respiratory syndrome (SARS) in Hong Kong. Environ. Health Perspect. **112**(15), 1550–1556 (2004)
12. Lofgren, E.T., Halloran, M.E., Rivers, C.M., Drake, J.M., Porco, T.C., Lewis, B., Yang, W., Vespignani, A., Shaman, J., Eisenberg, J.N.S., Eisenberg, M.C., Marathe, M., Scarpino, S.V., Alexander, K.A., Meza, R., Ferrari, M.J., Hyman, J.M., Meyers, L.A., Eubank, S.: Mathematical

models: a key tool for outbreak response. Proc. Natl. Acad. Sci. USA **111**(51), 18,095–18,096 (2014)
13. Ma, J., Earn, D.J.D.: Generality of the final size formula for an epidemic of a newly invading infectious disease. Bull. Math. Biol. **68**(3), 679–702 (2006)
14. Poletto, C., Pelat, C., Levy-Bruhl, D., Yazdanpanah, Y., Boelle, P.Y., Colizza, V.: Assessment of the Middle East respiratory syndrome coronavirus (MERS-CoV) epidemic in the Middle East and risk of international spread using a novel maximum likelihood analysis approach. Eurosurveillance **19**(23), 20824 (2014)
15. Ruan, S., Wang, W.: Dynamical behavior of an epidemic model with a nonlinear incidence rate. J. Differ. Equ. **188**(1), 135–163 (2003)
16. UN: World Population Prospects: The 2015 Revision, Key Findings and Advance Tables. Technical Report, United Nations, Department of Economic and Social Affairs, Population Division (2015)
17. WHO Ebola Response Team: Ebola Virus Disease in West Africa - The First 9 Months of the Epidemic and Forward Projections. New Engl. J. Med. **371**(16), 1481–1495 (2014)

Real-Time Assessment of the International Spreading Risk Associated with the 2014 West African Ebola Outbreak

Ana Pastore-Piontti, Qian Zhang, Marcelo F.C. Gomes, Luca Rossi, Chiara Poletto, Vittoria Colizza, Dennis L. Chao, Ira M. Longini, M. Elizabeth Halloran and Alessandro Vespignani

Abstract The 2014 West African Ebola Outbreak is the largest Ebola virus disease (EVD) epidemic ever recorded, not only in number of cases but also in geographical extent. Unlike previous EVD outbreaks, the large number of cases observed in major cities with international airports raised the concern about the possibility of exportation of the infection in countries around the world. Starting in July 2014,

A. Pastore-Piontti · Q. Zhang · A. Vespignani (✉)
Northeastern University, Boston, MA, USA
e-mail: a.vespignani@neu.edu; alexves@gmail.com

A. Pastore-Piontti
e-mail: a.pastoreypiontti@neu.edu

Q. Zhang
e-mail: qi.zhang@neu.edu

M.F.C. Gomes
Fiocruz, Rio de Janeiro, Brazil
e-mail: marcelo.gomes@fiocruz.br

L. Rossi
ISI Foundation, Turin, Italy
e-mail: luca.rossi@isi.it

C. Poletto · V. Colizza
Sorbonne Universities, UPMC Univ Paris 06, UMR-S 1136,
Institut Pierre Louis d'Epidemiologie et de Sante Publique, F-75013 Paris, France
e-mail: chiara.poletto@inserm.fr

V. Colizza
e-mail: vittoria.colizza@inserm.fr

D.L. Chao
Institute for Disease Modeling, Intellectual Ventures, Bellevue, WA, USA
e-mail: dennisc@intven.com

I.M. Longini
Department of Biostatistics, University of Florida, Gainesville, FL, USA
e-mail: ilongini@ufl.edu

M.E. Halloran
Fred Hutchinson Cancer Research Center, Seattle, WA, USA
e-mail: betz@fhcrc.org

G. Chowell and J.M. Hyman (eds.), *Mathematical and Statistical Modeling for Emerging and Re-emerging Infectious Diseases*,
DOI 10.1007/978-3-319-40413-4_4

we used the Global Epidemic and Mobility model to provide a real-time assessment of the potential international spread of the EVD epidemic. We modeled the unfolding of the outbreak in the most affected countries, considered different scenarios reflecting changes in the disease dynamic, and provided estimates for the probability of observing imported cases around the world for 220 countries. The model went through successive calibrations as more surveillance data were available, providing projections extending from a few weeks to several months. The results show that along the entire course of the epidemic the probability of observing cases outside of Africa was small, but not negligible, from September to November 2014. The inflection point of the epidemic occurred in late September and early October 2014 with a consistent longitudinal decrease in new cases, thus averting the status quo epidemic growth that could have seen hundreds of exported cases at the global scale in the following months.

Keywords Ebola · Epidemic · West Africa · Large scale model · International spread · Agent-based model · Computational model

1 Introduction

The Ebola Virus Disease (EVD) is caused by infection with a virus of the family Filoviridae, genus Ebolavirus [1]. The EVD causes an acute, serious illness, which is often fatal if is not treated. It is thought that fruit bats are the natural Ebola virus hosts, and that the virus is introduced into the human population through close contact with bodily fluids of infected animals such as fruit bats and monkeys. The EVD then spreads through human to human via direct contact with blood, secretions, and/or other bodily fluids of dead or living infectious people [2]. Gene sequencing of the virus causing the 2014 West African (2014 WA) outbreak showed 98 % homology with the Zaire Ebola virus, with a 55 % case fatality ratio (CFR) across the recently affected countries [3]. Unfortunately at the start of the outbreak there were no licensed treatments available for EVD, and severely ill patients could only be cared for with intensive supportive care. In August 2015, the preliminary assessment of the ring vaccination trial of the EVD vaccine candidate rVSV-ZEBOV provided a 100 % (95 % CI 74.7–100) efficacy [4, 5].

As in previous outbreaks, the current one started in a remote area of Guinea, during December of 2013, although the exact place is uncertain. Soon afterwards, in early 2014, there were cases of Ebola in the neighboring countries of Liberia (March 2014) and Sierra Leone (May 2014), affecting their capital cities. The West African region was affected by an Ebola epidemic that for the first time extended across three countries simultaneously: Guinea, Liberia and Sierra Leone. On July 20, 2014, a passenger infected with the Ebola virus, traveling from Liberia to Nigeria, started an outbreak in Lagos. In total 20 people were infected in Nigeria, where the outbreak was successfully contained [6].

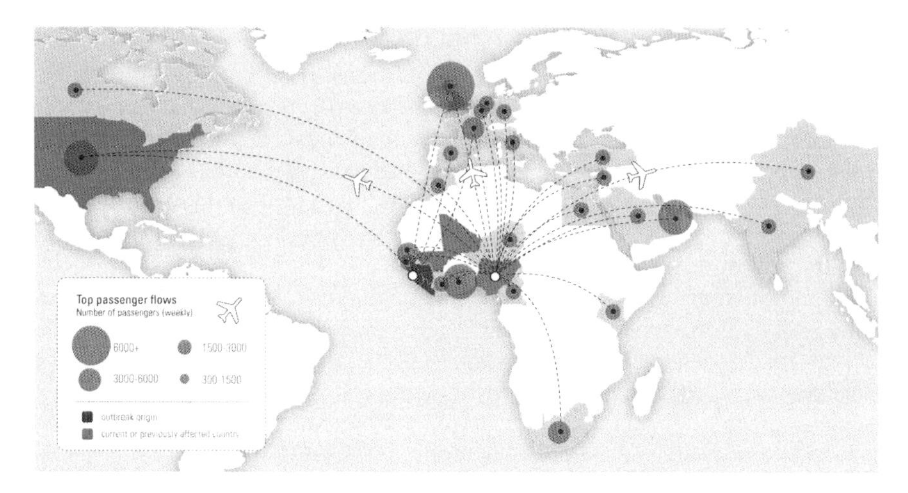

Fig. 1 Air traffic connections from West African countries to the rest of the world. Guinea, Liberia and Sierra Leone are not well connected outside the region. Nigeria, in contrast, being the most populous country in West Africa, with more than 166 million people, is well connected to the rest of the world. For historical reasons, all these countries have the strongest ties with European countries.

Unfortunately, it was not until July/August 2014 that the international community started to realize the catastrophic dimension of the epidemic [7]. In August 2014, more and more cases were observed in large cities such as Conakry, Freetown, Monrovia and Lagos, raising the concern about the possible internationalization of the outbreak, as these urban areas have major international airports (see Fig. 1). While importation of cases should not generate large outbreaks in countries where prompt isolation of cases in appropriate health care facilities occurs, it was clear that a quantitative analysis of the risk of internalization of the epidemic outside West Africa was needed to inform public health policies and country preparedness worldwide.

To better understand the potential international dissemination of the EVD outbreak, we proposed a computational framework to model the short-term disease dynamic behavior and provided a real-time quantitative assessments of the risk of EVD case importation across the world. The quantitative analysis is based on large-scale computer simulations of the 2014 WA EVD outbreak that generate stochastic outputs of the epidemic spread worldwide, yielding, among other measures, the case importation events at a daily resolution for 3,362 subpopulations in 220 countries. Specifically, we used the Global Epidemic and Mobility model (GLEAM) that integrates high-resolution data on human demography and mobility on a worldwide scale in a metapopulation stochastic epidemic model [8–10]. The disease dynamics within each population considers explicitly that EVD transmissions occur in the general community, in hospital settings, and during funeral rites [11]. We considered different scenarios that simulated the mitigation efforts on the ground. For parameter inference, we used a Monte Carlo likelihood analysis to select an ensemble of disease dynamic models executed with 3,000,000 simulations sampling the disease model space and the surveillance data on the 2014 WA EVD outbreak at various points in time. The selected models allowed us to generate numerical stochastic simulations of the EVD epidemic at the local (within West African countries) and global level. In September 2014, analyses on the risk of international spread of the outbreak focused on the analysis of the sheer volume of international passenger traffic across countries [12, 13]. We used an approach that fully couples the specific etiology of the disease, the local dynamics of the outbreak in the affected countries, and the individuals mobility worldwide.

Within this framework, we evaluated the progression of the epidemic in West Africa and its international spread under three different scenarios, namely status quo, marginal containment and containment, accounting for the different temporal dynamics that the EVD outbreak could follow depending on success of the containment interventions. The status quo scenario simply assumes that the epidemic grows at the same exponential rate observed in August 2014. while the other two scenarios consider partial and full control of the epidemics respectively. In the two intervention containment scenarios, as the outbreak evolved, we considered that the control policies were successfully reducing the transmissibility to a nearly sub-critical and sub-critical values, just as it actually happened after September 2014.

As the outbreak progressed, we were able to assess the risk of the internationalization of the epidemic in real-time, which allowed us to perform a longitudinal analysis throughout the months between September 2014 to February 2015 at a worldwide level. This analysis provided possibles outcomes, from the possibility of observing hundreds of exported cases by January 2015 in the status quo scenario, to just a few cases in the case of containment. In terms of international spreading risk, we found that the probability of case exportation was extremely low (upper bound less than 5 % by the end of September 2014) for non-African countries, including the most connected countries to Africa, such as the United Kingdom (UK), Belgium, France and the United States (US), which receive 40 % of the total traffic of passengers from West Africa to the rest of the world. We also found that this probability would have increased month by month if the outbreak were not contained. In our study we considered the effects of travel restrictions, considering an 80 % airline traffic reduction from and to the West African countries affected by the outbreak [14]

2 Methods

In this section we provide a description of the data and the data-driven computational framework that we used to provide a quantitative analysis of the development of the EVD outbreak in West Africa.

2.1 Global Epidemic and Mobility Model

The Global Epidemic and Mobility (GLEAM) model is a stochastic and individual based epidemic model that combines real-world data and computational techniques allowing us to perform in-silico simulation of the spatial spreading of a disease at a global level. GLEAM is based on a meta-population network approach where the world is divided into geographical regions connected by a network of interactions given by population traffic flows from transportation and mobility infrastructures. The model's technical details and the algorithms underpinning the computational implementation are extensively reported in the literature [8–10, 15]. Using real demographics, the model divides the world population into geographic census areas that are defined around transportation hubs and connected by mobility fluxes; this process effectively defines an infectious disease meta-population network model [16–18].

The subpopulations of the model correspond to geographical census areas defined around transportation hubs obtained using a Voronoi-like tessellation of the Earth's surface by assigning each cell of the grid to the closest transportation hub (generally airports or major urban areas) taking into account distance constraints. The population of each census area is obtained by integrating data from the high-resolution population database of the *Gridded Population of the World* project of the Socioeconomic Data and Application Center at Columbia University (SEDAC) [19]. The model counts more than 3,300 census areas in about 220 different countries (numbers may vary by the year considered according to changes in the databases, often because of countries' conflicts).

The mobility among sub-populations integrates the mobility by global air travel (obtained from the International Air Transport Association [20] and the Official Airline Guide [21] database) with the short-scale mobility between adjacent sub-populations, which represents the daily commuting patterns of individuals. Commuting and short-range mobility considers data from 80,000 administrative regions from countries in 5 different continents. The model also considers the modeling of mobility through different validated approaches [9, 22]. GLEAM simulates the number of daily passengers traveling worldwide by using the real data obtained from the airline transportation databases, which contain the number of available seats on each airline connection in the world among the indexed airports. The short range commuting flows are accounted for by defining effective mechanistic sub-population mixing [10]. The time step of the model is set to one day.

The disease model within each subpopulation assumes a compartmental classification of the disease under study. The epidemic evolution is modeled using an individual dynamics where transitions are mathematically defined by chain binomial and multinomial processes [23] to preserve the discrete and stochastic nature of the processes. Each sub-population's disease dynamic is coupled with the other sub-population's through the simulated travel and commuting patterns of disease carriers. The disease model used for this study is specific to the EVD and follows the compartmentalization used by Legrand et al. [11]. The model works in discrete time steps, representing a full day, to computationally implement the air travel, the compartmental transitions (where the force of infection takes into account both the infection dynamics and the short-range movement of individuals), and the partial aggregation of the results at the desired level of geographic resolution. The model is fully stochastic and from any nominally identical initialization (initial conditions and disease model) generates an ensemble of possible epidemic evolutions for epidemic observables, such as newly generated cases, time of arrival of the infection, and number of traveling carriers.

2.2 Disease Dynamic Model

In order to study the dynamics of the disease, we used a compartmental classification of the stages of the disease. We considered two different models of increasing detail. One parsimonious model assumes an SEIR compartmental structure where individuals are classified as it follows: susceptible individuals S who can acquire the infection; exposed individuals E that will become infectious at a rate $\epsilon = 1/7$ days^{-1}; infectious individuals I that can transmit the disease; removed individuals R where the infectious individuals move at a rate $\gamma = 1/10$ days^{-1}. The R compartment includes the individuals that can no longer transmit the disease because either they have recovered or died. The transition probabilities were chosen for consistency with the more refined model adopted in our analysis. The second model, based on Legrand et al. [11], contains features specific to EVD transmission. Individuals are classified in the following way: susceptible individuals S, who can acquire the disease after contact with infectious individuals, exposed individuals E who are infected but do not transmit the disease and are asymptomatic, infectious individuals I who can transmit the disease and are symptomatic, hospitalized infectious individuals H, dead individuals F that can infect through the burial ceremonies, and recovered or removed individuals R. In both models, individuals in the exposed state are allowed to follow usual mobility patterns and travel internationally. At the same time we also considered two variations of these models: (i) the EVD cases are identified after the first connecting flight; (ii) the EVD cases are able to travel to their final destination. These models provide a minimum and maximum for the probability of case importation in each country, whose spread depends on whether the transportation system of a country act as a traffic gateway or a destination hub. These models presented similar outcomes and we only report the results for (ii). In Fig. 2, we show a schematic representation of the model and the transitions between compartments. In Table 1 we report in detail the transition probabilities used in this study.

From the proportion of hospitalized cases θ, one can obtain the hospitalization rate θ_1 for the infectious compartment I. This can be done by assuming that θ corresponds to the fraction of instantaneous transitions from compartment I to the hospitalized compartment H, over all transitions originating from I. A similar construction is done to obtain the compartment specific death rates δ_1 and δ_2. For the calculation of δ_1, the fatality rate for non-hospitalized infected individuals, we consider that the CFR δ equals the fraction of transitions from compartment I to F with respect to all

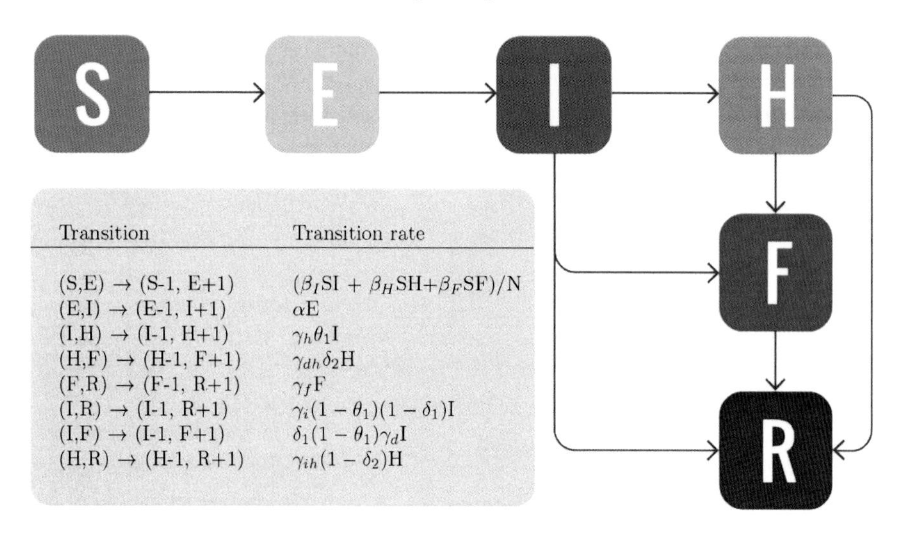

Fig. 2 Schematic representation of the compartmental model with susceptible individuals, S; exposed individuals, E; infectious cases in the community, I; hospitalized cases, H; dead but not yet buried, F; and individuals no longer transmitting the disease, R. Model parameters are: β_I, transmission coefficient in the community; β_H, transmission coefficient at the hospital; β_F, transmission coefficient during funerals. θ_1 is computed so that θ% of infectious cases are hospitalized. Compartment specific δ_1 and δ_2 are computed so that the overall case-fatality ratio is δ. The mean incubation period is given by α^{-1}; γ_h^{-1} is the mean duration from symptom onset to hospitalization; γ_{dh}^{-1} is the mean duration from hospitalization to death; γ_i^{-1} is the mean duration of the infectious period for survivors; γ_{ih}^{-1} is the mean duration from hospitalization to end of infectiousness for survivors; and finally, γ_f^{-1} is the mean duration from death to burial

Table 1 The time spent in each compartment corresponds to the mean time reported in the different references and used by the Legrand et al. study [11]

Transition parameters	Value (Ref.)
Mean duration of incubation period ($1/\alpha$)	7 days [26–28]
Mean time from onset to hospitalization ($1/\gamma_h$)	5 days [29]
Mean time from onset to death ($1/\gamma_d$)	9.6 days [29]
Mean time from onset to end of infectiousness for survivors ($1/\gamma_i$)	10 days [28, 30]
Mean time from death to traditional burial ($1/\gamma_f$)	2 days [11]
Proportion of cases hospitalized, θ	80 % [29]
Rate of transition from infectious to hospitalized (θ_1)	0.67
Case fatality ratio, δ	55 %
δ_1	0.54
δ_2	0.53
Mean time from hospitalization to end of infectiousness for survivors ($1/\gamma_{ih}$)	5 days
Mean time from hospitalization to death ($1/\gamma_{dh}$)	4.6 days

θ_1 is computed in order to obtain the given proportion, θ%, of infectious individuals hospitalized. δ_1 and δ_2 are computed in order to have an overall case fatality ratio δ. δ_1 and δ_2 are fatality ratio parameters associated with the different compartments. For details on how to compute each one of them see Ref. [11]

transitions that do not correspond to hospitalization. The same is done for δ_2, the fatality rate for hospitalized individuals, where we take δ equal to the fraction of transitions H to F, with respect to all transitions from compartment H.

The expression for the basic reproductive number R_0 is obtained following the method of Dieckmann & Heesterbeek [24, 25]. Legrand et al. [11] showed that this parameter can be written as the sum of three terms for this model: a term that accounts for the transmissions in the community, R_I, a second term that accounts for transmissions within hospitals, R_H, and a third that takes into account the infections from dead individuals, R_F. As the outbreak has been developing for several months, we consider that any containment measure is already in place. Therefore any reduction in the transmissibility in each setting is already incorporated in the corresponding effective transmission rate in each compartment, β_I, β_H and β_F. As shown in Ref. [11], the relationship between each compartment's specific reproduction rate and transmissibility is given by

$$\begin{aligned} R_0 &= R_I + R_H + R_F, \\ R_I &= \frac{\beta_I}{\Delta}, \\ R_H &= \frac{\theta \beta_H}{\gamma_{dh}\delta_2 + \gamma_{ih}(1-\delta_2)}, \\ R_F &= \frac{\delta \beta_F}{\gamma_F}, \end{aligned} \tag{1}$$

where the parameter $\Delta = \gamma_h\theta_1 + \gamma_d\delta_1(1-\theta_1) + \gamma_i(1-\theta_1)(1-\delta_1)$.

The modeling of the 2014WA Ebola outbreak was a challenging task because of the lack of information about the epidemic itself (i.e. number of cases or their location). We also faced the lack of updated information about health structure (number of hospitals and care givers) and demographics, just to mention a few.

Back in August 2014, the only regularly updated dataset was provided by the World Health Organization. From the *Disease Outbreaks News* (DONs) [31] at the beginning of the outbreak, and later through the *Situation Reports*, it was possible to construct a time series for the number of cases and deaths from EVD in West Africa. Despite the fact that the disease was already evolving for several months, for our assessment we only considered data after July 7, 2014. We chose this particular date because it was when the DONs and Situation Reports became periodic (twice a week) and consistent on the cases and dates of reports for the different countries. Using the compartmental model described above that includes the hospital and funeral settings, we first modeled the short term behavior of the disease dynamics.

2.3 Real-Time Model Calibration

We considered Guinea, Liberia and Sierra Leone as the countries officially affected by the EVD outbreak. In order to calibrate the model we used the WHO Disease outbreak News [31] at the very beginning of the outbreak and later the Situation Reports [6] provided by the WHO. From the available datasets we built a time-line tracking the number of cases occurring in each of these countries. It is worth noting that the data provided in these reports was constantly updated and revised, meaning that the number of cases reported were retrospectively changed according to new data and reports.

We assumed as the free parameters of the model those defining the transmissibility of EVD in each considered setting. For the remaining parameters we assumed initially the values reported in Table 1, together with results found across the literature for past outbreaks [11, 32, 33]. After the publication of the data from the WHO collaboration team [34, 35] we used these results to calibrate our model to the ongoing West African outbreak. In order to estimate the transmissibility components, we explored R_0 in the interval $[0.2, 4.2]$, generating for each sampled point a statistical ensemble of 1,000 identically initialized Monte Carlo simulations of the epidemic spread at the local and global level. We performed a Latin hypercube sampling of the model space defined by the vector $\mathbf{P}(R_I, R_H, R_F)$. The simulations were initialized with data on the number cases provided by the WHO reports in the three most affected countries during the week of July 6, 2014. For each ensemble, it is possible to estimate the likelihood function $\mathscr{L}(\mathbf{P}|\mathbf{x})$, where $\mathbf{x} = (x_{t_0}, \ldots, x_{t_N})$ indicates the number of cases, according to the WHO reports, during the time interval spanning from t_0 to t_N. As long as the new stable surveillance data are added to the WHO reports, the calibration time interval could also be extended. It should be noted that the vector $\mathbf{P}$ defines for each set of values a different global epidemic model through the non-parametric definition of the infection spread across different sub-populations. In other words, while the local transmission model has the same structure, the coupling among sub-populations is defined by a different non-parametric mechanistic approach. Consider the model with the maximum likelihood $\mathscr{L}(\hat{\mathbf{P}}|\mathbf{x})$, we have considered the likelihood region defined by the 1/10 relative likelihood function in defining the parameters range and selected models that satisfy

$$\frac{\mathscr{L}(\mathbf{P}|\mathbf{x})}{\mathscr{L}(\hat{\mathbf{P}}|\mathbf{x})} > \frac{1}{10} \tag{2}$$

This approach has the advantage of not assuming a best model but rather selecting the likelihood of each proposed model. The reference parameters are given by the model with highest likelihood. We were aware that a more rigorous statistical analysis such as Markov Chain Monte Carlo approaches would provide a more rigorous analysis of the prior in the parameter space. However given the computational cost of the modeling approach we decided to implement a more parsimonious analysis able to provide results in real time.

We first selected an ensemble of status quo models $\mathscr{E}^c$ (no change of transmissibility in time) in the parameter space $\mathbf{R_I} \times \mathbf{R_H} \times \mathbf{R_F}$ for each country c, based on the reported data for the country c with $t_0 =$ August 9, 2014 and $t_N =$ August 20, 2014, where $c \in \mathscr{C} = \{\text{Guinea}, \text{Liberia}, \text{SierraLeone}\}$. The ensemble of status quo models for the West Africa is the union of ensembles for these three countries, i.e., $\mathscr{E}^{WA} = \bigcup_{c \in \mathscr{C}} \mathscr{E}^c$. It must be noted that the transmissibility in the various settings is difficult to determine as different partitions of the transmissibility can provide similar growth rates for the epidemic, thus providing similar likelihood. The identifiability issue is taken into account by the likelihood approach that considers in the portfolio of viable models all the parameter combinations likely to reproduce the empirical data [36].

2.4 Containment Scenarios

In August 2014, we observed a sustained local transmission of EVD in Guinea, Liberia and Sierra Leone. The estimates of the transmissibility indicated a West African reproductive number R_0 ranging from 1.5 to 2.0. This transmissibility was in the range of estimates in previous outbreaks [11]. Considering the data available at early stages of the outbreak, we projected the status quo dynamics of the disease and provided a first assessment on the risk of internationalization of the 2014 WA EVD outbreak [37]. In September 2014, however the situation began to change rapidly. The growth rate of the disease decreased, and in each country the dynamics reached an inflection point after which the number of new cases started to consistently decrease. However, the inflection point and slow down of the epidemic in the different countries occurred at different times. The change in the behavior of the disease and the rapidly evolving situation thus prompted the need for constant updates of the models and their projections.

To better reflect the effects of the interventions, we considered two alternative scenarios in addition to the original *Status quo* scenario. The first alternative scenario, *Marginal containment*, considers an effective reduction in the transmission such that $R_0' \simeq 1$. The second scenario, *Containment*, considers that full control of the epidemic is achieved, with an effective reproductive number definitely subcritical $R_0' < 1$.

These alternative scenarios are introduced after a period of exponential growth, that we kept to describe the initial phase of the outbreak. To simulate the decrease in the basic reproductive number due to the control interventions, we considered that the transmissibility decreases in each infectious compartment linearly over a period of two weeks. In order to limit the number of free parameters we consider that the transmissibility β changes linearly according to

$$\beta'(t) = \left(1 - \xi \frac{(t - t_0)}{\Delta t}\right) \beta, \tag{3}$$

where ξ accounts for the reduction of R_0, $\xi = 1 - \frac{R_0'}{R_0}$, Δt is the period of time needed to achieve a basic reproductive number R_0', and t_0 is the starting date of the interventions. We also provided a sensitivity analysis using alternative decaying functions.

To analyze the effects of interventions, for each country c we define the one-dimension parameter space of intervention time $\mathbf{T}_0^c$ and re-run simulations based on the selected parameters in $\mathbf{R_I} \times \mathbf{R_H} \times \mathbf{R_F}$ but with sampling $\mathbf{T}_0^c$. The different starting date for the interventions used in this secondary calibration of the model ranged between September 15th and December 29th 2014, in steps of one week. For each model with different intervention times, we apply the same rule of calibration to select an ensemble of best intervention dates. In this way, we could receive ensembles of disease containment models for the marginal containment scenario $\mathscr{E}_{\text{marg}}^c$ and the containment scenario $\mathscr{E}_{\text{cont}}^c$. With such selected ensembles of models, we were able to project disease dynamics behavior in long-term under three scenarios.

This modeling approach to the containment and epidemic inflection point assume the effective reduction of transmissibility but does not provide any information on the role and effectiveness of specific interventions. Furthermore it cannot be easily linked to specific data on ebola treatment units admission, safe burial implementation and their geographical heterogeneity. In order to overcome this limits more detailed microsimulations approaches shall be used [38].

3 Results

By using the modeling approach as described in Sect. 2, we modeled the short term behavior of the outbreak in Guinea, Liberia and Sierra Leone, and quantified the probability of observing cases of Ebola around the world. In this section, we report our projections of both local EVD epidemic in West African countries and the risk of case importation in the rest of world.

3.1 Local Transmission of EVD

In Fig. 3 we show the time series for the three countries individually and for the aggregated region of West Africa, under the different scenarios considered through the months of July 2014 to February 2015. The red dots represent the data (cumulative number of cases) from the WHO reports, while the gray dots represent data made available after the calibration was done. The shaded areas show the 95 % reference range (RR) of the stochastic fluctuations for the selected models. In the figure one can readily observe how the actual course of the epidemic separates from the status quo behavior by mid-September 2014 for Guinea and Liberia, and in December 2014 for Sierra Leone.

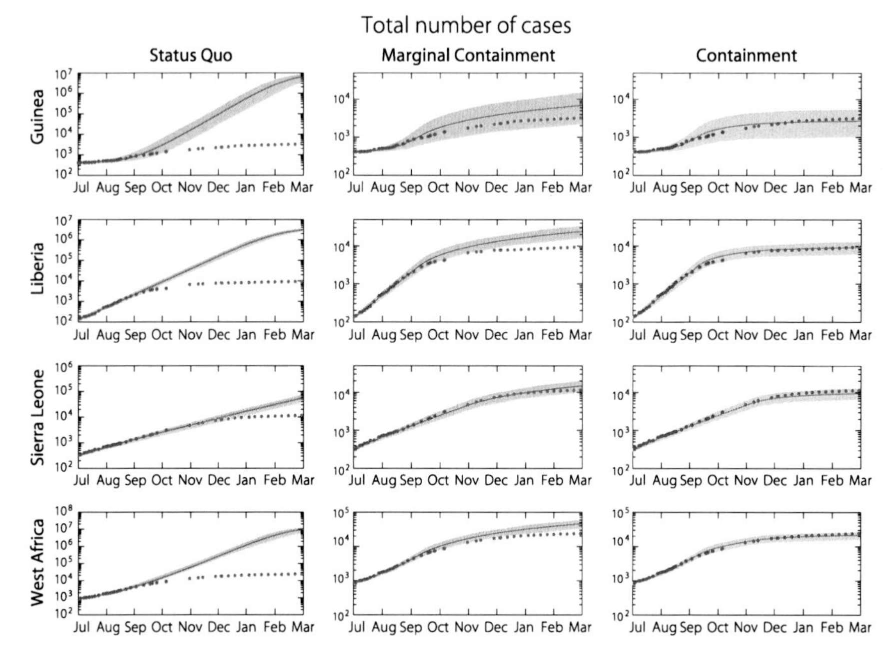

Fig. 3 Cumulative number of cases of EVD for the three most affected countries and for the aggregation of them. The plots show the results for the different scenarios considered: Status Quo, Marginal containment and Containment. The *dots* correspond to the data from the official WHO reports. The *red dots* were used for the model calibration. The *gray dots* are experimental data points received after the calibration of the model, while the *shaded areas* represent the 95 % reference range due to the fluctuations of the stochastic microsimulations of the selected models

From August 2014 to March 2015, we performed several calibrations of the model. For each one of them we used the data available at that time and implemented the methodology described in Sect. 2.3. The first calibration was done using data from the beginning of July until mid August 2014. At that time the outbreak was considered to be growing at an exponential rate in West Africa. After our second calibration the epidemic started to consistently deviate from the exponential growth behavior's. In Fig. 4 we show the number of EVD cases as a function of time for West Africa for the different re-calibrations of the model. The dots represent the data points obtained from the WHO reports. The red dots were used in the original calibration of the model. The gray dots correspond to data received after the first calibration was done. Each shaded area corresponds to the projections of the model for the different re-calibrations of it. Although we only show the results for the aggregation of the three countries, we performed the same analysis for each country individually and used the corresponding selected models for the projections.

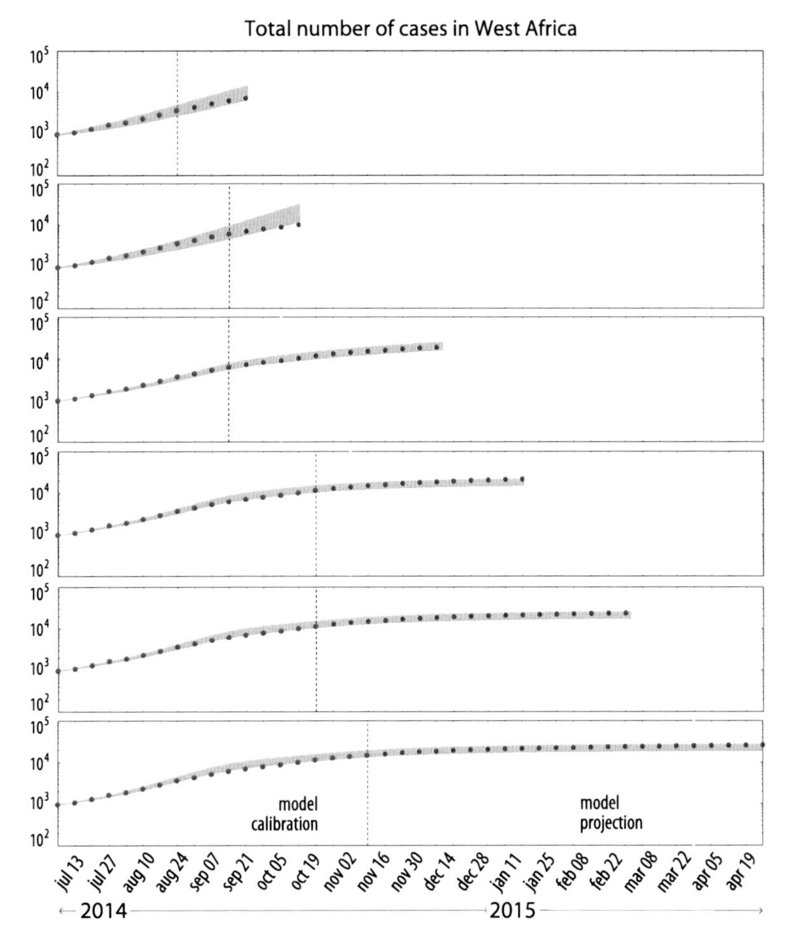

Fig. 4 Time series for the cumulative number of EVD cases in West Africa. The *dots* correspond to the data from the official WHO reports. The *red dots* were used for the original model calibration. The *gray dots* are experimental data points received after the calibration of the model, and are reported for the purpose of comparing with the model projections. The *shaded areas* correspond to the 95 % reference range due to the fluctuations of the stochastic microsimulations of the selected models

3.2 Assessing the International Spread of EVD

Once we performed the calibration of the model and the local projections, we use the selected models to simulate the international spread of EVD. This set of simulations allowed us to track the importation of Ebola cases to other countries around the world from West Africa. Through the simulations we could specifically track the number of passengers traveling daily worldwide on each airline connection in the world. The airline network used in the modeling of the international spread of EVD is based on the tickets booked by the passengers. This means that the network accounts for the origin of the individuals and their final destination. In order to provide a list of countries that could be experiencing the importation of cases of EVD we keep track of every single exposed individual traveling to the different countries at a daily scale. We quantified the risk of international spread as the probability of observing an exposed individual arriving in a given country, in a given month.

In Fig. 5 we provide a list of 10 countries with the largest risk of observing imported cases of EVD and their corresponding probabilities during the months of September, October and November 2014. Outside Africa, the countries with the largest risk of EVD case importation were the ones having strong historical tights with the affected region like United Kingdom, Belgium, France and USA. The results showed that, in general, the probability of observing cases in these countries decreases month to month, with the exception of United Kingdom. This result is due to the fact that this country receives most of its passenger from Sierra Leone. From Fig. 3 we can see that the outbreak was following the status quo scenario until the end of November and therefore potentially exporting more cases than the other countries where the epidemic was being mitigated. At the present time, we know that Nigeria, Senegal, Spain, United States, Mali, United Kingdom and Italy have observed EVD cases. Some of these cases were due to health care workers that were evacuated for medical aid or were returning from West Africa. In Fig. 5 we have included some of these countries to show that they rank among the ones with the larger probability of case importation. The results shown consider that some airlines decided, at that time, to interrupt flights to the most affected countries. We simulate this considering an 80 % air traffic reduction (ATR) from and towards West Africa [14]. In Table 2 we provide the mean number of imported cases, along with the minimum and maximum number

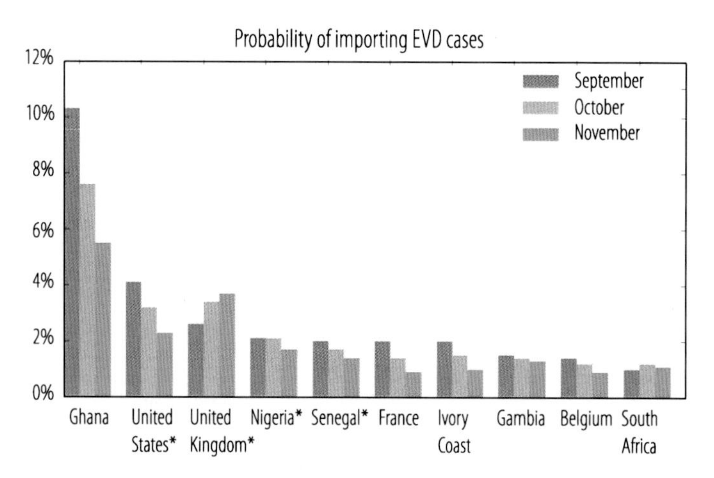

Fig. 5 Top10 countries at risk of EVD case importation during the months of September, October and November of 2014. The risk is assessed as the probability that a country will experience at least one case importation by that date, conditional of no presenting cases before that. The countries marked with an asterisk (*) presented imported cases of EVD during the outbreak

Table 2 Mean number of expected EVD imported cases (as well as minimum and maximum number of cases) for the top 10 countries with higher importation probabilities, during the months of September, October and November 2014

Country at risk	September	October	November
Ghana	0.11 [0–3]	0.08 [0–3]	0.05 [0–3]
United States	0.04 [0–3]	0.03 [0–3]	0.02 [0–2]
United Kingdom	0.03 [0–2]	0.03 [0–3]	0.04 [0–3]
Nigeria	0.02 [0–2]	0.02 [0–2]	0.02 [0–2]
Senegal	0.02 [0–2]	0.02 [0–2]	0.01 [0–2]
France	0.02 [0–2]	0.01 [0–2]	0.01 [0–2]
Ivory Coast	0.02 [0–2]	0.01 [0–2]	0.01 [0–2]
Gambia	0.01 [0–2]	0.01 [0–2]	0.01 [0–2]
Belgium	0.01 [0–2]	0.01 [0–2]	0.01 [0–2]
South Africa	0.01 [0–2]	0.01 [0–2]	0.01 [0–2]

We include in the list countries that observed imported cases in those months to support the results of our model, as those countries were ranking among the top of the possible ones importing cases

possible of cases, that the top 10 countries could have observed during the period September-November 2014. As the probability of importing cases is very low in general, we highlight that the 95 % confidence interval is generally bounded by 3 cases for the countries with higher risk of importation.

We can also look at the outbreak in a retrospective way and perform a longitudinal analysis, month to month, of the evolution of the outbreak. We quantify the probability of observing n imported cases of EVD at a worldwide level between the months of September 2014 and February 2015 for the three different scenarios described in Sect. 3.1. In Fig. 6 we show the monthly number of cases that could have been observed for the different scenarios, including $n = 0$, that is no import cases at all. We observe that in the status quo scenario not only does the probability of observing imported cases increases with time, but also the probability of observing more than one case increases, reaching hundreds of cases per month by January 2015. As soon as the containment measures are considered, the probability of observing cases around the world decreases and the number of possible exported cases decreases as well. We can perform an analogous analysis at the country level. In Fig. 6 we include the results month to month for United States, shows a similar behavior.

4 Discussion

During the months from August through November 2014 the WA EVD outbreak was posing a threat for the entire world. By defining a multimodel inference analysis, we modeled the short term behavior of the outbreak within West Africa and continuously updated and re-calibrated it as more data became available.

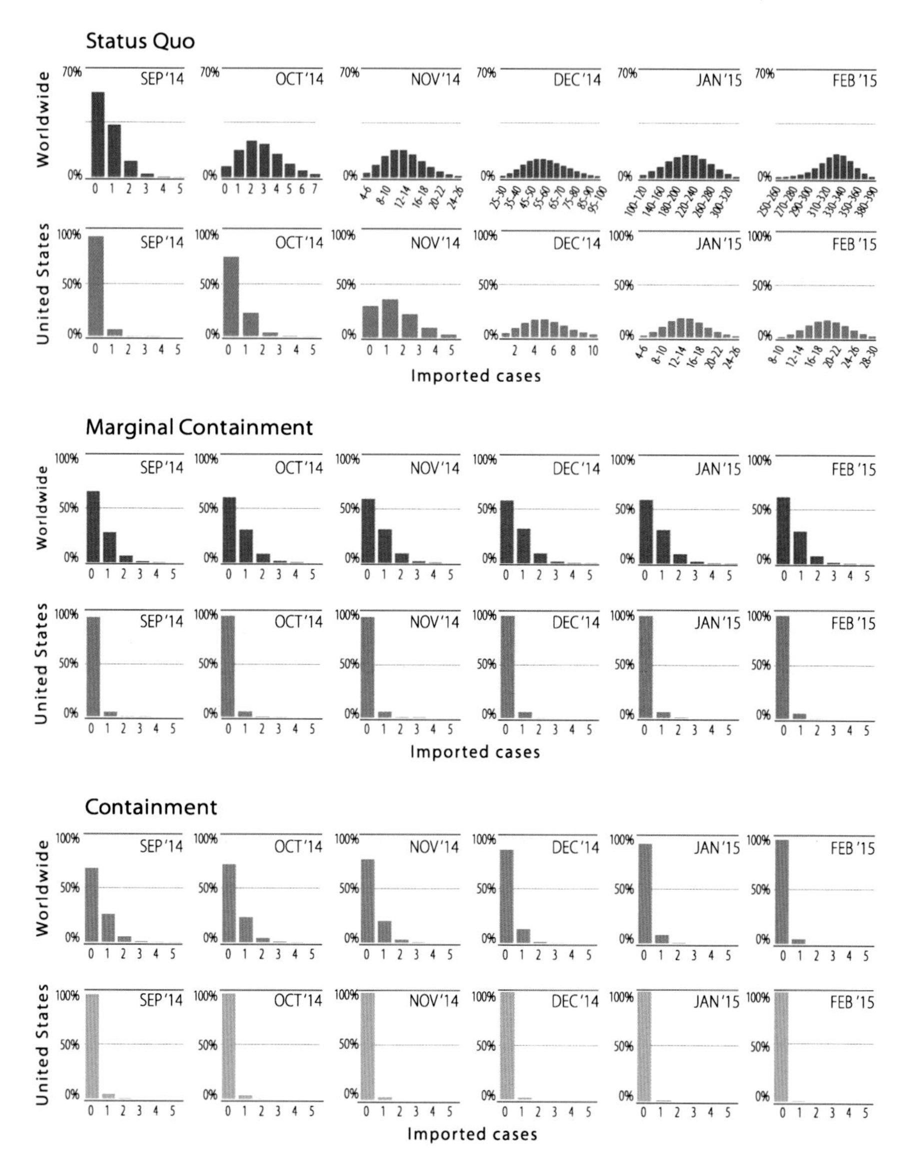

Fig. 6 Monthly number of imported cases projected at worldwide level and for United States. For each month we report the projections in the three different scenarios for the local spreading dynamics in West Africa. From *top* to *bottom*: status quo, marginal containment and containment

It is important to stress that the presented modeling analysis has been motivated by the need for a rapid assessment of the EVD outbreak trends and contains assumptions and approximations unavoidable in the real time analysis of a major public health crisis. A first confounding factor in obtaining the provided estimates for the transmissibility is the likely underreporting of cases and deaths in the affected countries. We have provided a sensitivity analysis that assumes a 50 % underreporting in the data about hospitalizations and deaths. In this case, the transmissibility estimate extends the range of allowed values up to $R_0 = 2.5$. Although this analysis does not drastically alter the picture offered by the baseline analysis, it is clear that a more precise understanding of the underreporting of cases is needed to increase the accuracy of the results. Another approximation contained in the model concerns the demographic analysis of traveling individuals. Although we use very detailed data about traffic flows and airline scheduling, there is very scant information about the sociodemographic features of traveling individuals. The introduction of heterogeneity due to income and household type in the traveling patterns would therefore increase the accuracy of the projections. Furthermore, the modeling approach does not include the specific implementation of the identification and isolation of cases and the quarantine of contacts, that would be relevant in discussing optimal containment strategies and that could provide a more detailed picture of the local transmission and EVD case generation [38].

Notwithstanding the previous limitations, the retrospective analysis of the outbreak is indicating that the picture emerging from the presented modeling approach is in a good agreement with the real-world epidemic evolution. In this perspective the real-time modeling effort could represent valuable additional information and situational awareness by comparing empirical data with the different scenario assumptions. In conclusion, the results provided here are encouraging in advocating for the use of data-driven computational frameworks with consideration of human mobility in providing real-time forecast and assessment of epidemic outbreaks.

Acknowledgments We acknowledge funding from DTRA-1-0910039 and MIDAS-National Institute of General Medical Sciences U54-GM111274. The funders had no role in study design, data collection and analysis, decision to publish, or preparation of the manuscript. MFCG acknowledges CNPq-Brazil fellowship 314164/2014-6. We thank Nicole Samay for her invaluable help in the editing and preparation of the figures of the manuscript.

References

1. Feldmann, H., Geisbert, T.W.: Lancet **377**, 849–62 (2011)
2. World Health Organization. Ebola key facts. http://www.who.int/mediacentre/factsheets/fs103/en/
3. ECDC: Outbreak of Ebola virus disease in West Africa. Third update (2014). Accessed 1 Aug 2014
4. Ebola ça Suffit Ring Vaccination Trial Consortium. BMJ **351**, h3740 (2015)
5. Henao-Restrepo, A.M., Longini, I.M., Egger, M., Dean, N.E., Edmunds, W.J., Camacho, A., Carroll, M.W., Doumbia, M., Draguez, B., Duraffour, S., et al.: Lancet **386**(9996), 857–866 (2015)
6. World Health Organization: Ebola Situation Report. http://www.who.int/csr/disease/ebola/situation-reports/archive/en/. Accessed 15 Dec 2015

7. World Health Organization: Statement on the 1st meeting of the IHR Emergency Committee on the 2014 Ebola outbreak in West Africa. http://www.who.int/mediacentre/news/statements/2014/ebola-20140808/en/. Accessed 15 Dec 2015
8. Balcan, D., Hu, H., Goncalves, B., Bajardi, P., Poletto, C., et al.: BMC Med. **7**, 45 (2009)
9. Balcan, D., Colizza, V., Goncalves, B., Hu, H., Ramasco, J.J., et al.: Proc. Natl. Acad. Sci. **106**, 21484–21489 (2009)
10. Balcan, D., Goncalves, B., Hu, H., Ramasco, J.J., Colizza, V., et al.: J. Comput. Sci. **1**, 132–145 (2010)
11. Legrand, J., Grais, R., Boelle, P., Valleron, A., Flahault, A.: Epidemiol Infect **135**, 610 (2007)
12. Brockmann, D., Schaade, L., Verbee, L.: 2014 Ebola Outbreak. Worldwide Air-Transportation, Relative Import Risk and Most Probable Spreading Routes. http://rocs.hu-berlin.de/projects/ebola/
13. Mekaru, S.: Ebola 2014: A Rapid Threat Assessment. The Disease Daily. (2014). http://healthmap.org/site/diseasedaily/article/ebola-2014-rapid-threat-assessment-8514
14. Poletto, C., Gomes, M.F. C., Pastore y Piontti, A., Rossi, L., Bioglio, L., Chao, D. L.,Longini, I. M., Halloran, M. E., Colizza, V., Vespignani, A.: Euro Surveill **19**(42), 20936 (2014). http://dx.doi.org/10.2807/1560-7917.ES2014.19.42.20936
15. Tizzoni, M., Bajardi, P., Poletto, C., Ramasco, J.J., Balcan, D., et al.: BMC Med. **10**, 165 (2012)
16. Rvachev, L.A., Longini, I.M.: Math. Biosci. **75**, 3–22 (1985)
17. Flahault, A., Valleron, A.: Math. Popul. Stud. **3**, 161–171 (1992)
18. Colizza, V., Barrat, A., Barthelemy, M., Valleron, A.J., Vespignani, A.: PLOS Med. **4**, e13 (2007)
19. GPWv3: Gridded Population of the World. Socio Economic Data and Aplications Center at Columbia University (2014)
20. IATA: International Air Transport Association (2014)
21. OAG: Official Airline Guide (2014)
22. Simini, F., Gonzalez, M.C., Maritan, A., Barabasi, A.L.: Nature **484**, 96–100 (2012)
23. Halloran, M.E., Longini, I.M., Struchiner, C.J.: Design and Analysis of Vaccine Studies, pp. 63–84. Springer Science + Business Media, New York (2009)
24. Diekmann, O., Heesterbeek, J.: Mathematical Epidemiology of Infectious Diseases: Model Building, Analysis and Interpretation. Wiley, Chichester (2000)
25. van den Driessche, P., Watmough, J.: Math. Biosci. **180**, 29–48 (2002)
26. Bwaka, M., Bonnet, M., Calain, P., Colebunders, R., Roo, A.D., et al.: J. Infect. Dis. **179**, S1–S7 (1999)
27. Ndambi, R., Akamituna, P., Bonnet, M., Tukadila, A., MuyembeTamfum, J., et al.: J. Infect. Dis. **179**, S8–S10 (1999)
28. Dowell, S., Mukunu, R., Ksiazek, T., Khan, A., Rollin, P., et al.: J. Infect. Dis. **179**, S87–S91 (1999)
29. Khan, A., Tshioko, F., Heymann, D., Guenno, B.L., Nabeth, P., et al.: J. Infect. Dis. **179**, S76–S86 (1999)
30. Rowe, A., Bertolli, J., Khan, A., Mukunu, R., Muyembe-Tamfum, J., et al.: J. Infect. Dis. **179**, S28–S35 (1999)
31. World Health Organization: Disease Outbreaks News. http://www.who.int/csr/don/archive/disease/ebola/en/
32. Chowell, G., Hengartner, N., Castillo-Chavez, C., Fenimore, P., Hyman, J.: J. Theor. Biol. **229**, 119–126 (2004)
33. Ndanguza, D., Tchuenche, J.M., Haario, H.: Afr Mat **24**, 55–68 (2011)
34. WHO Ebola Response Team: N Engl J Med **371**:1481–1495 (2014)
35. WHO Ebola Response Team: N. Engl. J. Med **372**:584–587 (2015)
36. Weitz, J.S., Dushoff, J.: Sci. Rep. **5**, 8751 (2015)
37. Gomes, M.F.C., Pastore y Piontti, A., Rossi, L., Chao, D., Longini, I., Halloran, M.E., Vespignani, A.: PLOS Currents Outbreaks, edn. 1. 2014 Sep 2. (2014). doi:10.1371/currents.outbreaks.cd818f63d40e24aef769dda7df9e0da5
38. Merler, S., Ajelli, M., Fumanelli, L., Gomes, M.F.C., Pastore y Piontti, A., Rossi, L., Longini, I.Jr, Halloran, M.E., Vespignani, A.: Lancet Infect. Dis. **15**(2), 204–211 (2015)

Modeling the Case of Early Detection of Ebola Virus Disease

Diego Chowell, Muntaser Safan and Carlos Castillo-Chavez

Abstract The most recent Ebola outbreak in West Africa highlighted critical weaknesses in the medical infrastructure of the affected countries, including effective diagnostics tools, sufficient isolation wards, and enough medical personnel. Here, we develop and analyze a mathematical model to assess the impact of early diagnosis of pre-symptomatic individuals on the transmission dynamics of Ebola virus disease in West Africa. Our findings highlight the importance of implementing integrated control measures of early diagnosis and isolation. The mathematical analysis shows a threshold where early diagnosis of pre-symptomatic individuals, combined with a sufficient level of effective isolation, can lead to an epidemic control of Ebola virus disease.

Keywords Ebola virus disease · Pre-symptomatic infection · Early detection · Point-of-care testing

---

Diego Chowell* and Muntaser Safan* both the authors contributed equally to this chapter

D. Chowell (✉) · M. Safan · C. Castillo-Chavez (✉)
Arizona State University, Tempe, AZ, USA
e-mail: dchowell@asu.edu

C. Castillo-Chavez
e-mail: ccchavez@asu.edu

M. Safan
e-mail: muntaser.safan@asu.edu

M. Safan
Mansoura University, Mansoura, Egypt

M. Safan
Umm Al-Qura University, Mecca, Saudi Arabia

G. Chowell and J.M. Hyman (eds.), *Mathematical and Statistical Modeling for Emerging and Re-emerging Infectious Diseases*,
DOI 10.1007/978-3-319-40413-4_5

1 Introduction

The Ebola viral strains are re-emerging zoonotic pathogens and members of the Filoviridae family consisting of five distinct species: *Bundibugyo, Cotes d'Ivoire, Reston, Sudan*, and *Zaire* with a high case-fatality rate in humans [1]. Filoviruses are long filamentous enveloped, non-segmented, single-stranded viruses, consisting of a negative-sense RNA genome [2]. Each Ebola species genome encodes seven linearly arranged genes: nucleoprotein (NP), polymerase cofactor (VP35), matrix protein (VP40), glycoprotein (GP), replication-transcription protein (VP30), matrix protein (VP24), and RNA-dependent RNA prolymerase (L) [2]. While there are no proven effective vaccines or effective antiviral drugs for Ebola, containing an outbreak relies on contact tracing and on early detection of infected individuals for isolation and care in treatment centers [2]. The most recent Ebola outbreak in West Africa, which began in December 2013, due to the Zaire strain, demonstrated several weaknesses in the medical infrastructure of the affected countries, including the urgent need of effective diagnostics, which have a fundamental role in both disease control and case management.

The Ebola virus is transmitted as a result of direct contact with bodily fluids containing the virus [3]. The virus enters via small skin lesions and mucus membranes where it is able to infect macrophages and other phagocytic innate immune cells leading to the production of a large number of viral particles [2]. The macrophages, monocytes, and dendritic cells infected in the early stage of the disease serve to spread the virus throughout the organs, particularly in the spleen, liver, and lymph nodes [2]. Consequently, critically ill patients display intensive viremia [4]. Recognizing signs of Ebola viral disease is challenging because it causes common non-specific symptoms such as fever, weakness, diarrhea, and vomiting, and the incubation period typically lasts 5–7 days [3]. Therefore, functioning laboratories and effective point-of-care diagnostic tests are critically needed in order to minimize transmission, allow better allocation of scarce healthcare resources, and increase the likelihood of success of antiviral treatments as they are developed [5].

There is an ongoing effort in place to improve Ebola diagnostics, primarily to detect the disease early. Currently, the cost and difficulty of testing limit diagnostic facilities to small mobile laboratories or centralized facilities with turnaround times measured in days rather than in a few hours, meaning that diagnosis is largely used to confirm disease. Ebola diagnosis can be achieved in two different ways: measuring the host-specific immune response to infection (e.g. IgM and IgG antibodies) and detection of viral particles (e.g. ReEBOV Antigen Rapid Test Kit for VP40), or particle components in infected individuals (e.g. RT-PCR or PCR). The most general assay used for IgM and IgG antibody detection are direct ELISA assays. Considering the physiological kinetics of the humoral immune system as well as impaired antigen-presenting cell function as a result of viral hemorrhagic fever, antibody titers are low in the early stages and often undetectable in severe patients prior to death [6]. This leaves polymerase chain reaction (PCR) for antigen detection as a viable option for early diagnostic assays. PCR is a chemical reaction that amplifies pieces of a virus's genes floating in the blood by more than a millionfold, which makes detection of pre-symptomatic individuals likely identifiable. Indeed, a research article published in 2000, illustrates the power of this technology to detect Ebola virus in humans in the pre-symptomatic stage [7]. In this study, 24 asymptomatic individuals who had been exposed to symptomatic Ebola patients were tested using PCR. Eleven of the exposed patients eventually developed the infection. Seven of the 11 tested positive for the PCR assay. And none of the other 13 did.

In this chapter, we extend the work presented in [8]. Here, we have developed and analyzed a mathematical model to evaluate the impact of early diagnosis of pre-symptomatic individuals on the transmission dynamics of Ebola virus disease in West Africa, under the assumption that the disease is maintained possibly at very low levels due to the deficiencies in health systems and our incomplete understanding of Ebola infection as illustrated by the case of Pauline Cafferkey. Therefore, eliminating Ebola may require a more sustained and long-term control effort.

Table 1 Definition of model states

Variable	Description
$S(t)$	Number of susceptible individuals at time t
$E_1(t)$	Number of latent undetectable individuals at time t
$E_2(t)$	Number of latent detectable individuals at time t
$I(t)$	Number of infectious individuals at time t
$J(t)$	Number of isolated individuals at time t
$R(t)$	Number of recovered individuals at time t

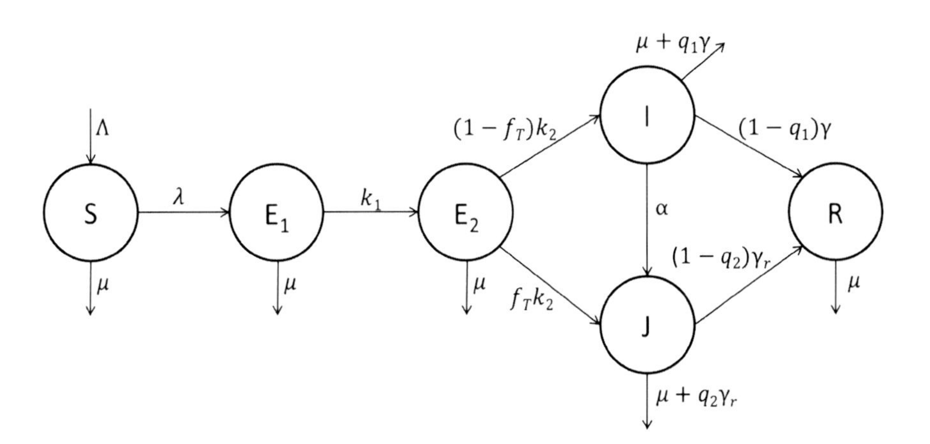

Fig. 1 Compartmental model showing the transition between model states

Table 2 Definition of model parameters

Parameter	Value	Unit	Description
Λ	17182	$\frac{population}{day}$	Recruitment rate
β	0.3335	day^{-1}	Mean transmission rate
μ	4.98×10^{-5}	day^{-1}	Natural death rate
κ_1	1/4	day^{-1}	Transition rate from undetectable to detectable latent state
κ_2	1/3	day^{-1}	Exit rate of latent detectable individuals by either becoming infectious or moving to isolation state
γ	1/6	day^{-1}	Removal rate of infectious individuals by either recovery or Ebola-induced death
γ_r	1/7	day^{-1}	Removal rate of isolated individuals by either recovery or Ebola-induced death
α	1/5	day^{-1}	Rate at which infectious individuals get isolated
f_T	$0.25 \in [0, 1]$	–	Fraction of latent detectable individuals who are diagnosed and get isolated
q_1	0.7	–	Probability that an infectious individual dies due to Ebola
q_2	0.63	–	Probability that an isolated individual dies due to Ebola
r	$0.35 \in [0, 1]$	–	Effectiveness of isolation
ℓ	$0.5 \in [0, 1]$	–	Relative transmissibility of isolated individuals with respect to infectious individuals

2 Model Formulation

The total population is assumed to be classified into six mutually independent subgroups: susceptible $S(t)$, non-detectable latent $E_1(t)$, detectable latent $E_2(t)$, infectious $I(t)$, isolated $J(t)$, and recovered $R(t)$ individuals. Table 1 shows the state variables and their physical meaning. The transition between all these states is shown in Fig. 1. And model parameters and their description are presented in Table 2. Parameter values have been obtained from previous studies [9, 10].

It is assumed that individuals are recruited (either through birth or migration) into the susceptible class at a rate Λ and die naturally with rate μ. Susceptible individuals get infected due to successful contacts with infectious or not perfectly isolated infected individuals at rate λ. As a consequence, they become latent undetectable, who develop their state of infection to become latent detectable at rate κ_1. We assume that the latent detectable class represent individuals whose viral load is above the detection limit of the PCR-based diagnostic test [7, 11]. Latent detectable individuals either are diagnosed and get isolated with probability f_T or develop symptoms to become infectious, who sequentially either get isolated at rate α, or are removed from the system by recovery or Ebola-induced death at rate γ. It is assumed here that Ebola-induced deaths occur for the infectious individuals with probability q_1. Similarly, isolated individuals leave their class at rate γ_r, by either dying due to Ebola with probability q_2, or they get recovered and become immune. It is assumed that isolation is partially effective so that successful contacts with susceptible individuals may lead to infection with probability r; this parameter is a measure of isolation effectiveness of infectious individuals. Thus, the force of infection is given by

$$\lambda(t) = \frac{\beta[I(t) + (1-r)\ell J(t)]}{N(t) - rJ(t)}. \tag{1}$$

The assumptions mentioned above lead to the following model of equations

$$\begin{aligned}
\frac{dS}{dt} &= \Lambda - \lambda S - \mu S,\\
\frac{dE_1}{dt} &= \lambda S - (\kappa_1 + \mu)E_1,\\
\frac{dE_2}{dt} &= \kappa_1 E_1 - (\kappa_2 + \mu)E_2,\\
\frac{dI}{dt} &= (1 - f_T)\kappa_2 E_2 - (\alpha + \gamma + \mu)I,\\
\frac{dJ}{dt} &= f_T \kappa_2 E_2 + \alpha I - (\gamma_r + \mu)J,\\
\frac{dR}{dt} &= (1 - q_1)\gamma I + (1 - q_2)\gamma_r J - \mu R
\end{aligned} \tag{2}$$

where

$$N(t) = S(t) + E_1(t) + E_2(t) + I(t) + J(t) + R(t)$$

is the total population size at time t. On adding all equations of system (2) together, we get

$$\frac{dN}{dt} = \Lambda - \mu N - q_1\gamma I - q_2\gamma_r J. \tag{3}$$

3 Model Analysis

3.1 Basic Properties

Since model (2) imitates the dynamics of human populations, all variables and parameters should be non-negative. Thus, following the approach shown in appendix A of [12], we show the following result.

Theorem 1 *The variables of model (2) are non-negative for all time.*

Lemma 1 *The closed set*

$$\Omega = \left\{(S, E_1, E_2, I, J, R) \in \mathbb{R}^6_+ : \frac{\Lambda}{\mu + q_1\gamma + q_2\gamma_r} \leq S + E_1 + E_2 + I + J + R \leq \frac{\Lambda}{\mu}\right\}$$

is positively invariant for model (2) and is absorbing.

Proof: Equation (3) implies that

$$\frac{dN}{dt} \leq \Lambda - \mu N, \tag{4}$$
$$\frac{dN}{dt} \geq \Lambda - (\mu + q_1\gamma + q_2\gamma_r)N. \tag{5}$$

It follows from (4) that

$$N(t) \leq \frac{\Lambda}{\mu} + \left(N(0) - \frac{\Lambda}{\mu}\right) e^{-\mu t} \tag{6}$$

and from (5) that

$$N(t) \geq \frac{\Lambda}{\mu + q_1\gamma + q_2\gamma_r} + \left(N(0) - \frac{\Lambda}{\mu + q_1\gamma + q_2\gamma_r}\right) e^{-(\mu + q_1\gamma + q_2\gamma_r)t}. \tag{7}$$

If we assume $N(0) > \Lambda/\mu$, then $dN/dt < 0$ and therefore (based on inequality (6)), $N(t)$ decreases steadily until reaching Λ/μ when t tends to ∞. Similarly, if we assume $N(0) < \Lambda/(\mu + q_1\gamma + q_2\gamma_r)$, then $dN/dt > 0$ and therefore (based on inequality (7)), $N(t)$ increases steadily until reaching a maximum at $\Lambda/(\mu + q_1\gamma + q_2\gamma_r)$ when t tends to ∞. It remains to check the case if $N(0)$ lies in the phase between $\Lambda/(\mu + q_1\gamma + q_2\gamma_r)$ and Λ/μ. To this end, both inequalities (6) and (7) are combined together to get

$$\frac{\Lambda}{\mu + q_1\gamma + q_2\gamma_r} + \left(N(0) - \frac{\Lambda}{\mu + q_1\gamma + q_2\gamma_r}\right) e^{-(\mu + q_1\gamma + q_2\gamma_r)t} \leq N(t) \leq \frac{\Lambda}{\mu} + \left(N(0) - \frac{\Lambda}{\mu}\right) e^{-\mu t}.$$

On taking the limit when t tends to ∞, we find that $N(t)$ remains within the same phase. Thus, the set Ω is positively invariant and absorbing.

3.2 Equilibrium Analysis

3.2.1 Ebola-Free Equilibrium and the Control Reproduction Number $\mathcal{R}_c$

It is easy to check that model (2) has the Ebola-free equilibrium

$$E_0 = \left(\frac{\Lambda}{\mu}, 0, 0, 0, 0, 0\right)' \tag{8}$$

where the prime " $'$ " means vector transpose.

The basic reproduction number, $\mathscr{R}_0$, is a measure of the average number of secondary cases produced by a typical infectious individual during the entire course of infection in a completely susceptible population and in the absence of control interventions [13, 14]. On the other hand, the control reproduction number, $\mathscr{R}_c$, quantifies the potential for infectious disease transmission in the context of a partially susceptible population due to the implementation of control interventions. When $\mathscr{R}_c > 1$, the infection may spread in the population, and the rate of spread is higher with increasingly high values of $\mathscr{R}_c$. If $\mathscr{R}_c < 1$, infection cannot be sustained and is unable to generate an epidemic. For our model, $\mathscr{R}_c$ is computed using the next generation matrix approach shown in [15]. Accordingly, we compute the matrices $\mathbf{F}$ (for the new infection terms) and $\mathbf{V}$ (for the transition terms) as

$$\mathbf{F} = \begin{pmatrix} 0 & 0 & \beta & (1-r)\ell\beta \\ 0 & 0 & 0 & 0 \\ 0 & 0 & 0 & 0 \\ 0 & 0 & 0 & 0 \end{pmatrix}, \quad \mathbf{V} = \begin{pmatrix} \kappa_1 + \mu & 0 & 0 & 0 \\ -\kappa_1 & \kappa_2 + \mu & 0 & 0 \\ 0 & -(1-f_T)\kappa_2 & \alpha + \gamma + \mu & 0 \\ 0 & -f_T\kappa_2 & -\alpha & \gamma_r + \mu \end{pmatrix}.$$

Thus, the control reproduction number is given by

$$\begin{aligned} \mathscr{R}_c = \rho(\mathbf{F}\mathbf{V}^{-1}) &= \frac{\kappa_1\kappa_2\beta[(1-f_T)(\mu+\gamma_r) + (1-r)\ell(\alpha + f_T(\gamma+\mu))]}{(\kappa_1+\mu)(\kappa_2+\mu)(\alpha+\gamma+\mu)(\gamma_r+\mu)} \\ &= \frac{\kappa_1\kappa_2\beta}{(\kappa_1+\mu)(\kappa_2+\mu)(\alpha+\gamma+\mu)}\left[1 - f_T + (1-r)\ell\left(\frac{\alpha}{\gamma_r+\mu} + f_T\frac{\gamma+\mu}{\gamma_r+\mu}\right)\right] \\ &= \mathscr{R}_0\left[1 - \frac{\alpha}{(\alpha+\gamma+\mu)}\right]\left[1 - f_T + (1-r)\ell\left(\frac{\alpha}{\gamma_r+\mu} + f_T\frac{\gamma+\mu}{\gamma_r+\mu}\right)\right] \end{aligned} \tag{9}$$

where ρ is the spectral radius (dominant eigenvalue in magnitude) of the matrix $\mathbf{F}\mathbf{V}^{-1}$ and

$$\mathscr{R}_0 = \frac{\kappa_1\kappa_2\beta}{(\kappa_1+\mu)(\kappa_2+\mu)(\gamma+\mu)} \tag{10}$$

is the basic reproduction number for the model.

The local stability of the Ebola-free equilibrium, E_0, for values of $\mathscr{R}_c < 1$ is established based on a direct use of Theorem 2 in [15]. We summarize our result in the following lemma.

Lemma 2 *The Ebola-free equilibrium E_0 of model (2) is locally asymptotically stable if and only if $\mathscr{R}_c < 1$.*

3.2.2 Ebola-Endemic Equilibrium

On putting the derivatives in the left hand side of (2) equal zero and solving the resulting algebraic system with respect to the variables $\bar{S}, \bar{E}_1, \bar{E}_2, \bar{I}, \bar{J}$, and $\bar{R}$, we obtain

$$\begin{aligned}
\bar{S} &= \frac{\Lambda}{\bar{\lambda}+\mu}, \\
\bar{E}_1 &= \frac{\Lambda}{\bar{\lambda}+\mu} \cdot \frac{\bar{\lambda}}{\kappa_1+\mu}, \\
\bar{E}_2 &= \frac{\kappa_1}{\kappa_2+\mu} \cdot \frac{\Lambda}{\bar{\lambda}+\mu} \cdot \frac{\bar{\lambda}}{\kappa_1+\mu}, \\
\bar{I} &= \frac{(1-f_T)\kappa_2}{\alpha+\gamma+\mu} \cdot \frac{\kappa_1}{\kappa_2+\mu} \cdot \frac{\Lambda}{\bar{\lambda}+\mu} \cdot \frac{\bar{\lambda}}{\kappa_1+\mu}, \\
\bar{J} &= \frac{\kappa_1}{\kappa_2+\mu} \cdot \frac{\Lambda}{\bar{\lambda}+\mu} \cdot \frac{\bar{\lambda}}{\kappa_1+\mu} \cdot \frac{\kappa_2}{\gamma_r+\mu}\left[f_T + (1-f_T)\frac{\alpha}{\alpha+\gamma+\mu}\right], \\
\bar{R} &= \frac{1}{\mu}[(1-q_1)\gamma I + (1-q_2)\gamma_r J]
\end{aligned} \tag{11}$$

where

$$\bar{\lambda} = \frac{\beta(I + (1-r)\ell\bar{J})}{\bar{N} - r\bar{J}} \tag{12}$$

is the equilibrium force of infection. On substituting from (11) into (12) and simplifying (with the assumption that $\lambda \neq 0$), we get

$$\bar{\lambda} = \frac{\mu(\mathscr{R}_c - 1)}{1 - Term} \tag{13}$$

where

$$Term = \frac{\kappa_1\kappa_2[q_1(1-f_T)\gamma(\gamma_r+\mu) + (r\mu + q_2\gamma_r)(f_T(\gamma+\mu)+\alpha)]}{(\kappa_1+\mu)(\kappa_2+\mu)(\alpha+\gamma+\mu)(\gamma_r+\mu)}.$$

Hence, the Ebola-endemic equilibrium is unique and we show the following lemma.

Lemma 3 *Model (2) has a unique endemic equilibrium that exists if and only if* $\mathscr{R}_c > 1$.

3.3 Normalized Sensitivity Analysis on $\mathscr{R}_c$

In considering the dynamics of the Ebola system (2), we conduct normalized sensitivity analysis on $\mathscr{R}_c$ to determine the impact of parameter perturbations on the transmission dynamics of the system. By computing the normalized sensitivity indices, we consider the percent change in the output with respect to a percent change in the parameter input. Those parameters with the largest magnitude of change impact the compartment model the most; the sign indicates whether the change produces an increase or a decrease on $\mathscr{R}_c$.

The normalized sensitivity indices for $\mathscr{R}_c$ are calculated by taking the partial derivative of $\mathscr{R}_c$ with respect to each parameter and multiply the derivative with the ratio of the parameter to $\mathscr{R}_c$. This value represents the percent change in $\mathscr{R}_c$ with respect to a 1 % change in the parameter value [16].

We use the parameters values from Table 2 to study the sensitivity of $\mathscr{R}_c$ to each parameter. We compute normalized sensitivity analysis on all parameters, but we just consider the impact of parameters that are the most sensitive: $\beta, r, \ell, \gamma_r, \gamma, \alpha$, and f_T. The other parameters (μ, κ_1, and κ_2) have a very low impact, namely less than 0.001 %. The numerical simulations to the sensitivity of $\mathscr{R}_c$ with respect to each of the most sensitive parameters are given in Table 3, for two different levels of isolation effectiveness ($r = 0.35$ and $r = 0.95$) and two values of f_T ($f_T = 0.25$ and $f_T = 0.75$), which is the fraction of pre-symptomatic individuals diagnosed and isolated. The other parameter values are kept as shown in Table 2.

In the case of high isolation effectiveness ($r = 0.95$), simulations show that both the removal rate, γ_r, of isolated individuals and the relative transmissibility parameter ℓ of isolated individuals with respect to infectious individuals are the least sensitive parameters (with 0.053 % change of $\mathscr{R}_c$), while the parameter of isolation effectiveness, r, is the most sensitive one, where a 1 % increase in r causes a 1.014 %

Table 3 Percent change in $\mathscr{R}_c$ with respect to a 1 % change in the parameter value, for a low and a high isolation effectiveness r, and a low and a high value of f_T, while keeping the other parameter values as presented in Table 2

	Parameter	β	r	ℓ	γ_r	γ	α	f_T
$f_T =$ 0.25	% change for $r = 0.35$	1 %	−0.23 %	0.423 %	−0.423 %	−0.382 %	−0.195 %	−0.119 %
	% change	1 % for $r = 0.95$	−1.014 %	0.053 %	−0.053 %	−0.445 %	−0.501 %	−0.306 %
$f_T =$ 0.75	% change for $r = 0.35$	1 %	−0.402 %	0.747 %	−0.747 %	−0.167 %	−0.086 %	−0.471 %
	% change for $r = 0.95$	1 %	−3.521 %	0.185 %	−0.185 %	−0.383 %	−0.431 %	−2.373 %

reduction in the value of $\mathscr{R}_c$. Also, the rate at which infectious individuals get isolated, α, and the fraction of pre-symptomatic individuals detected and isolated, f_T, impact negatively on the level of $\mathscr{R}_c$, where a 1 % percent increase in the value of f_T causes approximately a 0.31 % decline in the value of the reproduction number $\mathscr{R}_c$. Thus, as pre-symptomatic individuals are diagnosed and as isolation is highly effective, the number of available infectious individuals who are capable of transmitting Ebola decreases and therefore, the reproduction number decreases. Also, the removal (by recovery or Ebola-induced death) rate γ of infectious individuals affects negatively on $\mathscr{R}_c$. Hence, for the case of highly effective isolation, the parameters concerning early diagnosis and isolation have a significant impact on the reproduction number.

This percent impact of the parameters on $\mathscr{R}_c$ remains so as long as isolation is highly effective. However, if the effectiveness of isolation is low, in the sense that all parameter values are kept the same except the value of the parameter r, which is reduced to 0.35, then we get the results presented in Table 3. In this case, both the relative transmissibility ℓ and the removal rate of isolated individuals, γ_r, are the second most sensitive parameters, after β which is the most impactful one. Also, ℓ became more sensitive than r. The implication is that, when isolation is less effective, there exists the possibility for isolated people to make successful contacts with susceptible individuals and therefore the possibility of causing new infections increases. This causes an increase in the reproduction number. Also, it is noted that the effect of f_T and α is reduced, which means that diagnosing and isolating infected individuals becomes a weak strategy if the effectiveness of isolation is low.

On repeating the previous analyses, but this time for a higher value of f_T ($f_T = 0.75$), we obtain the results shown in Table 3. In comparison to the scenario when $f_T = 0.25$, the simulations show that increasing the fraction of pre-symptomatic individuals who are diagnosed and isolated, f_T, increases the percent impact of the parameters r, ℓ, γ_r, and f_T, and decreases the percent impact of the parameters γ and α, on the value of the control reproduction number $\mathscr{R}_c$.

3.4 Impact of Early Detection and Isolation on the Value of $\mathscr{R}_c$

To study the impact of early detection of pre-symptomatic individuals and isolation on the reproduction number, we first depict $\mathscr{R}_c$ as a function of f_T, for different levels of isolation effectiveness r. Figure 2 shows that the control reproduction number declines as the proportion, f_T, of pre-symptomatic individuals, who get diagnosed and isolated, increases. Simulations are done using parameter values from Table 2, but for three different values of r. It further shows that the curve corresponding to a low and an intermidate value of isolation effectivenes r (e.g. $r = 0.35$ for the solid curve and $r = 0.65$ for the dashed curve) hits $\mathscr{R}_c = 1$ at some critical value of f_T (say $f_T^\star$), while for the high value of r ($r = 0.95$), it never hits the critical threshold $\mathscr{R}_c = 1$, as the curve is totally below the critical threshold. This indicates that for a

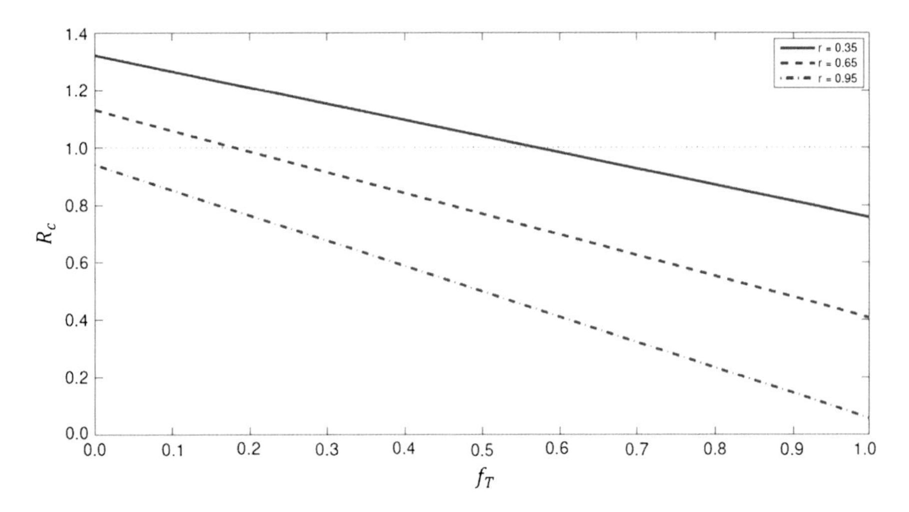

Fig. 2 Impact of early detection of pre-symptomatic individuals on the value of $\mathscr{R}_c$

high effectiveness of isolation, the control reproduction number is less than one and therefore the infection dies out. Analytically, the exact form of $f_T^\star$ is

$$f_T^\star = \left[1 + (1-r)\ell \frac{\alpha}{\gamma_r + \mu} - \frac{1}{\mathscr{R}_0}\left(1 + \frac{\alpha}{\gamma + \mu}\right)\right] / \left[1 - \frac{(1-r)\ell(\gamma + \mu)}{\gamma_r + \mu}\right]. \tag{14}$$

The critical proportion $f_T^\star$ represents the minimum proportion of pre-symptomatic individuals who are detected and get isolated to ensure an effective control of Ebola. This critical value remains feasible as long as the following inequality holds

$$(1-r)\ell < \frac{\gamma_r + \mu}{(\gamma + \mu)\mathscr{R}_0}. \tag{15}$$

If we keep all parameters fixed except r, then condition (15) could be rewritten in a more convenient form

$$r > 1 - \frac{\gamma_r + \mu}{\ell(\gamma + \mu)\mathscr{R}_0}. \tag{16}$$

This gives the minimum level of effectiveness of isolation required to obtain an isolation and early diagnosis-based control strategy for Ebola tranmission.

Now, we could also ask a similar question on the role of isolating infectious individuals to contain Ebola transmission. Figure 3 shows the impact of changing the rate at which infectious individuals get isolated, α, on $\mathscr{R}_c$, for the same three

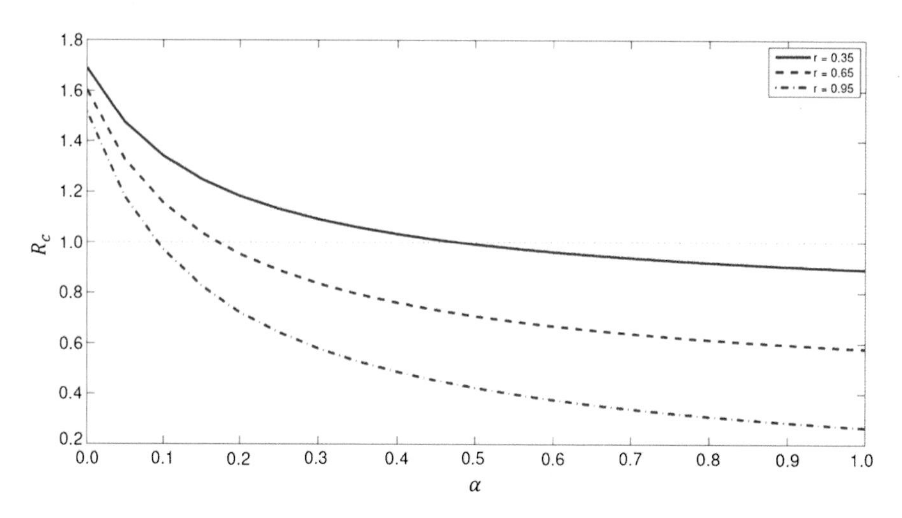

Fig. 3 Impact of isolating infectious individuals on the value of $\mathscr{R}_c$

different levels of isolation effectivenes, as used above. The analysis shows that it is possible to control the epidemic if and only if $\alpha > \alpha^{\star}$, where

$$\alpha^{\star} = \frac{[(1-f_T)(\gamma_r+\mu)(\gamma+\mu)+(1-r)\ell f_T(\gamma+\mu)^2]\mathscr{R}_0-(\gamma_r+\mu)(\gamma+\mu)}{(\gamma_r+\mu)-\ell(1-r)\mathscr{R}_0(\gamma+\mu)} \tag{17}$$

and with the implementation of condition (15).

4 Discussion and Conclusion

The Ebola epidemic has shown us major weaknesses not only in health systems in West Africa, but also in our global capacity to respond early to an outbreak with effective diagnostic capacities. After multiple outbreaks of infectious diseases, from severe acute respiratory syndrome (SARS) to Middle East respiratory syndrome coronavirus (MERS-CoV), we still do not have effective diagnostic tools to rapidly respond to a number of potential epidemics. The main reason why we lack of such diagnostic preparedness against infectious diseases is because of the lack of a financed global strategy that can be implemented ahead, rather than during an epidemic. This strategy must primarily focus on two critical aspects: First, a continuous interaction between the field to detect small outbreaks and collect samples, and reference laboratories with advanced sequencing tools to identify the pathogen. Second, the need of assay development for early diagnosis, their regulatory approval, and a plan of implementation in anticipation of an outbreak.

Here, motivated by some studies showing that PCR assay can detect Ebola virus in both humans and non-human primates during the pre-symptomatic stage [7, 11], we have developed and analyzed a mathematical model calibrated to the transmission dynamics of Ebola virus disease in West Africa to evaluate the impact of early diagnosis of pre-symptomatic infections. In the absence of effective treatments and vaccines, our results show the importance of implementing integrated control measures of early diagnosis and isolation. Importantly, our analysis identifies a threshold where early diagnosis of pre-symptomatic individuals, combined with a sufficient level of effective isolation, can lead to an epidemic control of Ebola virus disease. Furthermore, the need to incorporate vital dynamics is justified by our still limited understanding of Ebola infection including whether or not Ebola virus may persist among recovered individuals. The use of $\mathscr{R}_c$ in this context reflect our view that control measures should be sustainable and not just in response to an outbreak.

Acknowledgments We thank Benjamin Katchman for the helpful discussions about the different types of molecular diagnostics of Ebola.

References

1. Kugelman, J.R., Sanchez-Lockhart, M., Andersen, K.G., Gire, S., Park, D.J., Sealfon, R., Lin, A.E., Wohl, S., Sabeti, P.C., Kuhn, J.H., Palacios, G.F.: Evaluation of the potential impact of Ebola virus genomic drift on the efficacy of sequence-based candidate therapeutics (2015)
2. Beeching, N.J., Fenech, M., Houlihan, C.F.: Ebola virus disease. BMJ **349**, g7348 (2014)
3. Fauci, A.S.: Ebola–underscoring the global disparities in health care resources. N. Engl. J. Med. **371**(12), 1084–1086 (2014)
4. McElroy, A.K., Erickson, B.R., Flietstra, T.D., Rollin, P.E., Nichol, S.T., Towner, J.S., Spiropoulou, C.F.: Ebola hemorrhagic fever: novel biomarker correlates of clinical outcome. J. Infect. Dis. jiu088 (2014)
5. Fink, S.: Ebola drug aids some in a study in West Africa. The New York Times, 4 Feb 2015
6. Ippolito, G., Feldmann, H., Lanini, S., Vairo, F., Di Caro, A., Capobianchi, M.R., Nicastri, E.: Viral hemorrhagic fevers: advancing the level of treatment. BMC Med. **10**(1), 31 (2012)
7. Leroy, E.M., Baize, S., Volchkov, V.E., Fisher-Hoch, S.P., Georges-Courbot, M.C., Lansoud-Soukate, J., McCormick, J. B., : Human asymptomatic Ebola infection and strong inflammatory response. Lancet **355**(9222), 2210–2215 (2000)
8. Chowell, D., Castillo-Chavez, C., Krishna, S., Qiu, X., Anderson, K.S.: Modelling the effect of early detection of Ebola. Lancet Infect. Dis. **15**(2), 148–149 (2005)
9. Chowell, G., Nishiura, H.: Transmission dynamics and control of Ebola virus disease (EVD): a review. BMC Med. **12**, 196 (2014)
10. Fasina, F., Shittu, A., Lazarus, D., et al.: Transmission dynamics and control of Ebola virus disease outbreak in Nigeria, July to September 2014. Euro Surveill. **19**, 20920 (2014)
11. Qiu, X., Wong, G., Audet, J., et al.: Reversion of advanced Ebola virus disease in nonhuman primates with ZMapp. Nature **514**, 4753 (2014)
12. Thieme, H.R.: Mathematics in Population Biology. Princeton University Press, Princeton (2003)
13. Brauer, F., Castillo-Chavez, C.: Mathematical Models in Population Biologyand Epidemiology. Springer, Berlin (2011)
14. Anderson, R.M., May, R.M.: Infectious Diseases of Humans. Oxford University Press, Oxford (1991)

15. van den Driessche, P., Watmough, J.: Reproduction numbers and sub-threshold endemic equilibria for compartmental models of disease transmission. Math. Biosci. **180**, 29–48 (2002)
16. Caswell, H.: Matrix Population Models, 2nd edn. Sinauer Associates, Sunderland (2001)

Modeling Ring-Vaccination Strategies to Control Ebola Virus Disease Epidemics

Gerardo Chowell and Maria Kiskowski

Abstract The 2013-15 Ebola epidemic that primarily affected Guinea, Sierra Leone and Liberia has become the most devastating Ebola epidemic in history [1]. This unprecedented epidemic appears to have stemmed from a single spillover event in South Guinea in December 2013 and rapidly spread to neighboring Sierra Leone and Guinea in a matter of weeks. Here we employ a network-based transmission model to evaluate the potential impact of reactive ring-vaccination strategies in the context of the Ebola epidemic in West Africa. We model ring-based vaccination strategies that incorporate the radius of contacts that are vaccinated for each infectious individual, the time elapsed from individual infectiousness to vaccinating susceptible and exposed contacts, and the number of available vaccine doses. Our baseline spatial transmission model in which the ring vaccination strategy is investigated has been previously shown to capture Ebola-like epidemics characterized by an initial phase of sub-exponential epidemic growth. Here we also extend this baseline model to account for heterogeneous community transmission rates that may be defined as a scalable function of the distance between an infectious individual and each member of that individual's community. Overall, our findings indicate that reactive ring-vaccination strategies can effectively mitigate established Ebola epidemics. Importantly, we studied scenarios with varying number of weeks elapsed between the onset of symptoms and the day contacts are vaccinated and found that it is still beneficial to vaccinate contacts after the infectious period has elapsed. Our results indicate that while it is beneficial to vaccinate members of the community, the probability of extinction is not very sensitive to which contacts in the community are vaccinated unless transmission varies very steeply on the network distance between individuals. Both of

G. Chowell (✉)
School of Public Health, Georgia State University, Atlanta, GA, USA
e-mail: gchowell@gsu.edu

G. Chowell
Fogarty International Center, National Institutes of Health, Bethesda, MD, USA

M. Kiskowski (✉)
Department of Mathematics and Statistics,
University South Alabama, Mobile, AL, USA
e-mail: abyrne@southalabama.edu

G. Chowell and J.M. Hyman (eds.), *Mathematical and Statistical Modeling for Emerging and Re-emerging Infectious Diseases*,
DOI 10.1007/978-3-319-40413-4_6

these observations underscore the fact that vaccination can be effective by reducing transmission at the community level.

Keywords Mathematical epidemiology · Dynamical models · Agent-based models · Ebola virus (EBOV) · Ring vaccination · Reactive vaccination · Social networks · Infectious disease dynamics · Household transmission · Community transmission · Emergent dynamics · Reaction diffusion · Waves

Abbreviations

EVD Ebola virus disease

1 Introduction

The 2013-15 Ebola epidemic in Guinea, Sierra Leone and Liberia has become the most devastating Ebola epidemic in history [1]. While past Ebola outbreaks have never exceeded a few hundred cases [2], this epidemic has generated a total of 28295 reported cases including 11295 deaths as of September 23, 2015 [3]. Fortunately, only a few cases per week have been reported in limited areas of Guinea and Sierra Leone as of August 2015 [3]. The index case appears to have occurred in December 2013 in the forested area of Guéckédou in South Guinea and probably originated from human contact with an infected bat [4]. The Ebola virus reached neighboring Liberia and Sierra Leone in a matter of weeks and incidence rates rapidly increased over subsequent weeks, peaked in August 2014, and rapidly declined likely as a result of improved rates of case identification (e.g., contact tracing, diagnostic rates), treatment and isolation capacity as well as changes in population behavior that reduce contact rates [5].

During the course of the Ebola epidemic, mathematical modeling tools have been useful to: (1) evaluate the epidemic transmission potential [6–12], (2) project or forecast the trajectory of the epidemic under various hypothetical scenarios and forecasting time frames [13–21], (3) evaluate the impact of contact tracing [22, 23], assess the risk of international case importations [24, 25], and (4) assess the feasibility of Ebola vaccine trials [26, 27]. However, these modeling efforts were hampered by the limited availability of epidemiological data and the unprecedented scope of the epidemic.

Motivated by the recent ring vaccination trial of the r-VSV vectored Ebola vaccine conducted in Guinea [28], here we employed a network-based transmission model to evaluate the impact of reactive ring-vaccination strategies against Ebola epidemics. Reactive vaccination aims to vaccinate a community in response to an infection unfolding in the community. The entire community may be vaccinated (mass vaccination) or vaccination may target the most susceptible individuals (e.g. ring vaccination [23, 29–32]). Modeling targeted vaccination requires individual based models that can capture the contact structure of the community network [29, 30, 32, 33]. We recently developed a network model incorporating the effect of community mixing [34, 35]. This model was used to systematically analyze the effects of different levels of population mixing on Ebola transmission dynamics and was able to fit different observed regional growth dynamics by changing only the community mixing parameter [34]. In particular, this transmission model is able to generate Ebola-like epidemics that are characterized by sub-exponential growth that with control interventions levels off in just a few generations of the disease [36], and provides important insights on the level of control that would be required to contain Ebola epidemics [35]. The model predicted that in the absence of epidemic control, persistent outbreaks would propagate through a community as spatial waves of fixed size [35]. Given the importance of community mixing in this model, we sought to investigate the effect of targeted vaccination on the persistence of the epidemic.

We aimed to model vaccination strategies that start 6 months after the onset of the epidemic and incorporate variations in (1) the radius of contacts that are vaccinated for each infectious individual, (2) the time elapsed from individual infectiousness to vaccination and immunization of susceptible and exposed contacts, and (3) the size of the vaccine stockpile. While the original version of the model assumed homogenous infectious contact probabilities (e.g., household-community structure), here we extend the model to incorporate heterogeneous community transmission rates that may be defined as a scalable function of the distance between an infectious individual and each member of that individual's community.

2 Methods

We extended a network-based SEIR transmission model with household-community structure [34, 35] to model reactive ring-based vaccination strategies. We also adapted the underlying baseline transmission model to incorporate heterogeneously weighted contact infection probabilities throughout the network.

3 Household-Community Structure

As in a former implementation of the model, individuals are organized within households of size H (each household contains H individuals) and households are organized within communities of size C households (each community contains $C \times H$ individuals). Households are indexed $\{h_i, h_{i+1}, \ldots\}$ and a network distance η between two households h_i and h_j is defined as $\eta = |i - j|$. The i_{th} community is the community centered at the i_{th} household and contains all households within distance $R_c = (C - 1)/2$. Communities overlap; the extent of overlap between the i_{th} and

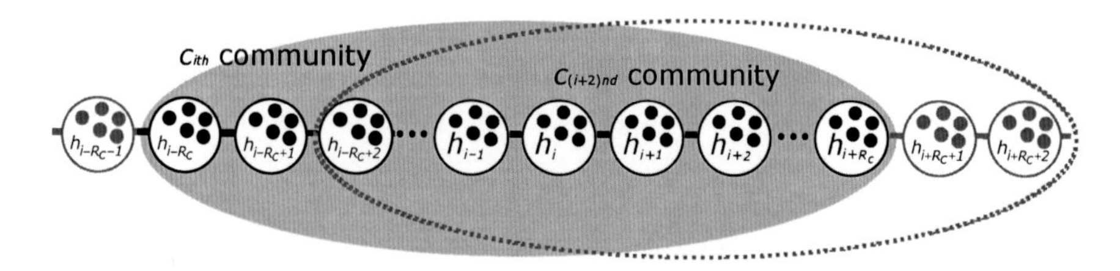

Fig. 1 A schematic of the c_{ith} **and** $c_{(i+2)nd}$ communities. Each household is indicated as a disk ($H = 5$ individuals are shown as smaller filled disks). The community size is $C = 2R + 1$ households. The community c_i centered at the i_{th} household contains the C households $\{h_{i-R_C}, h_{i-R_C+1}, \ldots, h_i, h_{i+1}, \ldots, h_{i+R_C}\}$ and is shown within the darker *gray ellipse*. The community c_{i+2} centered at the $(i + 2)_{nd}$ household contains the C households $\{h_{i-R_C+2}, h_{i-R_C+3}, \ldots, h_{i+2}, h_{i+3}, \ldots, h_{i+R_C+2}\}$ and is shown within the *outlined ellipse*. The network distance η of the i_{th} and the $(i + 2)_{nd}$ households is 2 and their communities each contain two households that the other community does not

j_{th} communities households decreases with the network distance of the i_{th} and j_{th} households (see Fig. 1). Network connectivity is identical for every individual.

4 SEIR-SV Transmission

Each household may be viewed as a complete graph of H nodes where each edge represents the rate of contact between any two household individuals. Likewise, each community may be viewed as complete graph of C nodes where each edge represents the rate of contact between community individuals.

Individuals in the network are assigned one of five states: ***S*** (susceptible), ***E*** (exposed), ***I*** (infectious), ***R*** (refractory) and ***V*** (vaccinated). Transition probabilities from susceptible (state ***S***) to exposed (state ***E***) depend on network structure and contact interactions between susceptible and exposed individuals:

$$
\begin{aligned}
p(S \to E) &= \textit{probability that a susceptible will become exposed} \\
&= (1 - \textit{probability of no exposures from any infected contacts}) \\
&= (1 - (1 - t_H)^{i_H} \cdot (1 - t_c)^{i_c}).
\end{aligned}
$$

where t_H and t_C are the rate of transmission of infection from a single infected individual to a single susceptible individual within a household or within the community, and i_H and i_C are the number of infectious household and community individuals in the network.

State transitions from exposed (state ***E***) to infectious (state ***I***) and from infectious (state ***I***) to refractory (state ***R***) occur independently of any network details:

$$p(E \rightarrow I) = \textit{probability that an exposed individual becomes infectious}$$
$$= 1/\gamma,$$

where γ is the average incubation period.

$$p(I \rightarrow R) = \textit{probability that an infectious individual will becomes refractory}$$
$$= 1/\lambda,$$

where λ is the average infectious period.

Compared to previous implementations of the model, the model is extended with a fifth state for vaccinated individuals (state V). Only susceptible individuals may transit to the vaccinated state ($S \rightarrow V$), and the sole effect of the transition is to remove those individuals from the pool of susceptibles. The transition rules depend on the details of a given vaccination program.

5 Homogeneous and Heterogeneous Transmission Rates on the Network

For any network configuration, transmission rates on the network are scaled to yield a given set of reproductive numbers R_{0H} and R_{0C}. The household reproductive number R_{0H} is the expected number of household contacts infected by a single infectious individual—if all other nodes of the network are susceptible, and likewise the community reproductive number R_{0C} is the expected number of infected community contacts.

In previous implementations of this model, we assumed homogenous infectious contact probabilities. For this case, an infected individual has an equal rate of transmission t_H with each household contact ($H-1$ household contacts in a fully susceptible network) which is equal to the average rate of transmission $\widehat{t_H}$ per contact. Likewise, an infected individual has an equal rate of transmission t_c with each community contact ($C \cdot H-1$ community contacts in a fully susceptible network), which is equal to the average rate of transmission $\widehat{t_c}$ per contact. Given that the expected lifetime of an infectious state is λ, and that the size of the household and community neighborhoods are $H \times 1$ and $H \times C$, respectively, the expected number of exposures resulting from an initial infected individual are:

$$R_{0H} \approx \lambda\, t_H \cdot (H - 1),$$
$$R_{0C} \approx \lambda\, t_C \cdot (C \cdot H - 1).$$

Even though saturation effects build over a single serial interval (this is why the equalities in the equation above are only approximate), solving for t_H and t_C above results in the rates of transmission (instantaneously/in the absence of saturation effects) corresponding to the reproductive numbers R_{0H} and R_{0C}:

$$t_H := \frac{R_{oH}}{\lambda(H-1)}, t_C := \frac{R_{oC}}{\lambda(C \cdot H - 1)}.$$

For heterogeneous transmission rates, the household and community networks may be considered a weighted complete graph where the weight of each edge $w_{\beta\theta}$ connecting nodes β and θ correspond to the contact rate of the nodes of β and θ. The expected number of household and community infections from a single infectious individual at node β are proportional to the product of the infectious interval λ and the sum of the transmission weights $t_{\beta i} = w_{\beta i}$ of all edges of the node β

Given household and community reproductive numbers (though certainly altering the longer term dynamics) may be fit by requiring that *average* transmission rates $\widehat{t_H}$ and $\widehat{t_C}$ satisfy the same equalities:

$$\widehat{t_H} := \frac{R_{oH}}{\lambda(H-1)}, \widehat{t_C} := \frac{R_{oC}}{\lambda(C \cdot H - 1)}.$$

For example, heterogeneous community transmission rates may be defined as a scalable function of the distance $\eta(g_t(\eta) = \alpha f(\eta))$ between an infectious individual and each other member of that individual's community. By applying symmetry and given the community radius $R_c = \frac{c-1}{2}$, a scalable average transmission rate $\widehat{t_C}$ may be computed as:

$$\widehat{t_C} = \frac{\textit{sum of all edge weights}}{\textit{number of edges}}$$

$$= \frac{\textit{sum of edge weights for nodes with positive distance} + \textit{sum of edge weights for nodes with zero distance}}{(C.H-1)}$$

$$= \frac{2(H\sum_{\eta=1}^{R_C} \alpha f(\eta)) + (H-1)\alpha f(0)}{(C.H-1)}$$

$$= \alpha \left(\frac{2(H\sum_{\eta=1}^{R_C} f(\eta)) + (H-1)f(0)}{(C.H-1)} \right)$$

By appropriate choice of α, the value of $\widehat{t_C}$ can be scaled so that $\widehat{t_C} = \frac{R_0 C}{\lambda(C.H-1)}$.

For a transmission-distance function that decreases linearly with distance, we use $g_t(\eta) = \alpha(R_c - \eta)$. The transmission rate decreases linearly from a maximal value to zero as the distance increases from 0 to R_c. For a flat transmission-distance function, we use $g_t(\eta) = \alpha$. For a transmission-distance function that decays exponentially, we use $g_t(n) = \alpha e^{(R_C - \eta)}$. The specific functions used in simulations are described in Fig. 2.

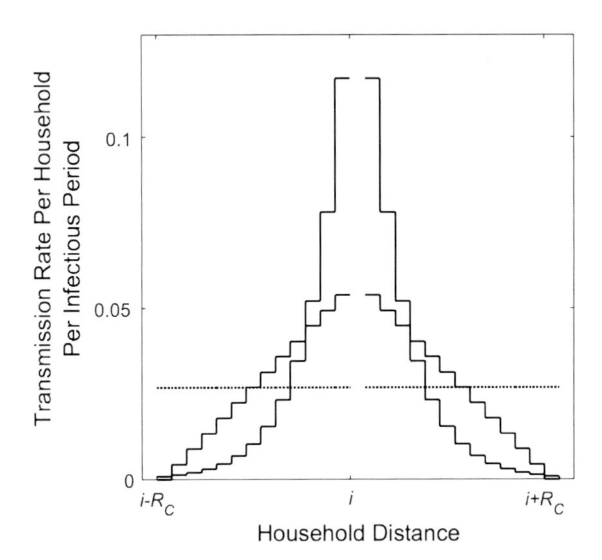

Fig. 2 Community transmission rate (per household, per infectious period) for different transmission-distance functions. The total cumulative transmission rate (area under the curves) is $R_{0C} = 0.7$ for each transmission distribution used for simulations: flat (*dotted plot*), linear (*black solid plot*) and exponential with base 1.5 (*gray solid plot*). For this figure, as in simulations, $R_C = 13$ ($C = 27$)

6 Parameter Values, Initial Conditions for Simulations and Details of a Simulated Vaccination Program

Simulations are initialized on day $s = 1$ with a single infectious individual within the network. As the infection spreads, the network grows dynamically so that the population is effectively infinite in size. We choose SEIR transmission parameter values corresponding to those matching early (putatively rural) epidemic dynamics in Guinea: $R_{0H} = 2.0$, $R_{0C} = 0.7$, $C = 27$ [32].

We model a vaccination program by vaccinating the susceptible and exposed contacts of infectious individuals located within a specified radius of the infected individual (ring vaccination). A given vaccination program is specified by 4 new parameters:

- t_{v0}: the day s of the outbreak that the vaccination program begins,
- R_v: the radius of contacts that are vaccinated for each infectious individual,
- w_v: the week that susceptible and exposed contacts become immune after an individual becomes infectious; equal to the sums of the delays of identifying an infectious individual, vaccinating contacts, and vaccinated contacts acquiring immunity
- v_{tot}: the total vaccine supply.

We approximate that the symptomatic period is equal to the infectious period. This means an exposed individual cannot be identified until that individual becomes infectious, so contacts are not vaccinated until $w_v \geq 0$ weeks after that individual is infectious. Likewise, all non-symptomatic (susceptible and exposed) contacts are vaccinated even though only susceptible individuals (state $\boldsymbol{S}$) transition to the vaccinated state (state $\boldsymbol{V}$). Exposed vaccinated individuals contribute to the total number of vaccines supplied. Once the total number of vaccinated individuals reaches v_{tot}, no further contacts are vaccinated.

In simulations, we model a vaccination program that is implemented after the epidemic establishes, at 180 days, and we measure the effect of a vaccination program over the next 180 days. An epidemic is defined as having ended when all exposed and infectious states have transitioned to refractory. Since the vaccination program begins on the 180th day of the simulation, we only simulate vaccination programs for epidemics that persist beyond the 180th day. Over the following six-month simulated time period, we measure the probability that the epidemic ends and the average cumulative number of infected individuals. Averages are calculated for N sets of 1000 s simulations and standard error is calculated as $\frac{\sigma}{\sqrt{N}}$ where σ is the standard deviation of N means of sets of 1000 simulations.

7 Results

7.1 Even Without Vaccination, Outbreaks Have a High Probability of Spontaneously Extinguishing Early on, a Lower Probability Thereafter

We first focus on transmission parameters and a transmission network that were selected in [35] to represent "rural Guinean dynamics". The household reproductive number is 2.0, the community reproductive number is 0.7, and the community transmission distribution is flat (homogeneous).

Even without vaccination, there is a high probability that an outbreak will extinguish spontaneously. Since this is due to stochastic fluctuations in the number of individuals infected by each infectious individual, this probability is especially high early during an outbreak when there are only a small number of infectious individuals. Figure 3a shows that for the parameters selected to represent "rural Guinean dynamics", the probability that the outbreak will extinguish the first month is approximately 40 % and decreases sharply thereafter. Once outbreaks have established for several months, they are fairly stable and spontaneously extinguish at an approximate rate of only ~0.02 outbreaks per month. Indeed, the data in Fig. 3a shows that if an outbreak persists beyond the first month, it has a probability of approximately 48/60 = 80 % to persist beyond six months.

As described in [35] after the initialization of an outbreak by a single infected individual, the number of infected individuals steadily increases within a community if the outbreak persists, creating a wave of fixed size that moves through communities.

Figure 3b shows the average number of infectious individuals per day for outbreaks aggregated by their duration where each curve corresponds to each of the bins in the histogram in Fig. 3a. In Kiskowski and Chowell (2015) [35] we focused on describing the dynamics of outbreaks that persist: after the initialization of an outbreak by a single infected individual, the number of infected individuals steadily increases

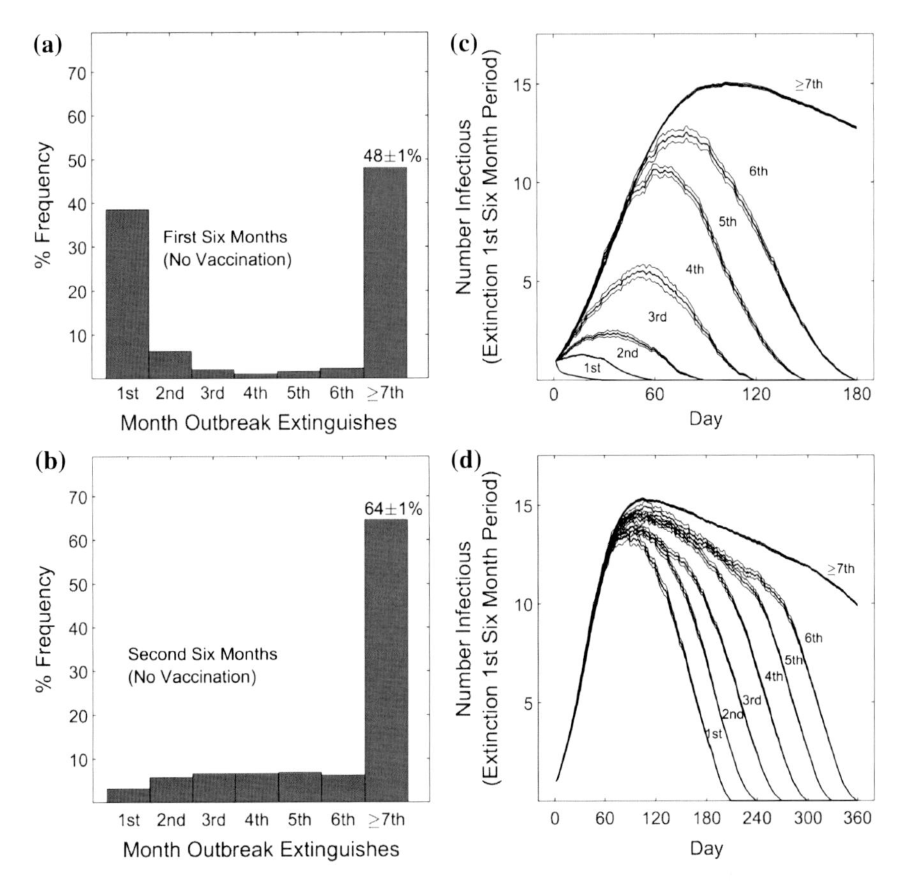

Fig. 3 Outbreak persistence without Vaccination. **a** The percent frequency that an outbreak spontaneously extinguishes versus simulation month for the (**a**) first or **b** second 6-month period. **c** The average number of infected individuals versus simulation day for simulations that spontaneously extinguished in each month of the (**c**) first or **d** second 6-month period. Simulations for the first 6-month period were initialized with a single infected individual on day 1 and were run for 180 days (6 months). Simulations for the second 6-month period were restricted to those with a single infected individual on day 1 that persisted for 180 days (6 months), and then were run for another 180 days. Frequencies and averages were calculated for $N = 10$ sets of 1000 simulations. Error bars show the standard error of $N = 10$ sets

within a community creating a wave of fixed size that moves through communities. Figure 3b shows that the dynamics of outbreaks that extinguish have the same initial dynamics as those that persist, but stochastically "peel off" from the dynamic of those that persist as the number of infectious individuals decrease stochastically to zero.

To study the effect of ring vaccination on outbreaks, we focused on the vaccination of outbreaks that have persisted for six months and thus have a lower probability of spontaneously extinguishing. Figure 3c shows the probability that an outbreak will extinguish in any of the months of a second 6-month period, given that it has already persisted for the first 6-month period. Overall, an outbreak that has persisted for six months has a 65 % chance of persisting another six months in the absence of vaccination and other control interventions. Figure 3d shows the average number of infectious individuals per day for each of the simulations binned by month extinguishing in Fig. 3c.

7.2 *Earlier Vaccination of Infected Individuals Increases the Probability that Outbreaks Will Extinguish Within Six Months*

Figure 4a shows the effect of a vaccination program on the number of infectious individuals. In this vaccination program, the program began after six months (on day 180) and 45 closest contacts of infectious individuals were vaccinated 1, 2, 4, or 8 weeks after an infectious individual became symptomatic. The panels in Fig. 5a–d show the effect that the vaccination program had on the duration of the outbreaks.

If the closest contacts of infected individuals are vaccinated within the first or second week (Fig. 5a, b), it is unlikely that the outbreak will persist longer than six months (<1 %). Even if the closest contacts are vaccinated at 4 or 8 weeks, the probability the outbreak persists for longer than six months is small (<10 %) or

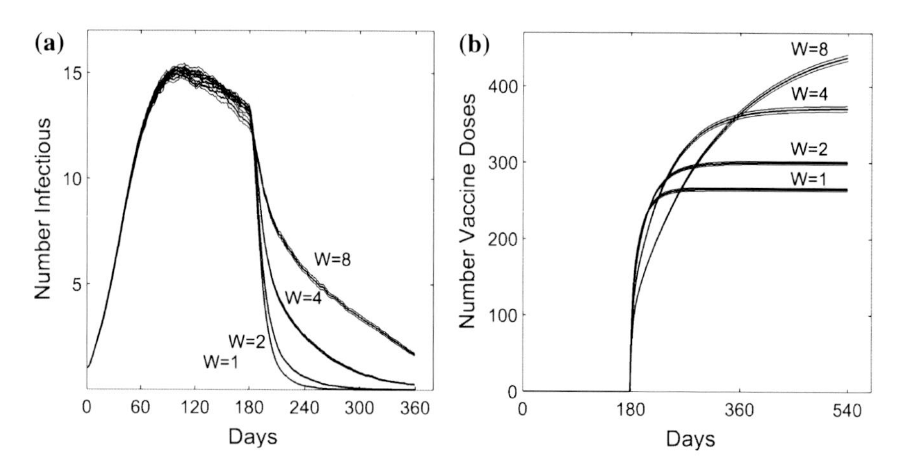

Fig. 4 Effect of vaccination week on outbreak dynamics. **a** Average number of infectious individuals and **b** average cumulative vaccines used versus day with vaccination after 1, 2, 4 or 8 weeks. Simulations were restricted to those with a single infected individual on day 1 that persisted for 180 days (6 months), and then were run for another 180 days. A vaccination program began in day 180. The 45 closest contacts of every infected individual were vaccinated (immunization rate =100 %) 1, 2, 4 or 8 weeks after the first day of infectiousness. Averages were calculated for $N = 10$ sets of 1000 simulations. Error bars show the standard error of $N = 10$ sets

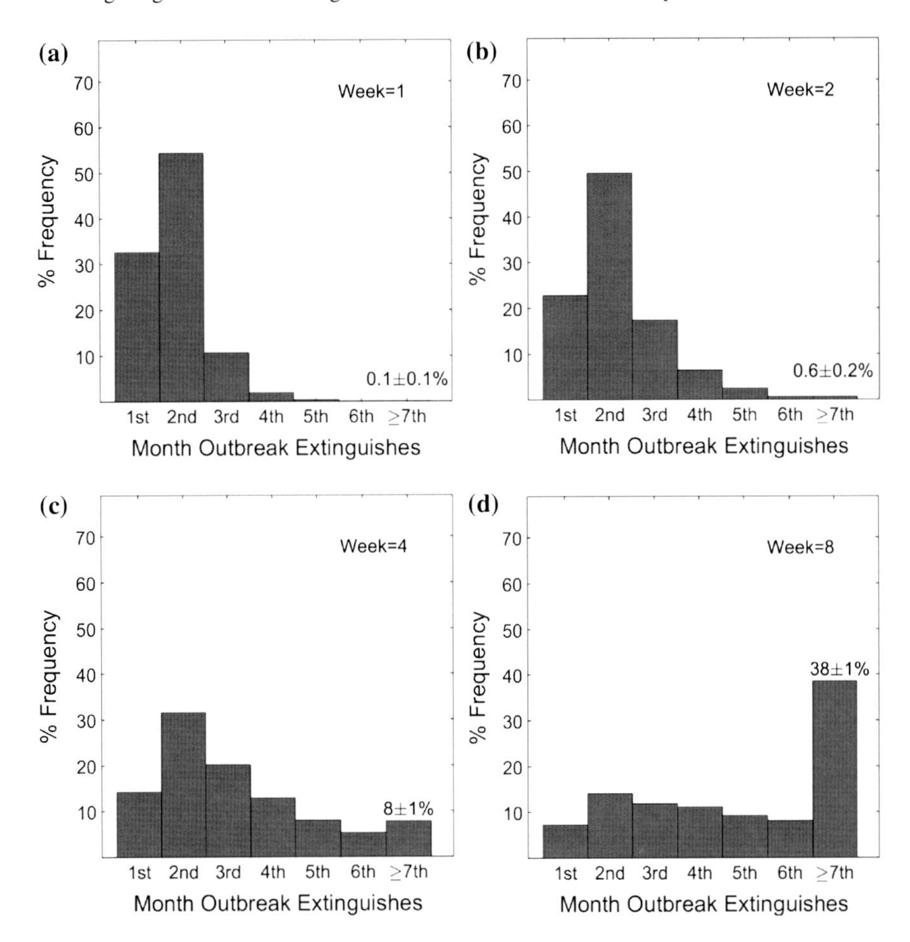

Fig. 5 Outbreak persistence with vaccination after 1, 2, 4 or 8 weeks. The percent frequency that an outbreak spontaneously extinguishes versus simulation month of the second 6-month period. The 45 closest contacts of every infected individual were vaccinated (immunization rate =100 %) **a** 1, **b** 2, **c** 4 or **d** 8 weeks after day infectious for the vaccination program described in Fig. 4. Averages were calculated for $N = 10$ sets of 1000 simulations. Error bars show the standard error of $N = 10$ sets

measurably reduced compared to the non-vaccination rate of 65 % (to 38 %). Although the average infectious period of an infectious individual is relatively shorter (5.6 days), the infection still circulates among contacts. As measured by the probability of the outbreak being extinguished, the vaccination program is more effective the fewer number of weeks elapse between the day that an individual becomes infectious. Figure 4b shows the average cumulative number of vaccines that are used in each vaccination program. Not only does the probability of ending the outbreak increase with earlier week vaccination as shown in Fig. 4a, but the average total number of vaccines needed to end the outbreak also decreases.

In simulations described so far (Figs. 4 and 5) we simulated a vaccination program in which the 45 closest contacts of each infectious individual have been vaccinated, representing a vaccination radius of 4 families ($45 = 4 \times 10 + 5$). We next consider whether simulations would predict an optimal radius for ring vaccination, especially in the context of limited vaccines. Figure 6a shows the probability of an outbreak persisting as a function of the number of vaccinated contacts ($=10 \times v_r + 5$) and

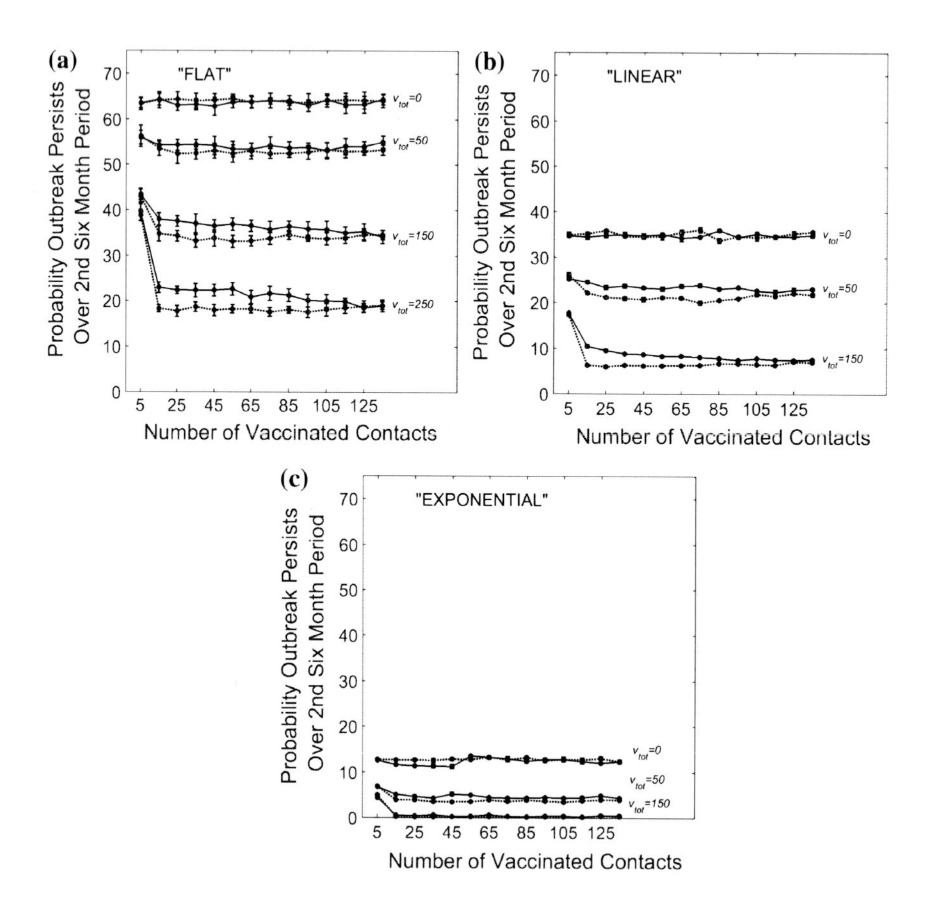

Fig. 6 Outbreak persistence versus vaccination radius and transmission structure, for a limited vaccine supply. The probability that an outbreak persists for the entire 6-month vaccination period versus the number of contacts vaccination for a transmission distribution that is **a** flat, or **b** varies linearly or **c** varies exponentially with radial distance from the infected contacts. For all simulations, simulations are restricted to outbreaks that persist through the first 6-month period and the vaccination program begins at 180 days. The number of contacts in the vaccinated pool of each infected individual is $5(1 + 2f)$, where $2f$ is the number of households vaccinated in the community. The infected contact's household is always in the vaccinated pool. For the *black plots*, the households in the vaccinated pool are chosen within a radius of $2f$, so that the vaccinated pool always includes the closest contacts. For the *gray plots*, the households are chosen randomly within the community (f households in the negative radial direction and f households in the positive radial direction). Averages were calculated for $N = 10$ sets of 1000 simulations. Error bars show the standard error of $N = 10$ sets

the vaccine supply v_{tot} for a transmission rate that is homogeneous throughout the community. In the context of unlimited vaccine supply, the probability of an outbreak persisting decreases monotonically with the radius of vaccination. In the context of limited vaccine supply, we find that there is always benefit in vaccinating the household (the number of vaccinated contacts is 5 when $v_r = 0$) and vaccinating *some* members of the community (i.e., with $v_r > 0$). This is particularly true as the vaccine supply increases; as the vaccine supply increases past 100 vaccines the marginal benefit of vaccinating community members is quite substantial. However, beyond choosing a positive vaccination radius, the persistence of the outbreak is not very sensitive to the chosen radius of vaccination. This lack of sensitivity to the vaccination radius in the context of a limited vaccine supply can be understood considering that, first, all members of the community have an equi-probable chance of being infected by an infectious contact (the transmission distribution is flat) so that the probability of transmission does not depend upon the radius within the community. Second, while vaccinating with a positive radius ensures that some vaccinated community members accumulate, ring vaccination with a small radius ensures a focused effort on communities in which infections are still actively circulating.

In a next set of simulations, we compare these results for networks with different community transmission structures. For all of these structures, the initial net community transmission probability is described by the same community reproductive number $R_{0C} = 0.7$. This represents the average number of community individuals that would be infected by a single infected individual in a naïve community. Even though they share this community reproductive number, outbreaks on the networks with a transmission rate that linearly decays with radius (Fig. 6b) or exponentially decays (Fig. 6c) have a much lower probability of persisting without any vaccination program (plots labeled $v_{tot} = 0$) and for any fixed vaccine supply (other values of v_{tot}). This is due to the increased transmission rates (and thus increased saturation effects) at smaller distances: infected individuals are more likely to infect individuals very close to them while these individuals find that the individuals closest to them are most likely to already be infected. While the vaccination program is more successful as the vaccine supply increases, we still do not find a strong sensitivity to the radius of vaccination. On the contrary, randomly vaccinating households appears to be slightly more effective than vaccinating the closest households. Since contacts are vaccinated two weeks after an individual becomes infectious, we speculate that by this time the infection has already spread to some extent through the community. Vaccinating only closest contacts may be less effective since some individuals are already exposed or infected, thus reducing the impact of vaccinating this pool.

8 Discussion

Motivated by the promising findings of the ring vaccination trial of the r-VSV vectored Ebola vaccine conducted in Guinea [28], we sought to evaluate the effectiveness of ring-vaccination strategies in controlling established Ebola-like epidemics by using a network-based transmission model previously employed to gain insights on the transmission dynamics of the 2013-15 Ebola epidemic in West Africa [34, 35]. We model a ring vaccination program that is characterized by the radius of the ring of vaccinated contacts, the time elapsed from individual infectiousness to start of vaccinating contacts and the development of their immunity, and the size of the vaccine stockpile. Overall, our findings indicate that reactive ring-vaccination strategies are effective at mitigating established Ebola epidemics. Importantly, while varying the number of weeks between the first day an individual becomes infectious and the day their contacts are vaccinated, we find that it is still beneficial to vaccinate contacts after the infectious period has elapsed. Likewise, while it is beneficial to vaccinate members of the community, the probability of extinction is not very sensitive to which contacts are vaccinated unless transmission depends very steeply on the network distance between individuals. Both of these observations underscore the fact that vaccination can be effective by reducing transmission at the community level and is in agreement with another ring-vaccination modeling study that captures varying levels of population clustering through a pair approximation model of Ebola transmission [37].

The baseline spatial transmission model employed here structures the population into communities of households to mimic the driving mechanisms of transmission of Ebola in West Africa [35], but we also adapted the spatial model to describe heterogeneous community transmission rates. In contrast to classic compartmental transmission models based on underlying homogenous mixing assumptions [38, 39], this spatially structured model has been able to successfully capture the qualitative patterns of epidemic growth observed in Guinea, Liberia and Sierra Leone [35]. Specifically, the simple household-community transmission model yields brief exponential growth during the first 2–3 generations of infections followed by sub-exponential epidemic growth during several disease generations. This is consistent with the local epidemic growth patterns observed for each of the EVD epidemics in the most affected countries in West Africa [36]. It is crucial to capture the appropriate spatial structure in models of disease transmission for epidemic forecasting because epidemic trajectories are highly sensitive to assumptions of contact structure [17, 34, 40–42].

Regardless of the outbreak duration, the initial dynamics of all outbreaks derived from the spatial model [34, 35] appear to be similar, with the number of infectious individuals initially increasing at comparable rates. Moreover, simulations indicate that extinguishing versus persistent outbreaks are initially identical. This may be more thoroughly tested with simulations continued from intermediate time points, to determine at what point in an outbreak the fate of an outbreak may be determined to be persistent or extinguishing. One prediction is that the probability of an outbreak spontaneously extinguishing is independent of the history of the epidemic, but depends only on the number of currently infectious individuals (a memoryless process). This is unlikely since the location of infected individuals, whether within saturated communities or surrounded by many available contacts, should affect the probability of persistence.

While the original version of the underlying spatial model employed in our study considered transmission probability at two scales: household and community level, in this paper we also analyzed a model incorporating heterogeneously distributed transmission rates across members of the community by using a scalable function of the distance between an infectious individual and members of that individual's community. We found that the outbreaks on the networks with a transmission rate that linearly or exponential decays with radius have a much lower probability of persisting without any vaccination program for any fixed vaccine supply. We have explained this as a result of the increased transmission rates (and thus increased saturation effects) at smaller distances. While the vaccination program is more successful as the vaccine supply increases, our results were not highly sensitive to the radius of vaccination. Vaccinating only closest contacts may be less effective than expected since some individuals may already be exposed or infected, thus reducing the impact of vaccinating this pool.

The relevance of these results to real world networks is limited by the relative simplicity of the network structure captured in our model. Yet, our model captures household and community structure that is important for describing Ebola transmission dynamics. Analysis of targeted vaccination in the context of more complex networks with long-range interactions and heterogeneity in the node degree are described in, for example, Refs. [43, 44]. Nevertheless, our model is useful to generate insights on transmission and control strategies for small communities or within subsets of larger networks in which the network may be characterized by relatively simplified interactions.

References

1. Team WHOER: Ebola Virus Disease in West Africa - The First 9 Months of the Epidemic and Forward Projections. New Engl. J. Med. **371**(16), 1481-1495, 22 Sep 2014
2. Chowell, G., Nishiura, H.: Transmission dynamics and control of Ebola virus disease (EVD): a review. BMC Med. **12**(1), 196 (2014)
3. Ebola response roadmap - Situation report - 23 Sep 2015. http://apps.who.int/ebola/current-situation/ebola-situation-report-23-september-2015. Accessed 27 Sep 2015
4. Baize, S., Pannetier, D., Oestereich, L., Rieger, T., Koivogui, L., Magassouba, N., et al.: Emergence of Zaire Ebola virus disease in Guinea–preliminary report. New Engl. J. Med. **371**(15), 1418–1425 (2014)
5. Chowell, G., Nishiura, H.: Characterizing the transmission dynamics and control of Ebola virus disease. PLoS Biol. **13**(1), e1002057 (2015)
6. Nishiura, H., Chowell, G.: Early transmission dynamics of Ebola virus disease (EVD), West Africa, March to August 2014. Euro surveillance: bulletin Europeen sur les maladies transmissibles = European communicable disease bulletin, vol. 19, no. 36 (2014)
7. Althaus, C.L.: Estimating the reproduction number of Zaire ebolavirus (EBOV) during the 2014 outbreak in West Africa. PLOS Curr. Outbreaks Ed. 1. doi:10.1371/currents.outbreaks.91afb5e0f279e7f29e7056095255b288 (2014)
8. Fisman, D., Khoo, E., Tuite, A.: Early epidemic dynamics of the West African 2014 Ebola outbreak: estimates derived with a simple two-parameter model. PLoS Curr. **6** (2014)
9. Towers, S., Patterson-Lomba, O., Castillo-Chavez, C.: Temporal variations in the effective reproduction number of the 2014 West Africa Ebola outbreak. PLOS Curr. Outbreaks (2014)

10. Camacho, A., Kucharski, A., Aki-Sawyerr, Y., White, M.A., Flasche, S., Baguelin, M., et al.: Temporal changes in Ebola transmission in Sierra Leone and implications for control requirements: a real-time modelling study. PLoS Curr. **7** (2015)
11. Alizon, S., Lion, S., Murall, C.L., Abbate, J.L.: Quantifying the epidemic spread of Ebola virus (EBOV) in Sierra Leone using phylodynamics. Virulence **5**(8), 825–827 (2014)
12. Volz, E., Pond, S.: Phylodynamic analysis of Ebola virus in the 2014 Sierra Leone epidemic. PLoS Curr. **6** (2014)
13. Pandey, A., Atkins, K.E., Medlock, J., Wenzel, N., Townsend, J.P., Childs, J.E., et al.: Strategies for containing Ebola in West Africa. Science **346**(6212), 991–995 (2014)
14. Yamin, D., Gertler, S., Ndeffo-Mbah, M.L., Skrip, L.A., Fallah, M., Nyenswah, T.G., et al.: Effect of Ebola progression on transmission and control in Liberia. Ann. Intern. Med. **162**, 11–17 (2014)
15. Meltzer, M.I., Atkins, C.Y., Santibanez, S., Knust, B., Petersen, B.W., Ervin, E.D., et al.: Estimating the future number of cases in the Ebola epidemic - Liberia and Sierra Leone. Morb. Mortal. Wkly. Rep. Surveill. Summ. **26**(63), 1–14 (2014)
16. Lewnard, J.A., Ndeffo Mbah, M.L., Alfaro-Murillo, J.A., Altice, F.L., Bawo, L., Nyenswah, T.G., et al.: Dynamics and control of Ebola virus transmission in Montserrado, Liberia: a mathematical modelling analysis. Lancet Infect. Dis. **14**(12), 1189–1195 (2014)
17. Merler, S., Ajelli, M., Fumanelli, L., Gomes, M.F., Piontti, A.P., Rossi, L., et al.: Spatiotemporal spread of the 2014 outbreak of Ebola virus disease in Liberia and the effectiveness of non-pharmaceutical interventions: a computational modelling analysis. Lancet Infect. Dis. **15**(2), 204–211 (2015)
18. Rivers, C.M., Lofgren, E.T., Marathe, M., Eubank, S., Lewis, B.L.: Modeling the impact of interventions on an epidemic of Ebola in Sierra Leone and Liberia. PLoS Curr **6** (2014)
19. Scarpino, S.V., Iamarino, A., Wells, C., Yamin, D., Ndeffo-Mbah, M., Wenzel, N.S., et al.: Epidemiological and viral genomic sequence analysis of the 2014 Ebola outbreak reveals clustered transmission. Clin. Infect. Dis. An official publication of the Infectious Diseases Society of America **60**(7), 1079–1082 (2015)
20. Drake, J.M., Kaul, R.B., Alexander, L.W., O'Regan, S.M., Kramer, A.M., Pulliam, J.T., et al.: Ebola cases and health system demand in Liberia. PLoS Biol. **13**(1), e1002056 (2015)
21. Fasina, F., Shittu, A., Lazarus, D., Tomori, O., Simonsen, L., Viboud, C., et al.: Transmission dynamics and control of Ebola virus disease outbreak in Nigeria, July to September 2014. Euro surveillance: bulletin Europeen sur les maladies transmissibles = European communicable disease bulletin, vol. 19, no. 40 (2014)
22. Webb, G., Browne, C., Huo, X., Seydi, O., Seydi, M., Magal, P.: A model of the: Ebola epidemic in West Africa with contact tracing. PLoS Curr. **7** (2014)
23. Browne, C., Gulbudak, H., Webb, G.: Modeling contact tracing in outbreaks with application to Ebola. J. Theor. Biol. **7**(384), 33–49 (2015)
24. Gomes, M.F., Piontti, A.P., Rossi, L., Chao, D., Longini, I., Halloran, M.E., et al.: Assessing the international spreading risk associated with the 2014 West African Ebola outbreak. PLOS Curr. Outbreaks (2014)
25. Bogoch, I.I., Creatore, M.I., Cetron, M.S., Brownstein, J.S., Pesik, N., Miniota, J., et al.: Assessment of the potential for international dissemination of Ebola virus via commercial air travel during the 2014 West African outbreak. The Lancet (2014)
26. Bellan, S.E., Pulliam, J.R.C., Pearson, C.A.B., Champredon, D., Fox, S.J., Skrip, L., et al.: The statistical power and validity of Ebola vaccine trials in Sierra Leone: a simulation study of trial design and analysis. Lancet Infect. Dis. **15**(6), 703–710 (2015)
27. Cooper, B.S., Boni, M.F., Pan-ngum, W., Day, N.P., Horby, P.W., Olliaro, P., et al.: Evaluating clinical trial designs for investigational treatments of Ebola virus disease. PLoS Med. **12**(4), e1001815 (2015)
28. Henao-Restrepo, A.M., Longini, I.M., Egger, M., Dean, N.E., Edmunds, W.J., Camacho, A., et al.: Efficacy and effectiveness of an rVSV-vectored vaccine expressing Ebola surface glycoprotein: interim results from the Guinea ring vaccination cluster-randomised trial. Lancet **386**(9996), 857–866 (2015)

29. Greenhalgh, D.: Optimal control of an epidemic by ring vaccination. Commun. Stat. Stoch. Models **2**(3), 339–363 (1986)
30. Muller, J., Schonfisch, B., Kirkilionis, M.: Ring vaccination. J. Math. Biol. **41**(2), 143–171 (2000)
31. Kretzschmar, M., van den Hof, S., Wallinga, J., van Wijngaarden, J.: Ring vaccination and smallpox control. Emerg. Infect. Dis. **10**(5), 832–841 (2004)
32. Tildesley, M.J., Savill, N.J., Shaw, D.J., Deardon, R., Brooks, S.P., Woolhouse, M.E., et al.: Optimal reactive vaccination strategies for a foot-and-mouth outbreak in the UK. Nature **440**(7080), 83–86 (2006)
33. Ferguson, N.M., Donnelly, C.A., Anderson, R.M.: The foot-and-mouth epidemic in Great Britain: pattern of spread and impact of interventions. Science **292**(5519), 1155–1160 (2001)
34. Kiskowski, M.: Three-scale network model for the early growth dynamics of 2014 West Africa Ebola epidemic. PLOS Curr. Outbreaks (2014). doi:10.1371/currents.outbreaks.b4690859d91684da963dc40e00f3da81
35. Kiskowski, M., Chowell, G.: Modeling household and community transmission of Ebola virus disease: epidemic growth, spatial dynamics and insights for epidemic control. Virulence **20**, 1–11 (2015)
36. Chowell, G., Viboud, C., Hyman, J.M., Simonsen, L.: The Western Africa Ebola virus disease epidemic exhibits both global exponential and local polynomial growth rates. PLoS Curr. **7** (2015)
37. Wells, C., Yamin, D., Ndeffo-Mbah, M.L., Wenzel, N., Gaffney, S.G., Townsend, J.P., et al.: Harnessing case isolation and ring vaccination to control Ebola. PLoS Negl. Trop. Dis. **9**(5), e0003794 (2015)
38. Anderson, R.M., May, R.M.: Infectious Diseases of Humans. Oxford University Press, Oxford (1991)
39. Hethcote, H.W.: The mathematics of infectious diseases. SIAM Rev. **42**(4), 599–653 (2000)
40. Sattenspiel, L., Dietz, K.: A structured epidemic model incorporating geographic mobility among regions. Math. Biosci. **128**(1–2), 71–91 (1995)
41. Newman, M.E.: Spread of epidemic disease on networks. Phys. Rev. E Stat. Nonlinear Soft Matter Phys. **66**(1 Pt 2), 016128 (2002)
42. Watts, D.J., Strogatz, S.H.: Collective dynamics of 'small-world' networks. Nature **393**(6684), 440–442 (1998)
43. Xu, Z., Zu, Z., Zheng, T., Zhang, W., Xu, Q., Liu, J.: Comparative analysis of the effectiveness of three immunization strategies in controlling disease outbreaks in realistic social networks. PloS One **9**(5), e95911 (2014)
44. Pastor-Satorras, R., Vespignani, A.: Immunization of complex networks. Phys. Rev. E Stat. Nonlinear Soft Matter Phys. **65**(3 Pt 2A), 036104 (2002)

Evaluating the Number of Sickbeds During Ebola Epidemics Using Optimal Control Theory

Eunok Jung, Jonggul Lee and Gerardo Chowell

Abstract Optimal control (OC) theory is a powerful tool to guide the design and implementation of control intervention strategies against epidemics. This technique defined control measures under a predetermined objective while minimizing the costs associated with the implementation of the control strategy. Here we use optimal control and epidemic modeling to explore the uncertainty in hospital bed capacity that would be needed to control an Ebola epidemic under different initial conditions, variation in the basic reproduction number, and associated costs to implement control measures. In particular, we focus on assessing the impact of effective isolation of infectious individuals in the health care setting because one key factor that facilitated the development of the Ebola epidemic in West Africa was the lack of public health surveillance systems to detect new outbreaks and the healthcare capacity that is needed to enforce infection control practices.

Keywords Epidemic model · Ebola · Optimal control · Hospital bed capacity · Infection control · Control measures

1 Introduction

The worst epidemic of Ebola virus disease (EVD) in West Africa appears to be finally ending after more than 20 months of Ebola transmission in the affected region [29]. A number of key factors allowed the Ebola virus to effectively spread and take hold in the populations of Guinea, Liberia, and Sierra Leona [6]. In particular, cases of EVD

E. Jung (✉) · J. Lee
Department of Mathematics, Konkuk University, Seoul, South Korea
e-mail: junge@konkuk.ac.kr

J. Lee
e-mail: jack9872@konkuk.ac.kr

G. Chowell
School of Public Health, Georgia State University, Atlanta, GA, USA
e-mail: gchowell@gsu.edu

G. Chowell and J.M. Hyman (eds.), *Mathematical and Statistical Modeling for Emerging and Re-emerging Infectious Diseases*,
DOI 10.1007/978-3-319-40413-4_7

were not reported until March 2014, several weeks after the first cases reportedly occurred in the forested area of Gueckedou in Guinea in December 2013. The World Health Organization declared the Ebola epidemic in West Africa a Public Health Emergency of International Concern on August 8th, 2014 [28] as the number of cases climbed across areas of West Africa [1, 11, 20, 21, 27]. The current size of the ongoing EVD epidemic has generated more than 22,495 cases of which 8981 have succumbed to the disease according to the World Health Organization as of September 30, 2015 [29].

A substantial amount of data has accumulated on the clinical and epidemiological characteristics of Ebola virus disease (EVD) transmission in humans during past outbreaks and the 2013–2015 Ebola epidemic in West Africa. These data are critical to parameterize models of Ebola transmission dynamics. For instance, the basic reproduction number, R_0, has been estimated for prior EVD outbreaks in Central Africa at approximately 2 using mathematical modeling and early phase outbreak trajectory data for the 1995 outbreak in Democratic Republic of Congo and the 2000 Uganda outbreak, respectively [5, 17]. Estimates of R_0 for the ongoing epidemic in West Africa are broadly consistent with those derived from prior outbreaks [1, 11, 21]. Also, the serial interval defined as the time from illness onset in primary case to illness onset in the secondary case has been estimated at about 15 days [10] while the case fatality ratio (CFR), calculated as the ratio of total EVD deaths to cases, has been estimated at about 70.8 % from the early phase of the epidemic in West Africa. Table 1 summarizes some key epidemiological parameters for EVD.

Optimal control (OC) theory is a powerful tool to guide the design and implementation of control intervention strategies against epidemics [18]. This technique defined control measures under a predetermined objective while minimizing the costs associated with the implementation of the control strategy. OC theory has been applied to various infectious diseases including tuberculosis (TB) [3, 4, 13, 25, 26], malaria [2, 19, 23], pandemic influenza [14–16] and avian influenza [12]. In this article, we use OC to explore the uncertainty in hospital bed capacity that would be needed to control an Ebola epidemic under different initial conditions, range of R_0 estimates, and associated costs to implement control measures. In particular, we focus on assessing the impact of effective isolation of infectious individuals in the health care setting because one key factor that facilitated the development of the Ebola epidemic in West Africa was the lack of public health surveillance systems to detect new outbreaks and the healthcare capacity that is needed to enforce infection control practices [8, 22].

2 Materials and Method

Our baseline model follows the SEIR-type transmission model structure that models the transmission dynamics of Ebola in the absence of control interventions or behavior changes. Our model incorporates hospital-based transmission that results from weak public health infrastructure in order to investigate the effect of isolation strategies using optimal control theory.

2.1 *Mathematical Model of EVD Transmission*

To consider the specific situation of the EVD outbreak in West Africa, we use a SEIR-type compartmental transmission model. In our model the host population is divided into six epidemiological classes as follows: susceptible individuals (S) who can get infected with Ebola by close contact with the virus; exposed latent individuals (E); infectious and symptomatic individuals (I) who can infect susceptible individuals; hospitalized individuals (J); recovered individuals (R); and Ebola deaths (D). Flowchart of EVD transmission between six epidemiological classes is shown in Fig. 1. Susceptible individuals are infected by contact with both infectious and symptomatic individuals and hospitalized individuals at a rate β. A factor l represents the relative infectivity of the hospitalized individuals (J). In other words, hospitalized infected individuals are assumed to be isolated at a rate $(1 - l)$. The mean incubation period is given by $1/k$ and α is the hospitalization rate. The mean infectious period in the absence of hospitalization and the mean period of hospital stay are $1/\gamma_1$ and $1/\gamma_2$, respectively. The case fatality proportion of EVD is denoted by f. Epidemic parameters and baseline values are given in Table 1. The governing model system of EVD transmission dynamics is described by the following set of nonlinear differential equations:

$$\begin{aligned}
\frac{dS}{dt} &= -\beta S(I + lJ)/N, \\
\frac{dE}{dt} &= \beta S(I + lJ)/N - kE, \\
\frac{dI}{dt} &= kE - (\alpha + \gamma_1)I, \\
\frac{dJ}{dt} &= \alpha I - \gamma_2 J, \\
\frac{dR}{dt} &= \gamma_1(1 - f)I + \gamma_2(1 - f)J, \\
\frac{dD}{dt} &= \gamma_1 f I + \gamma_2 f J,
\end{aligned} \tag{1}$$

where $N = S + E + I + J + R$.

The basic reproductive number, R_0, quantifies the average number of secondary cases generated by a primary case over its infectious period in a completely susceptible population during the early epidemic phase. In general, if $R_0 > 1$, an epidemic in a susceptible population is expected to occur. When $R_0 < 1$, the infection cannot sustain itself. R_0 depends on the infectious period, the probability of transmission

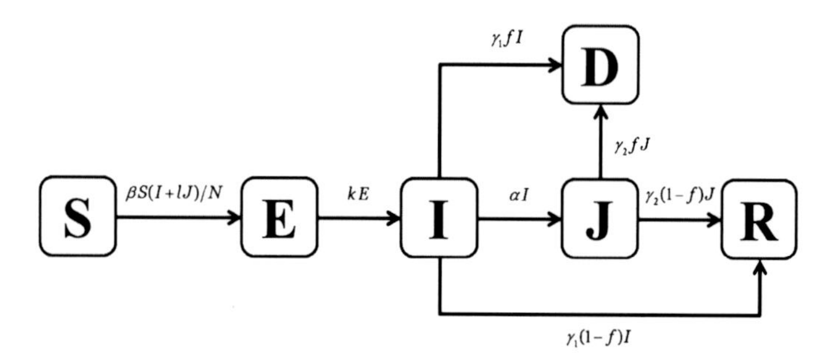

Fig. 1 Flowchart of EVD transmission between six epidemiological classes. S individuals get infected with Ebola by contact with I and J individuals at the rate β. l represents the relative infectiousness of J individuals in the healthcare setting. People in the E class move into the I class after the mean incubation period $1/k$. I individuals are hospitalized at the rate α. I and J individuals either die and recover at the rates γ_1 and γ_2, respectively, with the Ebola case fatality proportion denoted by f of EVD. Baseline values for the parameters are given in Table 1

Table 1 Parameters and baseline values

Symbol	Description	Value/Range	References
l	1 − isolation effectiveness	0.8	Assumed
$1/k$	Mean incubation period	11 days	[27]
α	Hospitalized rate	1/5	[27]
$1/\gamma_1$	Mean infectious period	5.6 days	[27]
$1/\gamma_2$	Mean period of hospitalization	7 days	[27]
f	Fatality rate	0.7	[27]
R_0	Basic reproductive number	1.6	[6]
β	Transmission rate	0.2857	Calculated from R_0
B	Weight constant	1000	Assumed
T	Simulated time	365 days	Assumed

per one contact, and the number of susceptible individuals contacted per unit time. For the Ebola model without controls, R_0 is calculated by the next generation method [9] as follows:

$$R_0 = \beta\left(\frac{1}{\gamma_1+\alpha} + \frac{\alpha}{\gamma_1+\alpha}\frac{l}{\gamma_2}\right). \tag{2}$$

We set the basic reproduction number of EVD at $R_0 = 1.6$ [6]. Hence, the transmission rate, β, can be calculated from Eq. (2).

2.2 *Optimal Control Strategy for Prevention of EVD*

In this section, we consider the EVD transmission model that incorporates a time-dependent control function. In this study, we focus on the effects of isolating hospitalized individuals. The Ebola model that incorporates isolation of hospitalized individuals is given by the following set of equations:

$$\begin{aligned}
\frac{dS}{dt} &= -\beta S\left(I + l(1-u(t))J\right)/N, \\
\frac{dE}{dt} &= \beta S\left(I + l(1-u(t))J\right)/N - kE, \\
\frac{dI}{dt} &= kE - (\alpha + \gamma_1)I, \\
\frac{dJ}{dt} &= \alpha I - \gamma_2 J, \\
\frac{dR}{dt} &= \gamma_1(1-f)I + \gamma_2(1-f)J, \\
\frac{dD}{dt} &= \gamma_1 f I + \gamma_2 f J,
\end{aligned} \tag{3}$$

where the time-dependent isolation control function $u(t)$ represents the effort of increasing the isolation effectiveness, $(1-l)$, for hospitalized individuals, $J(t)$. Hence, $u(t)J(t)$ turns up *the number of sickbeds at time* t.

Our goal is to minimize the number of infectious individuals, I, while keeping the cost associated with implementing the control low. Then the objective functional to be minimized is given as follows:

$$\mathscr{J} = \int_0^T \left(I + \frac{1}{2} B u^2 \right) dt, \tag{4}$$

where the parameter B is a weight constant and T is the simulated final time. We assume that the cost of implementing the control is in the quadratic form. The role of the weight constant, B, keeps a balance due to the size and importance between two parts of the objective functional. The optimal solution, $u^*(t)$, can be found by

$$\mathscr{J}(u^*) = \min_{\Omega} \mathscr{J}(u), \tag{5}$$

where $\Omega = \{u \in L^2 \mid 0 \le u \le 1\}$.

Here we use a 'relative cost' for the cost implementing the control. The relative total cost, TC, during the simulated time is then calculated as follows:

$$TC = \sum_{j=1}^{N} \frac{B}{2} u_j^2 \Delta t,$$

where the discrete value of u_j is defined by $u((j-1)\Delta t)$ for $j = 1, \ldots, N$. Parameters Δt and N represent the time step and the total number of time steps, respectively.

2.3 Characteristics of Optimal Control

Pontryagin's Maximum Principle [24] provides the necessary conditions to set up our OC problem by constraining the dynamic optimal problem into an unconstrained problem by minimizing pointwise a Hamiltonian, H, with respect to u as follows:

$$H = I + \frac{B}{2}u^2 + \sum_{i=1}^{6} \lambda_i g_i,$$

where g_i is the right hand side of the differential equation of the ith state variable. By applying Pontryagin's Maximum Principle and the existence result for OC pairs from Fleming and Rishel (1975), we obtain the following theorem.

Theorem 1 *Given optimal controls u^* and solutions $S^*, E^*, I^*, J^*, R^*, D^*$ of the corresponding state system, there exists adjoint variables $\lambda_1, \ldots, \lambda_6$ satisfying*

$$\begin{aligned}
\frac{\lambda_1}{dt} &= (\lambda_1 - \lambda_2)(\beta\,(I + l(1-u)J)\,/N),\\
\frac{\lambda_2}{dt} &= (\lambda_2 - \lambda_3)k,\\
\frac{\lambda_3}{dt} &= -1 + (\lambda_1 - \lambda_2)\beta S/N + \lambda_3(\alpha + \gamma_1) - \lambda_4\alpha - \lambda_5\gamma_1(1-f) - \lambda_6\gamma_1 f,\\
\frac{\lambda_4}{dt} &= (\lambda_1 - \lambda_2)\beta Sl(1-u)/N + \lambda_4\gamma_2 - \lambda_5\gamma_2 - \lambda_6\gamma_2 f,\\
\frac{\lambda_5}{dt} &= 0,\\
\frac{\lambda_6}{dt} &= 0,
\end{aligned} \tag{6}$$

and $\lambda_1(T) = \ldots = \lambda_6(T) = 0$, the transversality conditions. Furthermore

$$u^* = \min\left\{\max\left\{0, \beta l S^* \frac{J^*}{N^*}\frac{\lambda_2 - \lambda_1}{B}\right\}, 1\right\}. \tag{7}$$

Proof Corollary 4.1 of [24] gives the existence of an OC pair due to the convexity of integrand of J with respect to u, a priori boundedness of the state solutions, and the Lipschitz property of the state system with respect to the state variables. The form of the adjoint equations and transversality conditions are standard results from the Pontryagin's Maximum Principle [24]. We differentiate the Hamiltonian with respect to states, S, E, I, J, R, and D respectively:

$$\frac{d\lambda_1}{dt} = -\frac{\partial H}{\partial S}, \ldots, \frac{d\lambda_6}{dt} = -\frac{\partial H}{\partial D},$$

and then the adjoint system can be written as Eq. (6). By considering the optimality condition,

$$\frac{\partial H}{\partial u} = 0 \quad \text{at } u^*, \tag{8}$$

which can then be solved for the optimal solution, u^*, giving us:

$$\frac{\partial H}{\partial u} = Bu + \beta l S \frac{J}{N}(\lambda_1 - \lambda_2) = 0$$

at u^* on the set $\{t \mid 0 \leq u^*(t) \leq 1\}$. On this set,

$$u^* = \beta l S^* \frac{J^*}{N^*} \frac{\lambda_2 - \lambda_1}{B}.$$

Taking into account the bounds on controls, we obtain the characterization of u in (7). □

3 Results and Discussion

In this section, we present results for OC strategies for various weight constants, B, and investigate the impacts of cost, and initial size of infectious individuals, $I(0)$, hospitalization rate, α, and the basic reproductive number, R_0, on the maximum number of sickbeds.

3.1 Optimal Control Strategies for Various Weight Constants

We consider a broad range of weight constant, B, to investigate their sensitivity on OC results. The weight constant, B, varies from 1 to 12,000 and other parameters are given in Table 1. We chose the initial values of state variables for applying OC strategies as $(S, E, I, H, R, D) = (982114, 4496, 1000, 1155, 3371, 7865)$. These values are obtained by solving the model system without control (1) with the initial values, $(S, E, I, H, R, D) = (1000000, 0, 1, 0, 0, 0)$ for the simulated time, 279 (days). The following four ranges for B are analyzed:

- Range I: $1 \leq B < 1000$
- Range II: $1000 \leq B < 9000$
- Range III: $9000 \leq B < 10000$
- Range IV: $10000 \leq B < 12000$

Figure 2 displays optimal controls and the corresponding state variables as a function of time in the left and right six frames, respectively.

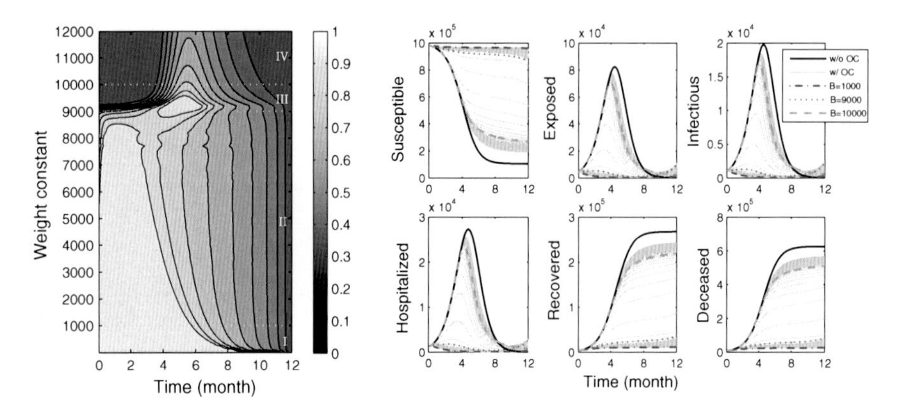

Fig. 2 Optimal controls and the corresponding state variables are displayed as a function of time in the *left* and *right six* frames, respectively. The weight constant B varies from 1 to 12000. The *dashed white lines* divides the weight constants into *four ranges* in the *left frame* (denoted by roman characters I–IV). As the level of OC increases, the *gray shades* vary smoothly from *black* to *white*. In the *right frame* the state variables without OC (w/o OC) are plotted by thick *black lines*. The state variables with OC (w/ OC), which are basically plotted by the thin *gray lines*, determined by three threshold values $B = 1000$, 9000, and 10000 are displayed by the *dot-dashed*, *dotted*, and *dashed line*, respectively

In general, as the weight constant B is smaller, that is, the relative unit cost of using control is cheaper, the longer the period of full OC from the beginning is employed. In the range I (blue region), optimal controls work fairly; keeping the epidemic free state during the entire simulated duration. OC strategies in the range II (green region) show no peak but the number of infectious individuals are slightly increased at the end of simulated time. The patterns of optimal controls in the range I and II show that the full effort from the beginning to the certain period is needed to protect the spread of EVD and then optimal controls are decreasing smoothly to zero (no effort). If the cost is too expensive, it is hard to implement the early intervention, which is the most important feature for the epidemic free state. Hence, OC strategies in the range III and IV are unable to control the EVD epidemic. In the range III the magnitude of epidemic peak for each curve is reduced to a certain degree. However, in the range IV, OC strategies do not work for extremely high cost levels. Overall, Fig. 2 shows that the pattern of OC strategy is sensitive to the weight constant, B, which is related to the cost of implementing the control.

Figure 3 illustrates the epidemic size, the maximum number of $u(t)J(t)$, and the relative TC as a function of the weight constant, B, in the top, middle, and bottom frames, respectively. Note that there are jumps in all three frames when $B \geq 9000$ (Range III & IV) because OC strategies do not work well. Let us ignore the cases in Range IV. In the top frame, the epidemic size is slowly increased as B is increased from 1 to 9000. On the other hand, TC is significantly increasing as almost a linear function. In contrast with epidemic size and TC, the number of $\max(uJ)$ does not

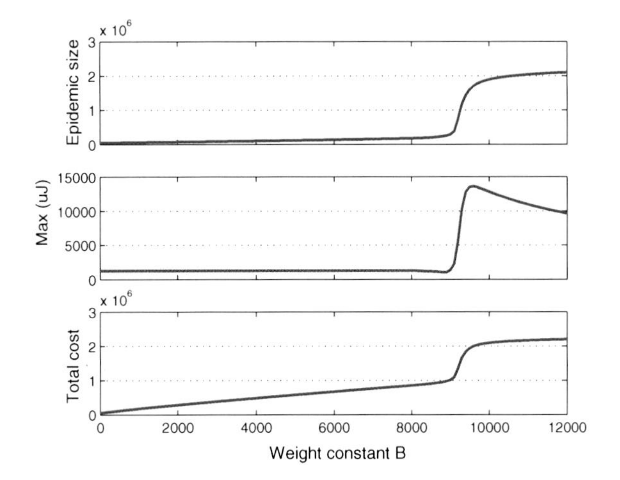

Fig. 3 The epidemic size, $\max(uJ)$, and TC as a function of the weight constant are displayed in the *top*, *middle*, and *bottom frames*, respectively. Baseline values of the parameters in this simulation are given in Table 1

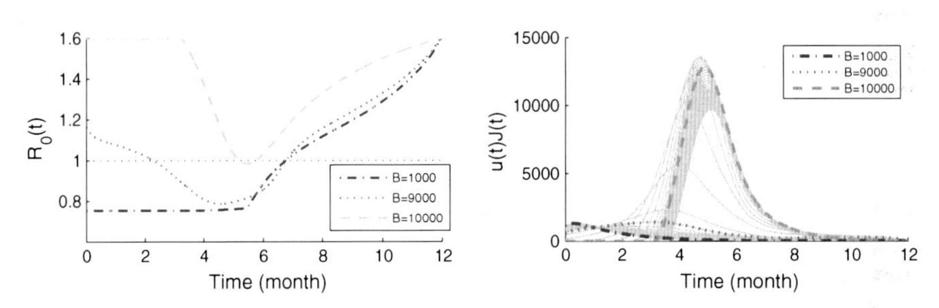

Fig. 4 The reproductive number, $R_0(t)$, and the number of perfectly isolated individuals in a hospital (sickbeds), $u(t)J(t)$, as a function time are displayed in the *left* and *right frames*, respectively. Baseline values of the parameters in this simulation are given in Table 1

vary when $B < 9000$. Surprisingly, *the maximum number of sickbeds,* $\max(uJ)$*, is not very sensitive to the relative TC* if OC strategy is applied.

Figure 4 depicts the reproductive number, $R_0(t)$, and the number of perfectly isolated individuals in a hospital (sickbeds), $u(t)J(t)$, as a function of time in the left and right frames, respectively. We define the time-dependent reproductive number using the quarantine control, $u(t)$, as follows:

$$R_0(t) = \beta\left(\frac{1}{\gamma_1+\alpha} + \frac{\alpha}{\gamma_1+\alpha}\frac{l(1-u(t))}{\gamma_2}\right). \tag{9}$$

The time-dependent reproductive numbers, $R_0(t)$, in the cases of $B = 1000$ (blue), 9000 (green), and 10000 (yellow) in the left frame of Fig. 4 have similar patterns that track the reversed curves of optimal controls in the left frame of Fig. 2. The value of $R_0(t)$ in $B = 1000$ is less than one until around seven month into the epidemic and then increases to1.6 as optimal controls approach zero at the end of the simulation. Note that the baseline $R_0(t)$ is 1.6 when OC is not applied (i.e., $u(t) = 0$). In the case with $B = 10000$, $R_0(t)$ is almost greater than or equal to 1 during the entire epidemic period. It confirms again that OC does not work for high cost levels associated with control efforts. Furthermore, the curves of $u(t)J(t)$ as a function of time in the right frame of Fig. 4 show that the number of sickbeds has a peak ($max(uJ)$) during the early period and then smoothly decreased to zero in the ranges of I and II ($1 \leq B < 9000$). On the other hand, if the relative cost is getting expensive, especially in the ranges of III and IV ($9000 \leq B \leq 12000$), then the number of sickbeds has a huge peak around 5 months into the epidemic.

3.2 Estimation of the Maximum Number of Sickbeds

One of main questions in this work is the following:

Can we estimate the maximum number of sickbeds for different epidemiological scenarios?

In the previous section, we already estimated the maximum number of sickbeds as a function of the weight constant, B. Now we investigate the impacts of the initial value of infectious individuals, $I(0)$, the hospitalized rate, α, and the basic reproductive number, R_0, on the maximum number of sickbeds, $max(uJ)$.

Figure 5 displays the $max(uJ)$ as a function of $I(0)$, α and R_0 in the left, middle and right frame, respectively. Parameters are chosen as the baseline values in Table 1. Note that the initial values are fixed as $(S, E, I, J, R, D)=(999000, 0, 1000, 0, 0, 0)$ for the comparisons between the simulation results. In the left frame, the $max(uJ)$ is an almost linear function of the initial number of infectious individuals, $I(0)$, except the extremely small initial values. When the $I(0)$ is varied from 1 to 1000, the values of $max(uJ)$ are in the range of [10, 300]. In the middle frame, the $max(uJ)$ is sensitively changed by the hospitalized rate, α, in the range of [200, 700]. On the other hand, interestingly, the $max(uJ)$ is not sensitive to the basic reproductive number, R_0: the $max(uJ)$ is an almost constant function of R_0.

In order to investigate the impacts of α and R_0 on the $max(uJ)$, the numbers of maximum sickbeds, $max(uJ)$, are depicted as the contours of α and R_0 in Fig. 6. The ranges for α and R_0 are chosen as [0.2, 0.9] and [1.6, 2], respectively. Figure 6 clearly illustrates that the $max(uJ)$ is sensitive to the hospitalized rate, α, while the $max(uJ)$ is not sensitive to the basic reproductive number, R_0. Overall, we can estimate the number of maximum sickbeds in the various scenarios if OC strategies are conducted.

In this article we have employed OC and a relatively simple compartmental model of Ebola transmission that incorporates varying levels of isolation of infectious individuals in the hospital $J(t)$, which is connected to the control parameter $u(t)$. This allowed us to illustrate the theoretical number of "sick beds" with affected Ebola patients at time t, which is given by $u(t)J(t)$. Our ultimate goal was to assess the

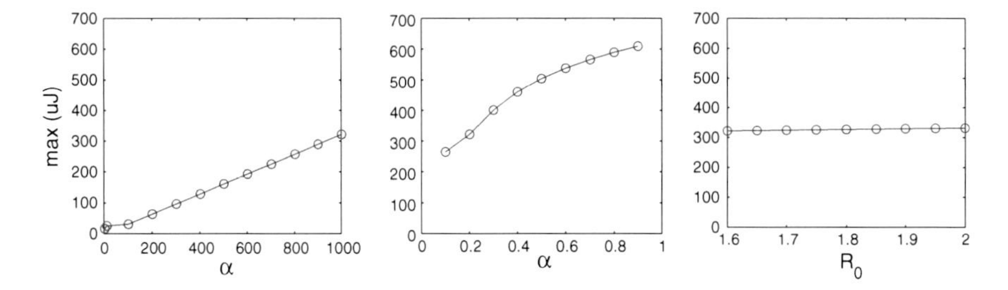

Fig. 5 Maximum values of sickbeds, $max(uJ)$, as a function of the initial infectious individuals, $I(0)$, the hospitalization rate, α, and the basic reproductive number, R_0 are displayed in the *left*, *middle* and *right frames*, respectively

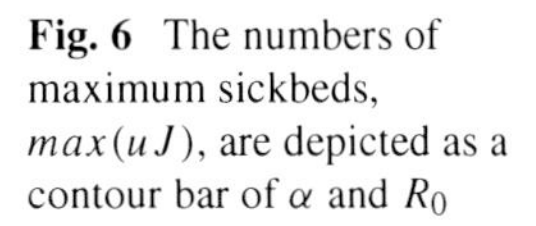

Fig. 6 The numbers of maximum sickbeds, $max(uJ)$, are depicted as a contour bar of α and R_0

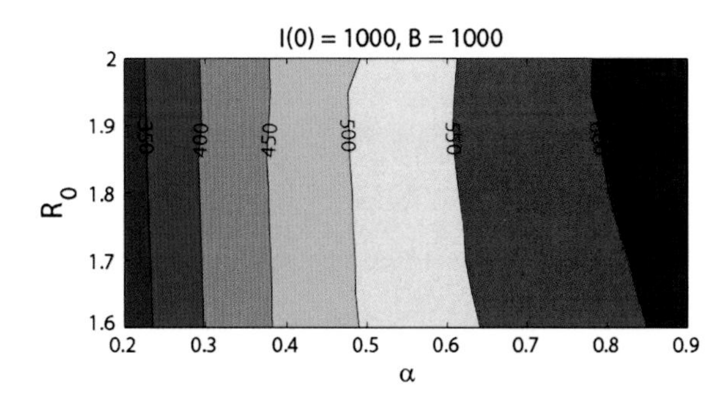

theoretical trade-off between minimizing the number of Ebola virus infectious individuals and the cost of implementing the control strategy.

Our simulation results derived from implementing OC strategies in Fig. 3 showed that the full control during the early period is key to ensure elimination of Ebola epidemics. However, this result should be interpreted with caution as it is sensitive to the inherent structural assumptions in our model (e.g., homogeneous mixing) which may not reflect Ebola transmission dynamics at the local scale [7].

We have also highlighted the sensitivity of the weight constant, B, which is related to the cost of implementing control. It was not surprising to observe that the epidemic size and the relative TC are sensitive to the weight constant, B. By contrast, the number of maximum sickbeds ($max(uJ)$) were not sensitive to the the weight constant, B that represents the relative cost implementing the control strategy. This result suggests that the maximum number of sickbeds can be estimated in the broad range of costs, when optimal quarantine strategy is conducted. Finally, we have also explored the sensitivities of the initial size of infectious individuals, $I(0)$, the hospitalized rate, α, and the basic reproductive number, R_0 on the values of $max(uJ)$ in Figs. 5 and 6. We observed that the numbers of $max(uJ)$ are increasing functions of $I(0)$ and α, while it is an almost constant function of R_0.

References

1. Althaus, C.L.: Estimating the reproduction number of Ebola virus (EBOV) during the 2014 outbreak in West Africa. PLOS Current, Outbreaks (2014)
2. Blayneh, K., Cao, Y., Kwon, H.D.: Optimal control of vector-borne diseases: treatment and prevention. Discret. Contin. Dyn. B **11**(3), 587–611 (2009)
3. Choi, S., Jung, E.: Optimal tuberculosis prevention and control strategy from a mathematical model based on real data. Bull. Math. Biol. 1–24 (2014)
4. Choi, S., Jung, E.: Optimal tuberculosis prevention and control strategy from a mathematical model based on real data. Bull. Math. Biol **76**(7), 1566–1589 (2014). doi:10.1007/s11538-014-9962-6, http://dx.doi.org/10.1007/s11538-014-9962-6
5. Chowell, G., Hengartner, N.W., Castillo-Chavez, C., Fenimore, P.W., Hyman, J.: The basic reproductive number of ebola and the effects of public health measures: the cases of congo and uganda. J. Theor. Biol. **229**(1), 119–126 (2004)
6. Chowell, G., Nishiura, H.: Transmission dynamics and control of ebola virus disease (evd): a review. BMC Med. **12**(1), 196 (2014)
7. Chowell, G., Viboud, C., Hyman, J.M., Simonsen, L.: The western africa ebola virus disease epidemic exhibits both global exponential and local polynomial growth rates. PLoS Currents **7** (2014)
8. del Rio, C., Mehta, A.K., Lyon, G.M., Guarner, J.: Ebola hemorrhagic fever in 2014: the tale of an evolving epidemic. Ann. Intern. Med. **161**(10), 746–748 (2014)
9. Diekmann, O., Heesterbeek, J.: Mathematical Epidemiology of Infectious Diseases, vol. 146. Wiley, Chichester (2000)
10. Fine, P.E.: The interval between successive cases of an infectious disease. Am. J. Epidemiol. **158**(11), 1039–1047 (2003)
11. Fisman, D., Khoo, E., Tuite, A.: Early epidemic dynamics of the west african 2014 ebola outbreak: estimates derived with a simple two-parameter model. PLOS Currents Outbreaks **6** (2014)
12. Jung, E., Iwami, S., Takeuchi, Y., Jo, T.C.: Optimal control strategy for prevention of avian influenza pandemic. J. Theor. Biol. **260**(2), 220–229 (2009)
13. Jung, E., Lenhart, S., Feng, Z.: Optimal control of treatments in a two-strain tuberculosis model. Discret. Contin. Dyn. Syst. Ser. B **2**(4), 473–482 (2002)
14. Lee, J., Kim, J., Kwon, H.D.: Optimal control of an influenza model with seasonal forcing and age-dependent transmission rates. J. Theor. Biol. **317**, 310–320 (2013)
15. Lee, S., Chowell, G., Castillo-Chávez, C.: Optimal control for pandemic influenza: the role of limited antiviral treatment and isolation. J. Theor. Biol. **265**(2), 136–150 (2010)
16. Lee, S., Golinski, M., Chowell, G.: Modeling optimal age-specific vaccination strategies against pandemic influenza. Bull. Math. Biol. **74**(4), 958–980 (2012)
17. Legrand, J., Grais, R., Boelle, P., Valleron, A., Flahault, A.: Understanding the dynamics of ebola epidemics. Epidemiol. Infect. **135**(04), 610–621 (2007)
18. Lenhart, S., Workman, J.T.: Optimal Control Applied to Biological Models (2007). http://books.google.com/books?hl=ko&lr=&id=NBcTXZK61doC&pgis=1
19. Makinde, O.D., Okosun, K.O.: Impact of chemo-therapy on optimal control of malaria disease with infected immigrants. Biosystems **104**(1), 32–41 (2011)
20. Meltzer, M.I., Atkins, C.Y., Santibanez, S., Knust, B., Petersen, B.W., Ervin, E.D., Nichol, S.T., Damon, I.K., Washington, M.L.: Estimating the future number of cases in the ebola epidemic–liberia and sierra leone, 2014–2015. MMWR Surveill. Summ. **63**(suppl 3), 1–14 (2014)
21. Nishiura, H., Chowell, G.: Early transmission dynamics of ebola virus disease (evd), west africa, march to august 2014. Eur. Surveill. **19**(36), 20,894 (2014)
22. Okeke, I.N.: Divining without seeds: the case for strengthening laboratory medicine in Africa. Cornell University Press, New York (2011)

23. Okosun, K.O., Ouifki, R., Marcus, N.: Optimal control analysis of a malaria disease transmission model that includes treatment and vaccination with waning immunity. Biosystems **106**(2), 136–145 (2011)
24. Pontryagin, L.S.: Mathematical Theory of Optimal Processes. CRC Press, Boca Raton(1987)
25. Silva, C.J., Torres, D.F.: Optimal control for a tuberculosis model with reinfection and post-exposure interventions. Math. Biosci. **244**(2), 154–164 (2013)
26. Whang, S., Choi, S., Jung, E.: A dynamic model for tuberculosis transmission and optimal treatment strategies in south korea. J. Theor. Biol. **279**(1), 120–131 (2011)
27. WHO Ebola Response Team: Ebola virus disease in west africa – the first 9 months of the epidemic and forward projections. New Engl. J. Med. **371**(16), 1481–1495 (2014). doi:10.1056/NEJMoa1411100;21
28. World Health Organization: Ebola virus disease update - west africa (2014). http://www.who.int/csr/don/2014_08_08_ebola/en/
29. World Health Organization: Ebola situation reports (2015). http://apps.who.int/ebola/ebola-situation-reports

Inverse Problems and Ebola Virus Disease Using an Age of Infection Model

Alexandra Smirnova, Linda DeCamp and Hui Liu

Abstract Parameter estimation problems in ordinary and partial differential equations constitute a large class of models described by ill-posed operator equations. A considerable number of such problems come from epidemiology and infectious disease modeling, with Ebola Virus Disease (EVD) being a very important example. While it is not difficult to find a solution of an SEIJCR ODE constrained least squares problem, this problem is extremely unstable and a number of different parameter combinations produce essentially the same case curve. This is a serious obstacle in the study of the Ebola virus epidemics, since reliable approximations of system parameters are important for the proper assessment of existing control measures as well as for the forward projections aimed at testing a variety of contact tracing policies. In this paper, we attempt a stable estimation of system parameters with the use of iterative regularization along with a special algorithm for computing initial values. The numerical study is illustrated by data fitting and forward projections for the most recent EVD outbreak in Sierra Leone and Liberia.

Keywords Parameter estimation · Ebola · West Africa · Epidemics · Differential equations · Inverse problem · Iterative regularization · Model fitting

A. Smirnova (✉) · L. DeCamp
Georgia State University, Atlanta, GA, USA
e-mail: asmirnova@gsu.edu

L. DeCamp
e-mail: ldecamp1@student.gsu.edu

H. Liu
University of North Carolina, Charlotte, NC, USA
e-mail: hliu34@uncc.edu

G. Chowell and J.M. Hyman (eds.), *Mathematical and Statistical Modeling for Emerging and Re-emerging Infectious Diseases*,
DOI 10.1007/978-3-319-40413-4_8

1 Introduction

The Ebola Virus Disease (EVD) outbreak in West Africa that began in early 2014 has received wide attention due to its scale, scope, location and alarming potential. The largest previous Ebola outbreak was in Uganda in 2000, with a total of 425 cases. The West African outbreak surpassed the size of that outbreak by the first week of June, 2014. The World Health Organization (WHO) declared the Ebola outbreak in West Africa a public health emergency on August 8th [1]. By the 21st of that month the case count exceeded the total of all other previous outbreaks combined—2,387 cases (Fig. 1). As of July 5, 2015 there have been 27,609 Ebola cases with 11,261 fatalities, and these numbers are widely believed to be underreported [2]. The areas hardest hit by the 2014 outbreak encompass about 428,945 km^2, more than 50 times the 8,000 km^2 comprising the three districts affected during the 2000 Uganda outbreak [3]. In addition, the three primarily affected countries suffer from a recent history of civil unrest, poverty and lack of health infrastructure [4, 5].

The Ebola Virus Disease initially came to notice of the world in 1976. Two months apart in time and 500 miles apart in distance, two outbreaks of this then unrecognized virus occurred in Sudan and Zaire (now Democratic Republic of Congo) [6, 7]. Ebola is known to affect humans and nonhuman primates (gorillas, chimpanzees, etc.) [8]. Human-to-human transmission results from direct contact through broken skin or mucous membranes with the blood, other bodily fluids or secretions of infected people. The incubation period, or the time interval from infection to onset of symptoms, is from 2 to 21 days. The patients become contagious once they begin to show symptoms [9]. They are not contagious during the incubation period. Individuals remain infectious as long as their blood and secretions contain the virus [10, 11].

The 2014–15 Ebola outbreak was first reported on March 23, 2014, by the WHO Regional Office for Africa. The report indicated a rapidly evolving outbreak of EVD with 29 fatalities from 49 cases as of March 22 [12]. Investigative journalism proposes that the first case was a young boy who died in December 2013 [13]. These first cases occurred in a region at the conflux of the borders of Guinea, Liberia and Sierra Leone (in a region that had not seen an Ebola outbreak before). There were no proven drugs

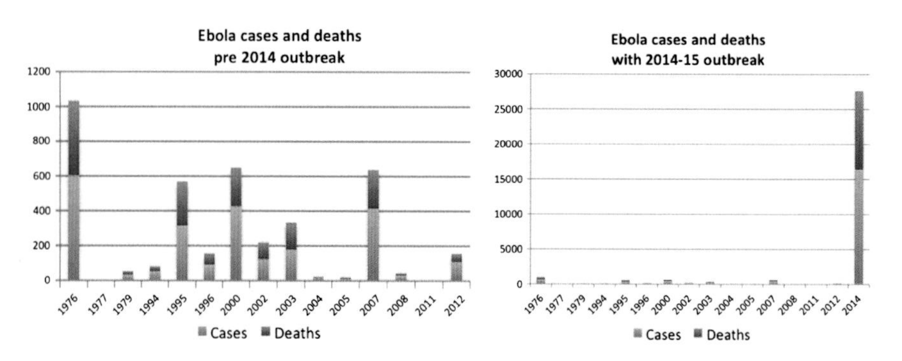

Fig. 1 Pre and post outbreak case and death counts [2]

or vaccines against EVD at the start of the outbreak. Given that the symptoms of the disease are similar to malaria, typhoid fever, hepatitis and other viral hemorrhagic fevers, identification of the true nature of the disease may have been delayed [1, 14]. EVD infections can only be confirmed through laboratory testing.

Researchers have investigated prior EVD outbreaks using compartmental models, stochastic processes and statistical methods. Parameters for transmission and periods of incubation, infectiousness and recovery were determined by fitting incidence data or using statistical tools [11, 15, 16]. Statistical models were also used to determine incubation periods or reproductive numbers [17–19]. In order to study the 2014–15 outbreak, both the Centers for Disease Control (CDC) and WHO developed models to forecast the progress of the EVD. The CDC utilized an SEIR model wherein the Infectious class is sub-categorized into three groups of isolation: Hospitalization, Effective Home Care (isolation characteristics), and Home With No Effective Isolation with each subcategory having a differing rate of transmission determined by goodness of fit to cumulative data as of August 28, 2014. The periods for incubation and time to recovery or death were determined from previous outbreaks by probability distribution of the data [20]. The WHO used data gathered from the current outbreak to identify parameter values by employing gamma distributions to fit the data. The WHO's estimates for the incubation period, time to recovery, and reproductive numbers are similar to values found for other outbreaks. To determine future case numbers the WHO utilized two methods: (a) data through September 14, 2014 was log transformed and fitted with resultant parameters used for projections and (b) a stochastic branching process model was used to estimate the incidence rate and projections were based upon it [21]. In [22], a family of logistic patch models for use in EVD analysis and future projections has been validated. The ability of each model to predict epidemic data was compared based on forecasting errors, parameter distributions and parameter confidence intervals.

There is uncertainty as to whether those who recover from Ebola can subsequently be reinfected [23]. Apart from susceptible and infected humans, most models include the exposed class, $E(t)$, since the virus is only transmitted through contacts with actively symptomatic infected individuals [24, 25]. Where no vaccine is available, the isolation of infected and the quarantine of exposed individuals are the only control measures enforced. Various SEQIJ (Susceptible-Exposed-Quarantined-Infected-Isolated) models incorporate these dynamics. Some quarantine models also include hospitalized, recovered, and contaminated deceased classes [24, 26].

Compared to previously known viral diseases, the Ebola outbreak in West Africa has some unique characteristics that affect its modeling and parameter identification (Table 1):

1. The disease is transmitted to susceptible humans from both infectious humans and improper handling of the deceased.
2. An adequate model needs to incorporate the principal features of contact tracing activities (identification, isolation, efficiency).

Table 1 Parameters for Model with Contact Tracing [10, 20, 26–28]

Parameter	Definition	Baseline value	Source
N	Total population, Liberia (now 4.397×10^6)	4×10^6	[26, 29]
	Total population, Sierra Leone (now 6.205×10^6)	6×10^6	[26, 29]
κ	Average number of contacts traced per infected individual before and after 10/01/2014	0, before	[26]
		10, after	[26]
π	Probability a contact traced infected human is isolated without infecting others	0.4–0.6	[26]
ω	Probability a contact traced individual is infected	0.1	[26]
$1/\gamma$	Average time from symptoms onset to recovery	30 days	[10, 28]
$1/\nu$	Average time from symptoms onset to death	8 days	[26, 27]
$1/\sigma$	Average incubation period	9 days	[10, 27, 28]
β	Transmission rate from infectious humans	TBD	[20, 26]
ε	Transmission rate from contaminated deceased	TBD	[20, 26]
$1/\alpha$	Average time from symptoms onset to isolation	TBD	[20, 26]
$1/\psi$	Average time until deceased is properly handled	TBD	[20, 26]

3. The current outbreak is an evolving event; the data will, of necessity, be quickly outdated and subject to correction (very noisy) caused by such issues as differing reporting periods, retroactive re-classifications, and non-reporting.

To account for contact tracing activities, a new SEICJR (Susceptible-Exposed-Infected-Contaminated Deceased-Isolated Infectious-Removed) model has been developed by G. Webb and his group [26]. The last two classes, $J(t)$ and $R(t)$, decouple from $I(t)$ and $C(t)$ and their values, though they are not explicitly present in the system, can also be evaluated from it:

$$\frac{dS}{dt} = -\beta S(t)\frac{I(t)}{N} - \varepsilon S(t)\frac{C(t)}{N}, \tag{1}$$

$$\frac{dE}{dt} = \beta S(t)\frac{I(t)}{N} + \varepsilon S(t)\frac{C(t)}{N} - \sigma E(t), \tag{2}$$

$$\frac{dI}{dt} = \sigma E(t) - (\alpha + \gamma + \nu)I(t) - \kappa(\alpha I(t) + \psi C(t))\pi\omega, \tag{3}$$

$$\frac{dC}{dt} = \nu I(t) - \psi C(t). \tag{4}$$

This compartmental model classifies the population and describes movement between the compartments. (1) The Susceptible class (S) can be infected by Ebola virus following a contact with infectious or contaminated deceased classes; (2) members of the Exposed class (E) have been infected by the Ebola virus but are not yet infectious;

(3) the Infectious class (I) can infect others, and human population in this class will either recover or move to the Contaminated deceased; (4) the Contaminated deceased class (C) may transmit the disease during funerals or from improper handling. In the above model, parameters β, ε, α, and ψ need to be estimated from case data given by the cumulative clinical reported cases (K) [26]

$$K(t) = \int_0^t \Big(\alpha I(s) + \psi C(s)\Big) ds + K(0). \tag{5}$$

While it is not difficult to find a solution of the constrained least squares problem, this problem is extremely unstable and "lots of different values of $\beta, \varepsilon, \alpha$, and ψ fit". This is a serious obstacle in the study of Ebola virus, since reliable approximations of system parameters are important for the proper assessment of existing control measures as well as for the forward projections aimed at testing a variety of contact tracing policies. In this paper, we evaluate a stable estimation of system parameters with the use of iterative regularization along with a special algorithm for computing initial values, β_0, ε_0, α_0, and ψ_0. The paper is organized as follows. In Sect. 2, the severe ill-posedness of the underlying inverse problem is demonstrated. In Sect. 3, an algorithm for localizing the unknown parameters is introduced. The procedure of iterative regularization and experimental results for simulated data are presented in Sect. 4, followed by the results for real data [30] in Sect. 5. In Sect. 6, some future plans are outlined.

2 Ill-Posedness of the Least Squares Problem

In our first numerical experiment, we have attempted to study uniqueness and stability of parameters $\beta, \varepsilon, \alpha$, and ψ for Sierra Leone and Liberia using the information on cumulative cases up until September 23, 2014 [26]. Given the system of differential equations and real data, we minimized the cost functional with Matlab built-in functions lsqcurvefit (trust-region-reflective algorithm) and ode23s (stiff system solver).

The data sets for the two countries are given in Table 2. Case counts have been adjusted throughout this outbreak due to ongoing reclassification, follow up investigations and laboratory results. Under-reporting remains an acknowledged issue in World Health Organization's periodic situational reports. The data given here reflects the historical record of cumulative number of Ebola cases in Sierra Leone and Liberia as reported by WHO.

The total populations of 6 and 4 million were assumed for Sierra Leone and Liberia, respectively. As in [26], $K_0 = 16$, $S_0 = 6 \times 10^6$, $E_0 = 47$, $I_0 = 26$, $C_0 = 12$ for Sierra Leone, and $K_0 = 33$, $S_0 = 4 \times 10^6$, $E_0 = 40$, $I_0 = 22$, $C_0 = 12$ for Liberia. Common to both, $\gamma = 1/30$, $\nu = 1/8$, $\sigma = 1/9$, $\kappa = 0$ have been taken [26]. The last assumption, $\kappa = 0$, is due to the fact that before September 23, 2014, contact tracing (if occurred) was insufficient.

Table 2 Ebola Virus Disease Cumulative Case Data Used for Parameter Fitting [30]

Sierra Leone												
Date	5/27	5/30	6/5	6/7	6/17	6/23	6/30	7/2	7/6	7/8	7/12	7/14
Cases	16	50	81	89	97	158	239	252	305	337	386	397
Date	7/17	7/20	7/23	7/27	7/30	8/1	8/4	8/6	8/9	8/11	8/13	8/16
Cases	442	454	525	533	574	646	691	717	730	783	810	848
Date	8/18	8/20	8/26	8/31	9/6	9/13	9/14	9/19	9/21	9/23		
Cases	907	910	1026	1216	1361	1620	2673	1813	1940	2021		
Liberia												
Date	6/17	6/23	6/30	7/2	7/6	7/8	7/12	7/14	7/17	7/20	7/23	7/27
Cases	33	51	107	115	131	142	172	174	196	224	249	329
Date	7/30	8/1	8/4	8/6	8/9	8/11	8/13	8/16	8/18	8/20	8/26	8/31
Cases	391	468	516	554	599	670	786	846	972	1082	1378	1698
Date	9/5	9/8	9/14	9/17	9/21	9/23						
Cases	2046	2407	2710	3022	3280	3458						

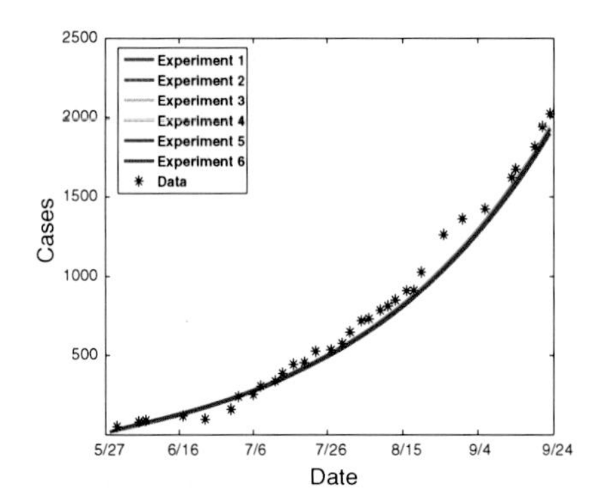

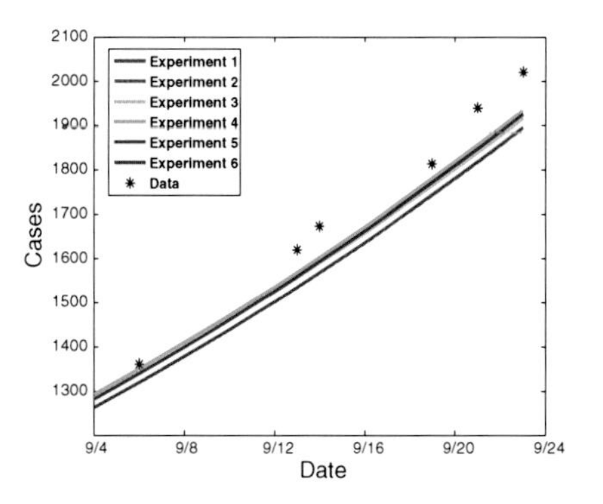

Fig. 2 Sierra Leone cases and reconstructions, May 27 to September 23, 2014

In the course of our simulations, we've used different initial values for the unknown parameters in the attempt to find global minimum setting the tolerance level of 10^{-15} for the solution and residual.

Demonstrated in the graphs and tables that follow, we obtained vastly varying values for each of the parameters yet all these six combinations produced virtually the same curve. In Fig. 2, all 6 experiments for Sierra Leone are plotted for the entire time period of 119 days and for a shorter 20 day period; the experimental curves are virtually indistinguishable and provide a very good fit for the real data listed in Table 2 [30]. The parameter values obtained and the initial values used are given in Table 3. The relative discrepancies between the data points and the curves generated are around 8 % and are also shown in Table 3.

Table 3 Sierra Leone: reconstructed parameter values with their associated initial values

Parameters obtained by a prepackaged optimization routine						
Experiment	β	ε	α	ψ	Relative discrepancy	R_0
1	3.7574E–01	1.5392E–01	4.8055E–01	2.9522E–02	7.7909E–02	1.608
2	4.2127E–03	5.4522E–01	1.0030E–01	1.9548E–01	8.8867E–02	1.364
3	1.1778E–03	5.8250E–01	8.9686E–02	2.1700E–01	8.9681E–02	1.358
4	6.7365E–02	3.3599E–01	4.4134E–01	4.5305E–02	8.8811E–02	1.658
5	4.0865E–01	1.3677E–01	4.8223E–01	2.7710E–02	8.6094E–02	1.601
6	2.6428E–01	5.8175E–02	5.7956E–02	6.5124E–01	8.5770E–02	1.274
Initial values used by optimization						
Experiment	β	ε	α	ψ	Relative discrepancy	R_0
1	1.6000E–01	1.0000E–01	1.0000E–01	1.0000E–01	5.9059E–01	1.103
2	5.0000E–03	6.0000E–01	8.0000E–02	8.0000E–02	4.5471E+01	3.955
3	1.2500E–03	6.0000E–01	1.8000E–01	1.2000E–01	2.0298E+00	1.851
4	2.5000E–02	3.0000E–01	1.0000E–01	1.5000E–01	6.1796E–01	1.065
5	2.8000E–01	2.0000E–01	1.0000E–01	1.0000E–01	7.9440E+00	2.052
6	1.0000E–01	8.0000E–05	8.0000E–02	1.6000E–01	8.9195E–01	0.420

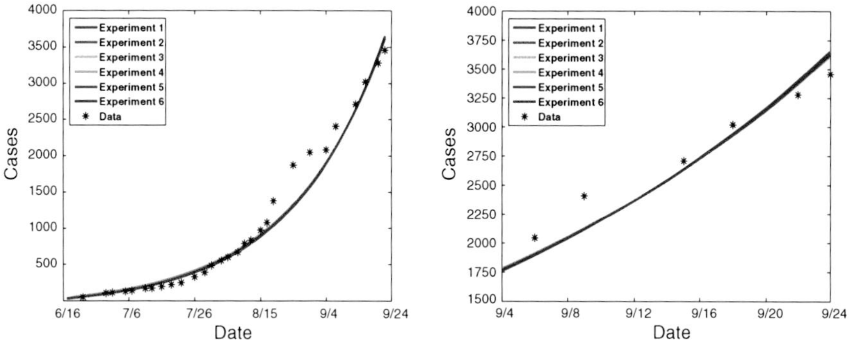

Fig. 3 Liberia cases and reconstructions, May 27 to September 23, 2014

Very similar results have been obtained when performing the experiments on data from Liberia. The associated reconstructed curve graphs for the six experiments are given in Fig. 3 for both the entire time frame, 98 days, and for a 20 day segment. Once again, different parameter values give virtually the same curve. The parameter values obtained and the initial values used are given in Table 4. The relative discrepancies, just under 11 % are also shown in Table 4.

The same non-uniqueness was observed when numerical experiments were conducted with our own code that implemented iteratively regularized Gauss-Newton algorithm [31, 32] for solving the least squares problem. Depending on a reference

Table 4 Liberia: reconstructed parameter values with their associated initial values

Parameters obtained by a prepackaged optimization routine

Experiment	β	ε	α	ψ	Relative discrepancy	R_0
1	1.7052E–01	5.3268E–01	1.8202E–01	1.7401E–01	1.1241E–01	1.625
2	1.7426E–02	5.6448E–01	3.6038E–01	6.5235E–02	1.1314E–01	2.119
3	3.0433E–01	6.6652E–01	1.2112E–01	7.3769E–01	1.1449E–01	1.493
4	4.7794E–01	1.1099E–01	1.9028E–01	5.6650E–01	1.1219E–01	1.441
5	2.8304E–01	3.0027E–01	2.0009E–01	1.2401E–01	1.1743E–01	1.634
6	6.8792E–01	1.1050E–06	3.3242E–01	3.8950E–02	1.1351E–01	1.402

Initial Values used by optimization

Experiment	β	ε	α	ψ	Relative discrepancy	R_0
1	3.0000E–01	3.1600E–01	1.8000E–01	1.8000E–01	1.3869E–01	1.535
2	2.0000E–07	4.0000E–01	3.0000E–02	3.0000E–02	4.2391E+00	8.850
3	2.0000E–06	2.0000E–02	6.0000E–02	1.5000E–02	9.5355E–01	0.763
4	1.0000E–02	1.0000E–02	4.0000E–01	3.0000E–01	9.5136E–01	0.025
5	5.0000E–10	2.0000E–02	2.0000E–09	6.6000E–01	9.5585E–01	0.024
6	3.0000E–02	6.0000E–06	6.0000E–01	4.0000E–01	9.5067E–01	0.040

element used in the penalty functional, the process converged to one local minimum or another.

While some of the parameter values displayed in Tables 3 and 4 can be ruled out based on the reproduction numbers they generate and/or other biological considerations, it is evident that the problem is extremely ill-posed and a sufficiently close initial approximation is required for "correct" parameters to be reconstructed. In the next section, we propose a strategy for computing β_0, ε_0, α_0, and ψ_0.

3 Computation of Initial Values

For the evaluation of initial values of system parameters, we propose the following method. From (5) one has

$$\frac{dK}{dt} = \alpha I(t) + \psi C(t) \tag{6}$$

with noisy values of $K(t)$ being available at finitely many non-uniformly distributed grid points (see Table 2). Hence it is reasonable to assume that

$$\psi_0 = \frac{K1_0 - \alpha_0 I_0}{C_0}, \tag{7}$$

where $K1_0$ is an approximation to the first derivative of $K(t)$ at $t = 0$ calculated by either finite differences or spline interpolation. Differentiating (6) and using ODE system (1)–(4), one concludes

$$\begin{aligned}\frac{d^2K}{dt^2} &= \alpha\frac{dI}{dt} + \psi\frac{dC}{dt}\\ &= \alpha\sigma E + (\psi\nu - \alpha(\alpha+\gamma+\nu))I - \psi^2 C.\end{aligned}$$

Taking into account (7), one arrives at the following quadratic equation for α_0

$$\begin{aligned}&I_0(I_0 + C_0)\alpha_0^2 + \left[-\sigma E_0 C_0 + I_0^2\nu + (\gamma+\nu)C_0 I_0 - 2I_0 K1_0\right]\alpha_0\\ &+ K2_0 C_0 - K1_0\nu I_0 + K1_0^2 = 0.\end{aligned}$$

In the above, $K2_0$ is an approximate value of the second derivative of $K(t)$ at $t = 0$. If one differentiates (6) once again, then from (1)–(4) one obtains

$$\begin{aligned}\frac{d^3K}{dt^3} &= \alpha\frac{d^2I}{dt^2} + \psi\frac{d^2C}{dt^2}\\ &= \alpha\sigma\frac{dE}{dt} + \left[\psi\nu - \alpha(\alpha+\gamma+\nu)\right]\frac{dI}{dt} - \psi^2\frac{dC}{dt}\\ &= \alpha\sigma S[\beta I + \varepsilon C]/N + \sigma[\psi\nu - \alpha(\alpha+\gamma+\nu) - \alpha\sigma]E\\ &\quad - \left\{[\psi\nu - \alpha(\alpha+\gamma+\nu)](\alpha+\gamma+\nu) + \psi^2\nu\right\}I + \psi^3 C.\end{aligned}$$

Introduce the notation

$$\begin{aligned}A := &\left\{K3_0 - \sigma[\psi_0\nu - \alpha_0(\alpha_0+\gamma+\nu) - \alpha_0\sigma]E_0 + \{\left[\psi_0\nu - \alpha_0(\alpha_0+\gamma+\nu)\right]\right.\\ &\left.\times(\alpha_0+\gamma+\nu) + \psi_0^2\nu\}I_0 - \psi_0^3 C_0\right\}N/(\alpha_0\sigma S_0),\end{aligned}$$

then one can set

$$\beta_0 = \frac{A - \varepsilon_0 C_0}{I_0}. \tag{8}$$

In the expression for A, constant $K3_0$ estimates the third derivative of $K(t)$ at $t = 0$. To approximate ε_0, it remains to differentiate (6) one more time. By (1)–(4),

$$\begin{aligned}\frac{d^4K}{dt^4} &= \alpha\frac{d^3I}{dt^3} + \psi\frac{d^3C}{dt^3}\\ &= \frac{\alpha\sigma[\beta I + \varepsilon C]}{N}\frac{dS}{dt} + \left\{\frac{\alpha\sigma\beta S}{N} - [\psi\nu - \alpha(\alpha+\gamma+\nu)](\alpha+\gamma+\nu) - \psi^2\nu\right\}\\ &\quad\times\frac{dI}{dt} + \left\{\frac{\alpha\sigma\varepsilon S}{N} + \psi^3\right\}\frac{dC}{dt} + \sigma[\psi\nu - \alpha(\alpha+\gamma+\nu) - \alpha\sigma]\frac{dE}{dt}.\end{aligned}$$

Applying all four equations of (1)–(4) and simplifying the identity, one derives

$$\frac{d^4K}{dt^4} = -\frac{\alpha\sigma S}{N^2}\{\beta^2 I^2 + 2\beta\varepsilon IC + \varepsilon^2 C^2\} + \frac{\beta S}{N}\{\alpha\sigma^2(E-I) - 2\alpha\sigma(\alpha+\gamma+\nu)I$$
$$+\sigma\psi\nu I\} + \frac{\varepsilon S}{N}\{\psi\sigma C(\nu-\alpha) + \alpha\sigma\nu I - \alpha\sigma C(\sigma+\alpha+\gamma+\nu)\}$$
$$-\left\{\left[\psi\nu - \alpha(\alpha+\gamma+\nu)\right](\alpha+\gamma+\nu) + \psi^2\nu\right\}[\sigma E - (\alpha+\gamma+\nu)I]$$
$$+\psi^3[\nu I - \psi C] - \sigma^2 E\left[\psi\nu - \alpha(\sigma+\alpha+\gamma+\nu)\right].$$

Illuminating β according to (8) and canceling quadratic terms, one gets the linear equation for ε_0 as follows

$$K4_0 = \frac{\varepsilon_0 S_0}{N}\left\{\alpha_0\sigma[\nu I_0 - \psi_0 C_0] + \alpha_0\sigma C_0(\alpha_0+\gamma+\nu) - \frac{\alpha_0\sigma^2 C_0 E_0}{I_0}\right\}$$
$$-\frac{\alpha_0\sigma S_0 A^2}{N^2} + \frac{A S_0}{I_0 N}[\alpha_0\sigma^2(E_0 - I_0) - 2\alpha_0\sigma(\alpha_0+\gamma+\nu)I_0 + \sigma\psi_0\nu I_0]$$
$$-\left\{[\psi_0\nu - \alpha_0(\alpha_0+\gamma+\nu)](\alpha_0+\gamma+\nu) + \psi_0^2\nu\right\}\{\sigma E_0 - (\alpha_0+\gamma+\nu)I_0\}$$
$$+\psi_0^3[\nu I_0 - \psi_0 C_0] - \sigma^2 E_0\left[\psi_0\nu - \alpha_0(\sigma+\alpha_0+\gamma+\nu)\right].$$

Here $K4_0$ denotes a numerical value of $\frac{d^4K}{dt^4}(0)$. While the proposed algorithm can offer some insight into how to approximate initial values, the method is far from ideal. Numerical differentiation of noisy data is a separate unstable problem. Computation of ε_0 and β_0 is even more difficult than solving for α_0 and ψ_0, since equations for ε_0 and β_0 contain higher order derivatives. The quadratic equation for α_0 may not have real solutions. At the same time, it can have two nonnegative real roots, generating two sets of initial vectors $[\beta_0, \varepsilon_0, \alpha_0, \psi_0]$ and resulting into two different solutions of the least squares problem.

The good news, however, is that in many cases this approach does work and does help to localize the unknown parameters β, ε, α, and ψ. Combined with an iterative regularization method, nonnegativity constraints, and *a posteriori* stopping rule, the above algorithm can become a valuable tool in the nonlinear optimization process. In the next section, we apply the proposed technique to stable parameter estimation from data sets for cumulative number of human cases in Sierra Leone and Liberia given in Table 2.

4 Regularization Algorithm and Experimental Results for Simulated Data

In this section we present a regularized algorithm for solving the parameter identification inverse problem. Its goal is to obtain the values of β, ε, α, and ψ given real data, d, on EVD cumulative clinical cases. This can be cast as a constrained least squares minimization

$$\min_{q,u} \frac{1}{2} ||K[q]u - d||^2 \quad \text{provided} \quad F(q,u) = 0, \tag{9}$$

where K is defined in (5), $q := [\beta, \varepsilon, \alpha, \psi]$, $u := [I, C]$, and the operator equation $F(q,u) = 0$ is given by (1)–(4). Suppose $u = u[q]$ is a (numerical) solution to (1)–(4). Introduce the notation

$$\Phi_i(q) := K_i[q]u[q] = \int_0^{t_i} \Big(\alpha I[q](s) + \psi C[q](s)\Big) ds + K(0), \quad i = 1, 2, \ldots, m, \tag{10}$$

a parameter-to-observation map. Then we get unconstrained least squares problem:

$$\min_q J(q) := \min_q \frac{1}{2} ||\Phi(q) - d||^2 = \min_q \frac{1}{2} (\Phi_i(q) - d_i)^2, \quad \Phi : \mathbb{R}^4 \to \mathbb{R}^m, \tag{11}$$

with m being the number of data points. The Jacobian matrix for Φ can be computed explicitly. Indeed,

$$\begin{aligned}
\frac{\partial \Phi_i}{\partial \beta} &= \int_0^{t_i} \left\{ \alpha \frac{\partial I[q](s)}{\partial \beta} + \psi \frac{\partial C[q](s)}{\partial \beta} \right\} ds, \\
\frac{\partial \Phi_i}{\partial \varepsilon} &= \int_0^{t_i} \left\{ \alpha \frac{\partial I[q](s)}{\partial \varepsilon} + \psi \frac{\partial C[q](s)}{\partial \varepsilon} \right\} ds, \\
\frac{\partial \Phi_i}{\partial \alpha} &= \int_0^{t_i} \left\{ I[q] + \alpha \frac{\partial I[q](s)}{\partial \alpha} + \psi \frac{\partial C[q](s)}{\partial \alpha} \right\} ds, \\
\frac{\partial \Phi_i}{\partial \psi} &= \int_0^{t_i} \left\{ C[q] + \alpha \frac{\partial I[q](s)}{\partial \psi} + \psi \frac{\partial C[q](s)}{\partial \psi} \right\} ds.
\end{aligned}$$

The partial derivatives of $I[q]$ and $C[q]$ with respect to $\beta, \varepsilon, \alpha$, and ψ can be computed from the corresponding ODE systems. For example, $\frac{\partial I[q]}{\partial \beta}$ and $\frac{\partial C[q]}{\partial \beta}$ satisfy

$$\frac{d}{dt}\left(\frac{\partial S}{\partial \beta}\right) = -\frac{SI}{N} - \frac{\beta I}{N}\frac{\partial S}{\partial \beta} - \frac{\beta S}{N}\frac{\partial I}{\partial \beta} - \frac{\varepsilon C}{N}\frac{\partial S}{\partial \beta} - \frac{\varepsilon S}{N}\frac{\partial C}{\partial \beta},$$
$$\frac{d}{dt}\left(\frac{\partial E}{\partial \beta}\right) = \frac{SI}{N} + \frac{\beta I}{N}\frac{\partial S}{\partial \beta} + \frac{\beta S}{N}\frac{\partial I}{\partial \beta} + \frac{\varepsilon C}{N}\frac{\partial S}{\partial \beta} + \frac{\varepsilon S}{N}\frac{\partial C}{\partial \beta} - \sigma\frac{\partial E}{\partial \beta},$$
$$\frac{d}{dt}\left(\frac{\partial I}{\partial \beta}\right) = \sigma\frac{\partial E}{\partial \beta} - (\alpha + \gamma + \nu)\frac{\partial I}{\partial \beta},$$
$$\frac{d}{dt}\left(\frac{\partial C}{\partial \beta}\right) = \nu\frac{\partial I}{\partial \beta} - \psi\frac{\partial C}{\partial \beta},$$

with homogeneous boundary conditions (since initial values in (1)–(4) do not depend on the system parameters). All other initial values and pre-estimated parameters are given in Sect. 2. The expression for Φ' yields $\nabla J = \Phi'^{*}(q)\Phi(q)$ and the approximation of the first term of the Hessian as $\nabla^2 J(q) \approx \Phi'^{*}(q)\Phi'(q)$. Then, iteratively regularized Gauss Newton (IRGN) method for the solution of (11) [31, 32] is given by

$$q_{k+1} = q_k + \lambda_k p_k, \quad \lambda_k > 0, \tag{12}$$

where search direction p_k solves

$$(\Phi'^{*}(q_k)\Phi'(q_k) + \tau_k I)p_k = -(\Phi'^{*}(q_k)(\Phi(q_k) - d) + \tau_k(q_k - q_0)). \tag{13}$$

In (13), τ_k is a regularizing sequence that converges to zero as k approaches infinity, and q_0 is a reference value for q computed by the algorithm suggested in Sect. 3. This particular version of IRGN algorithm is motivated by Tikhonov's variational regularization with stabilizer $\tau||q - q_0||^2$:

$$\min_q J_\tau(q) := \min_q ||\Phi(q) - d||^2 + \tau||q - q_0||^2, \quad \tau > 0. \tag{14}$$

If the above is understood in terms of Bayesian statistics, the penalty term in Tikhonov's regularization corresponds to the negative-log of the *prior* probability density, the fidelity term corresponds to the negative-log of the likelihood, and the regularized solution corresponds to the maximizer of the *posterior* probability density function, known as the *maximum a posteriori (MAP) estimator* of the solution [33–35].

To evaluate the performance of the proposed stabilizing algorithm we begin our numerical experiments with simulated data. To that end, we solve the corresponding forward problem using the system parameters reconstructed in [26] for Sierra Leone:

$$\beta = 0.3200, \quad \varepsilon = 0.0078, \quad \alpha = 0.1000, \quad \text{and} \quad \psi = 0.2000.$$

These parameters give a very good fit to the actual data prior to September 23, 2014. To be consistent with the real data environment, we assume that simulated data on cumulative EVD cases is discrete, and the values are available the same days when the real data is reported. To approximate $K1_0$, $K2_0$, $K3_0$, and $K4_0$, we spline the discrete values and get

$$K1_0 = 5.3113, \quad K2_0 = 0.0912, \quad K3_0 = -0.0769, \quad K4_0 = 0.$$

Based on the above estimates for the derivatives, we obtain complex valued β_0, ε_0, α_0, and ψ_0. Setting the imaginary parts to zero, we arrive at

$$\beta_0 = 0.1671, \quad \varepsilon_0 = 0.0927, \quad \alpha_0 = 0.1037, \quad \text{and} \quad \psi_0 = 0.2179.$$

As one can see, these values are rather close to the actual parameters. To strike a balance between fitting and penalizing, we use $\tau_k = \frac{\tau_0}{(1+k)^p}$ with $\tau_0 = 10^{-2}$ and $p = 4$, which is the largest value of p generating a convergent regularization process. Initially, the relative discrepancy (RD) is 7.70×10^{-1} and the relative error (RE) is 4.50×10^{-1}. After 75 steps, RD$= 1.19 \times 10^{-4}$ and RE$= 2.44 \times 10^{-2}$. The iterative solution

$$\beta_{75} = 0.3193, \quad \varepsilon_{75} = 0.0058, \quad \alpha_{75} = 0.0983, \quad \text{and} \quad \psi_{75} = 0.2077,$$

turns out to be a reasonable approximation to the exact parameters above. The basic reproduction numbers [26, 36] for the exact and computed solutions are virtually identical, $R_0 = 1.257581$ and $R_0 = 1.257956$, respectively. The condition number of the 4×4 matrix $\Phi'^*(q_k)\Phi'(q_k)$ is of order 10^{10} with stabilizing term reducing it to 10^6 early in the process. The stopping rule is not strictly enforced in the noise-free case. The goal is not to move beyond RD $= 10^{-4}$ to ensure that convergence is not destroyed by rounding errors.

At the next step of the experiment we add 3 % relative random noise to the simulated data. Due to instability of numerical differentiation, the estimated values of $K1_0$, $K2_0$, $K3_0$, and $K4_0$ change substantially:

$$K1_0 = 1.4161, \quad K2_0 = 1.9434, \quad K3_0 = -0.4264, \quad K4_0 = 0.$$

The last value is approximated by zero, since the data curve is restored through cubic spline interpolation. This accuracy appears to be sufficient in case of simulated data. For real data, we combine spline interpolation and finite differences, which result in nonzero values of $K4_0$. Less accurate derivatives give rise to less accurate complex valued β_0, ε_0, α_0, and ψ_0 with the real part of ε_0 being negative. Thus we approximate the initial values of system parameters by the following nonnegative real numbers:

$$\beta_0 = 0.2859, \quad \varepsilon_0 = 0, \quad \alpha_0 = 0.0012, \quad \text{and} \quad \psi_0 = 0.1154.$$

While τ_0 remains equal to 10^{-2} in case of noisy data, we have to switch to $p = 3$ to ensure convergence. We also try not to "do better than the data" (to prevent convergence to the "noisy" solution) and stop the iterative process when RD transitions through the 3 % level. As the result, we obtain

$$\beta_8 = 0.3196, \quad \varepsilon_8 = 0.0110, \quad \alpha_8 = 0.1016, \quad \text{and} \quad \psi_8 = 0.1508,$$

which gives RE$= 1.25 \times 10^{-1}$, RD$= 2.89 \times 10^{-2}$, and the basic reproduction number of $R_0 = 1.264207$. It is not surprising that the impact of noise is substantial, since

$$\Phi'^*(q_8)\Phi'(q_8) = \begin{pmatrix} 0.8555 & 0.6153 & -0.8886 & -0.0127 \\ 0.6153 & 0.4426 & -0.6392 & -0.0091 \\ -0.8886 & -0.6392 & 0.9240 & 0.0135 \\ -0.0127 & -0.0091 & 0.0135 & 0.0003 \end{pmatrix}$$

with the first and the third lines dangerously close to being proportional. For this part of the experiment, the condition number of $\Phi'^*(q_k)\Phi'(q_k)$ is also of order 10^{10} and it is reduced to $10^3 - 10^5$ with regularization. To summarize, a numerical analysis of the model with simulated data, while showing some potential, clearly demonstrates all the challenges that follow from instability of the Gauss-Newton process and of the numerical differentiation task.

5 Numerical Analysis for Real Data

In this section we present experimental results for real data [30] displayed in Table 2 for Sierra Leone and Liberia covering the EVD outbreak up until September 23, 2014. To ensure stability of the iterative process, we take $\tau_k = \frac{\tau_0}{(1+k)^p}$ with $\tau_0 = 10^{-2}$, $p = 1$ for Sierra Leone, and $p = 2$ for Liberia (the largest value of p for which convergence is observed). A rather aggressive stopping rule is used to avoid overfitting that would be unacceptable, since cumulative EVD cases are considerably underreported and the problem is very ill-posed. Specifically, we stop iterations (12)–(13) after the first transition of the relative discrepancy (RD) through the 10 % level, $RD := \frac{||\Phi(q_k)-d_\delta||}{||d_\delta||} = 0.1$, where d_δ is noisy data.

Until the stopping moment is reached, the condition number of $\Phi'^*(q_k)\Phi'(q_k)$ in (13) would normally change from 10^{11} to 10^9 with regularization bringing it down to 10^3 or 10^2 for $p = 1$. For $p = 2$, the condition number of $\Phi'^*(q_k)\Phi'(q_k) + \tau_k I$ ranges from 10^4 to 10^3. In case of Sierra Leone data, the matrix $\Phi'^*(q_k)\Phi'(q_k)$ at the computed solution is

$$\Phi'^*(q_5)\Phi'(q_5) = \begin{pmatrix} 0.2438 & 0.1036 & -0.2380 & -0.3571 \\ 0.1036 & 0.0440 & -0.1011 & -0.1518 \\ -0.2380 & -0.1011 & 0.2326 & 0.3487 \\ -0.3571 & -0.1518 & 0.3487 & 0.5231 \end{pmatrix}$$

which illustrates even better than condition numbers how unstable the model is.

For the Sierra Leone data, experiments have been conducted with $m = 119$ (see Table 2). To avoid numerical differentiation at the end point, we approximate derivatives at $t = 1$ (after one day) by the following values

$$K1_0 = 12.84, \quad K2_0 = -2.853, \quad K3_0 = 0.6373, \quad K4_0 = -0.02529.$$

These values give rise to two sets of initial approximations:

$$\beta_0 = -18.23, \quad \varepsilon_0 = 39.10, \quad \alpha_0 = 0.2684, \quad \psi_0 = 0.4887, \quad \text{and}$$

$$\beta_0 = -0.7193, \quad \varepsilon_0 = 1.1001, \quad \alpha_0 = 0.3354, \quad \psi_0 = 0.3434.$$

If one replaces β_0 with zero and uses the first set, the process turns out to be divergent. If β_0 is replaced with zero in the second set, then after 5 iterations (as dictated by the stopping rule) we get

$$\beta_5 = 0.0255, \quad \varepsilon_5 = 1.1071, \quad \alpha_5 = 0.2666, \quad \text{and} \quad \psi_5 = 0.2914,$$

which yield the basic reproduction number [26, 36] of $R_0 = 1.178$. The first graph in Fig. 4 illustrates the data fit for the cumulative human cases that have been used to reconstruct parameters. The second graph in Fig. 4 shows future projections generated by these parameters and their comparison to the actual data for the period from 5/27/14 to 6/17/15 (with the forecasting time being from 9/23/14 to 6/15/15) as well as to the projections obtained with parameter values from [26]. The values estimated in [26] are $\beta = 0.3200$, $\varepsilon = 0.0078$, $\alpha = 0.1000$, and $\psi = 0.2000$ ($R_0 = 1.258$). Note that the main goal of looking at future projections obtained with different sets of parameters is to provide some (very limited) evidence on the reliability of computed values of β, ε, α, and ψ, rather than to actually predict future cases. Therefore we do not adjust control parameters κ, π, and ω to fit the data. Instead we continue using $\kappa = 0$ and make the comparison based on the reconstructions of β, ε, α, and ψ only.

In case of Liberia, $m = 98$ and the approximate values of the derivatives are

$$K1_0 = 1.859, \quad K2_0 = 3.652, \quad K3_0 = -1.301, \quad K4_0 = 0.02729.$$

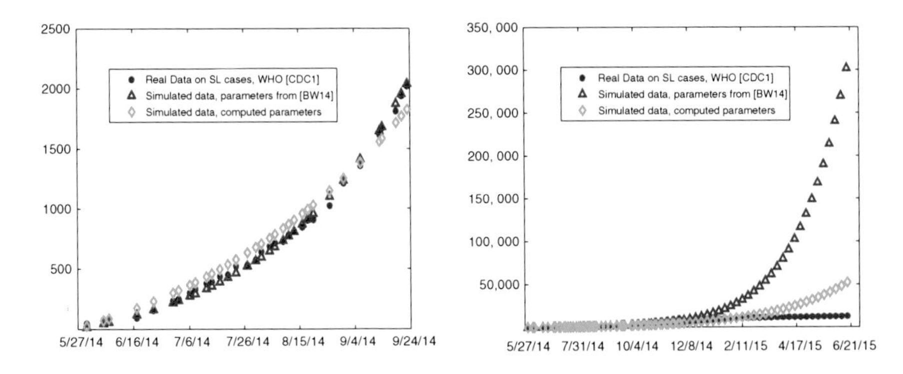

Fig. 4 Data fitting and future projections for Sierra Leone

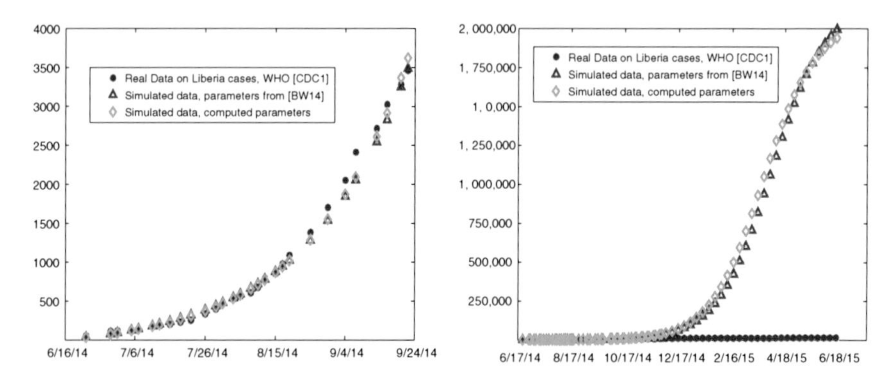

Fig. 5 Data fitting and future projections for Liberia

The quadratic equation for α_0 ends up having two complex conjugate roots so that

$$\beta_0 = 0.3836 \pm 0.0624i, \quad \varepsilon_0 = -2.5364 \mp 1.5768i,$$

$$\alpha_0 = 0.0220 \mp 0.2364i, \quad \text{and} \quad \psi_0 = 0.1147 \pm 0.4334i.$$

Using initial values $\beta_0 = 0.3836$, $\varepsilon_0 = 0$, $\alpha_0 = 0.0220$, and $\psi_0 = 0.1147$, after 15 iterations we arrive at

$$\beta_{15} = 0.4416, \quad \varepsilon_{15} = 0.0700, \quad \alpha_{15} = 0.1774, \quad \text{and} \quad \psi_{15} = 0.1528,$$

with $R_0 = 1.486$. The first graph in Fig. 5 shows the data fit for the cumulative human cases in Liberia that have been used to reconstruct the above parameters. The second graph in Fig. 5 gives future data projections with these parameters and compares them to the actual data for the period from 6/17/14 to 6/17/15 (with the forecasting time being from 9/23/14 to 6/15/15) as well as to projections obtained with parameter values from [26]. The values estimated [26] are $\beta = 0.3000$, $\varepsilon = 0.3160$, $\alpha = 0.1800$, and $\psi = 0.1800$ ($R_0 = 1.535$).

6 Discussion and Future Plans

As one can see in the second graph of Fig. 4, for Sierra Leone the green line (future projections based on computed parameters) stays relatively close to the red line (the actual data) until approximately the beginning of March, 2015. Then the simulated curve deviates from the actual one, and on 6/17/15 it predicts a bit over 50,000 cumulative cases instead of 12,965, which CDC gives based on WHO Situational Reports [CDC2]. This projection can be viewed as quite good considering that in reality the fit can even be better, since WHO data is known to be underreported (and our stopping rule does take this into account).

On the other hand, for Liberia the green line in the second graph of Fig. 5 gets very far away from the red curve, estimating the number of cases on 6/17/15 to be at 2 millions (half of the country population), while CDC [30] shows 10,666. Of course, this can simply be the matter of less accurate initial approximations in case of Liberia that caused convergence to the "wrong" solution. Or it can be the result of poor balance between accuracy and stability in the regularization algorithm. However, we must also keep in mind that by the first week of November 2014, "Liberia has seen a major falloff in new Ebola cases, with only about 50 emerging per day, versus 500 per day at its peak" due to "the amount of money and professionals that have poured into the country and the efforts of the nation's government and populace to slow its spread" [37]. At that same time, Sierra Leone was not showing "similar signs of progress". "The World Health Organization declared the end of the Ebola outbreak in Liberia on May 9, 2015 after 42 days (two incubation periods) had passed since the last Ebola patient was buried. On May 13, 2015, CDC changed the country classification for Liberia to a country with former widespread transmission and current, established control measures" [38].

While the claim about 500 cases per day at the peak of the outbreak may or may not be accurate (that depends on how many cases we assume to be under-reported), the falloff in new Ebola cases in Liberia was, indeed, considerable in November 2014, and that is when the forecasting curves begin to deviate substantially in the second graph of Fig. 5. As of September 23, 2014, Sierra Leone officially had 2,021 cases (see Table 2). By June 17, 2015, the number has grown to 12,965. For Liberia, these numbers are 3,458 and 10,666, respectively. All this indicates that control measures have gradually become very effective in Liberia, and the model which does not take them into consideration (we set $\kappa = 0$ in our experiments as mentioned in Sect. 2) cannot be used for long term forward projections. At the same time, in Sierra Leone it has taken longer for the control measures to take their effect, and that can be the reason for a better forecast that our parameters give in its case.

We will test this conjecture in our future work by assuming exponential rate of decay for the two transmission rates β and ε [10], $\beta(t) = \beta_0 \exp(-\zeta(t-\eta))$ and $\varepsilon(t) = \varepsilon_0 \exp(-\rho(t-\mu))$ and fitting against larger data sets, and by reconstructing the required coefficients to account for the impact of control measures. We will also explore other models that incorporate a combination of control measures to see how they can help with estimating future cases.

Acknowledgments This work is supported by NSF under grant (DMS-1112897). The authors would like to express their special gratitude to the unknown referee for his/her helpful comments and corrections to the preliminary version of this paper.

References

1. World Health Organization: Statement on the 1st meeting of the IHR Emergency Committee on the 2014 Ebola outbreak in West Africa. Accessed 6 Oct 2015. http://www.who.int/mediacentre/news/statements/2014/ebola-20140808/en/
2. World Health Organization: Ebola Situation Report - 8 July 2015. Accessed 13 July 2015. http://apps.who.int/ebola/current-situation/ebola-situation-report-8-july-2015
3. Mylne, A., Brady, O., Huang, Z., Pigott, D., Golding, N., Kraemer, M., Hay, S.: A comprehensive database of the geographic spread of past human Ebola outbreaks. Scientific Data **1** (2014)
4. UNEP/GRID: Africa Population Distribution Database 2000 Population Density (2015). Accessed 8 May 2015. http://na.unep.net/siouxfalls/globalpop/africa/afpopd00.gif
5. World Health Organization: Country Profiles. Accessed 5 Aug 2015. http://www.who.int/countries/en/
6. Report of a WHO/International Study Team and others 1978 Ebola haemorrhagic fever in Sudan. Bull. World Health Organ. **21**, 247–270 (1976)
7. Ebola haemorrhagic fever in Zaire, 1976. Bull. World Health Organ. **21**, 271–293 (1978)
8. Pourrut, X., Kumulungui, B., Wittmann, T., Moussavou, G., Dlicat, A., Yaba, P., Nkoghe, D., Gonzalez, J., Leroy, E.: The natural history of Ebola virus in Africa. Microbes Infect. **7**(7), 1005–1014 (2005)
9. World Health Organization: Frequently asked questions on Ebola virus disease. Accessed 5 Aug 2015. http://www.who.int/csr/disease/ebola/faq-ebola/en/
10. Althaus, C.L.: Estimating the reproduction number of Zaire ebolavirus (EBOV) during the 2014 outbreak in West Africa. PLOS Currents Outbreak (2014). Accessed 2 Sept 2014
11. Chowell, G., Hengartner, N.W., Castillo-Chavez, C., Fenimore, P.W., Hyman, J.M.: The basic reproductive number of Ebola and the effects of public health measures: the cases of Congo and Uganda. J. Theor. Biol. **229**, 119–126 (2004)
12. World Health Organization: Outbreak News; Ebola virus disease in Guinea. Accessed 19 Mar 2015. http://www.afro.who.int/en/clusters-a-programmes/dpc/epidemic-a-pandemic-alert-and-response/outbreak-news/4063-ebola-hemorrhagic-fever-in-guinea.html
13. Grady, D., Finkaug, F.: Tracing Ebolas Breakout to a 2-Year-Old in Guinea. New York Times, August 10, A1 (2014)
14. World Health Organization: Factors that contributed to undetected spread of the Ebola virus and impeded rapid containment. Accessed 5 Aug 2015. http://www.who.int/csr/disease/ebola/one-year-report/factors/en/
15. Lekone, P., Finkenstädt, B.: Statistical inference in a stochastic epidemic SEIR model with control intervention: Ebola as a case study. Biometrics **62**, 1170–1177 (2006)
16. Legrand, J., et al.: Understanding the dynamics of Ebola epidemics. Epidemiol. Infect. **135**, 610–621 (2007)
17. Eichner, M., Dowell, S., Firese, N.: Incubation period of Ebola hemorrhagic virus subtype Zaire. Osong Public Health Res. Perspect. **2**, 3–7 (2011)
18. Ferrari, M., Bjornstad, O., Dobson, A.: Estimation and inference of R0 of an infectious pathogen by a removal method. Math. Biosci. **198**, 14–26 (2005)
19. White, L., Pagano, M.: A likelihood-based method for real-time estimation of the serial interval and reproductive number of an epidemic. Stat. Med. **27**, 2999–3016 (2008)
20. Meltzer, M., Atkins, C., Santibanez, S., Knust, B., Petersen, B., Ervin, E., Nichol, S., Damon, I., Washington, M.: Estimating the future number of cases in the Ebola epidemic Liberia and Sierra Leone, 2014–2015. CDC Centers for Disease Control and Prevention, vol. 63, pp. 1–14 (2014). Accessed 26 Sept 26
21. Ebola virus disease in West Africa the first 9 months of the epidemic and forward projections. New Engl. J. Med. **371**, 1481–1495 (2014)
22. Pell, B., Baez, J., Phan, T., Gao, D., Chowell, G., Kuang, Y.: Patch Models of EVD Transmission Dynamics. In: Chowell-Puente, G., Hyman, J.M. (eds.) Springer Series "Mathematical Modeling for Emerging and Re-emerging Infectious Diseases". (2015)

23. Wong, G., Kobinger, G.P., Qiu, X.: Characterization of host immune responses in Ebola virus infections. Expert Rev. Clin. Immunol. **10**, 781–790 (2014)
24. Fisman, D., Khoo, E., Tuite, A.: Early epidemic dynamics of the West African 2014 Ebola outbreak: Estimates derived with a simple two-parameter model. PLOS Currents Outbreak (2014). Accessed 8 Sept 2014
25. Weitz, J.S., Dushoff, J.: Modeling post-death transmission of Ebola: challenges for inference and opportunities for control. Sci. Rep. **5**, 8751 (2015)
26. Browne, C.J., Huo, X., Magal, P., Seydi, M., Seydi, O., Webb, G.: A Model of the 2014 Ebola Epidemic in West Africa with Contact Tracing. arXiv:1410.3817v2 [q-bio.PE]
27. Legrand, J., Grais, R.F., Boelle, P.Y., Valleron, A.J., Flahault, A.: Understanding the dynamics of Ebola epidemics. Epidemiol. Infect. **135**(4), 610–621 (2007)
28. Rivers, C., Lofgren, E., Marathe, M., Eubank, S., Lewis, B.: Modeling the impact of interventions on an epidemic of Ebola in Sierra Leone and Liberia. PLOS Currents Outbreak (2014). Accessed 6 Nov 2014 (revised)
29. United Nations Department of Economic and Social Affairs: Revision of the World Urbanization Prospects (2014)
30. Centers for Disease Control and Prevention: Ebola Outbreak in West Africa - Reported Cases Graphs (2014). http://www.cdc.gov/vhf/ebola/outbreaks/2014-west-africa/cumulative-cases-graphs.html
31. Bakushinsky, A.B.: Iterative methods for nonlinear operator equations without regularity. New approach. Dokl. Russian Acad. Sci. **330**, 282–284 (1993)
32. Bakushinsky, A.B., Kokurin, MYu.: Iterative Methods for Ill-Posed Operator Equations with Smooth Operators. Springer, Dordrecht (2005)
33. Calvetti, D., Somersalo, E.: Introduction to Bayesian Scientific Computing. Springer, New York (2007)
34. Kaipio, J., Somersalo, E.: Statistical and Computational Inverse Problems. Springer, New York (2005)
35. Vogel, C.R.: Non-convergence of the L-curve regularization parameter selection method. Inverse Probl. **12**, N4, 535–547 (1996)
36. van den Driessche, P., Watmoughb, J.: Reproduction numbers and sub-threshold endemic equilibria for compartmental models of disease transmission. Math. Biosci. **180**, N12, 29–48 (2002)
37. Sheets, C.A.: Ebola Deadly Outbreak: Why Is Liberia Improving While Sierra Leone Continues To Battle New Cases? International Business Times. http://www.ibtimes.com/ebola-deadly-outbreak-why-liberia-improving-while-sierra-leone-continues-battle-new-1725305
38. Centers for Disease Control and Prevention: Ebola Outbreak in West Africa - Outbreak Distribution Map (2014). http://www.cdc.gov/vhf/ebola/outbreaks/2014-west-africa/distribution-map.html
39. Pattyn, S.R.: Ebola virus haemorrhagic fever. International Colloquium on Ebola Virus Infection and other Haemorrhagic Fevers. Elsevier/North-Holland Biomedical Press, Amsterdam (1977)

Assessing the Efficiency of Movement Restriction as a Control Strategy of Ebola

Baltazar Espinoza, Victor Moreno, Derdei Bichara and Carlos Castillo-Chavez

Abstract We formulate a two-patch mathematical model for Ebola Virus Disease dynamics in order to evaluate the effectiveness of travel restriction (*cordons sanitaires*), mandatory movement restrictions between communities while exploring their role on disease dynamics and final epidemic size. Simulations show that **strict** restrictions in movement between high and low risk areas of closely linked communities may have a deleterious impact on the overall levels of infection in the total population.

Keywords Ebola · Epidemic model · Patch model · Spatial model · Transmission dynamics

1 Introduction

Ebola virus disease (EVD) is caused by a genus of the family *Filoviridae* called *Ebolavirus*. The first recorded outbreak took place in Sudan in 1976 with the longest most severe outbreak taking place in West Africa during 2014–2015 [35]. Studies have estimated disease growth rates and explored the impact of interventions aimed at reducing the final epidemic size [12, 24, 25, 32]. Despite these efforts, research that improves and increases our understanding of EVD and the environments where it thrives is still needed [29].

B. Espinoza · V. Moreno · D. Bichara (✉) · C. Castillo-Chavez
Simon A. Levin Mathematical, Computational and Modeling Science Center, Arizona State University, Tempe, AZ 85287, USA
e-mail: derdei.bichara@asu.edu

B. Espinoza
e-mail: bespino6@asu.edu

V. Moreno
e-mail: Victor.M.Moreno@asu.edu

C. Castillo-Chavez
e-mail: ccchavez@asu.edu

G. Chowell and J.M. Hyman (eds.), *Mathematical and Statistical Modeling for Emerging and Re-emerging Infectious Diseases*,
DOI 10.1007/978-3-319-40413-4_9

This chapter is organized as follows: Sect. 2 reviews past modeling work; Sect. 3 introduces a single Patch model, its associated basic reproduction number $\mathscr{R}_0$, and the final size relationship; Sect. 4 introduces a two-Patch model that accounts for the time spent by residents of Patch i on Patch j; Sect. 5 includes selected simulations that highlight the possible implications of policies that forcefully restrict movement (*cordons sanitaires*); and, Sect. 6 collects our thoughts on the relationship between movement, health disparities, and risk.

2 Prior Modeling Work

Chowell et al. [12] estimated the basic reproduction numbers for the 1995 outbreak in the Democratic Republic of Congo and the 2000 outbreak in Uganda. Model analysis showed that control measures (education, contact tracing, quarantine) if implemented within a reasonable window in time could be effective. Legrand et al. [24] built on the work in [12] through the addition of hospitalized and dead (in funeral homes) classes within a study that focused on the relative importance of control measures and the timing of their implementation. Lekone and Finkenstädt [25] made use of an stochastic framework in estimating the mean incubation period, mean infectious period, transmission rate and the basic reproduction number, using data from the 1995 outbreak. Their results turned out to be in close agreement with those in [12] but the estimates had **wider** confidence intervals.

The 2014 outbreak is the deadliest in the history of the virus and naturally, questions remain [11, 15, 23, 27, 28, 32, 33]. Chowell et al. [11] recently introduced a mathematical model aimed at addressing the impact of early detection (via sophisticated technologies) of pre-symptomatic individuals on the transmission dynamics of the Ebola virus in West Africa. Patterson-Lomba et al. [33] explored the potential negative effects that restrictive intervention measures may have had in Guinea, Sierra Leone, and Liberia. Their analysis made use of the available data on Ebola Virus Disease cases up to September 8, 2014. The focus on [33] was on the dynamics of the "effective reproduction number" R_{eff}, a measure of the changing rate of epidemic growth, as the population of susceptible individuals gets depleted. R_{eff} appeared to be increasing for Liberia and Guinea, in the initial stages of the outbreak in densely populated cities, that is, during the period of time when strict quarantine measures were imposed in several areas in West Africa. Their report concluded, in part, that the imposition of enforced quarantine measures in densely populated communities in West Africa, may have accelerated the spread of the disease. In [15], the authors showed that the estimated growth rates of EVD cases were growing exponentially at the national level. They also observed that the growth rates exhibited polynomial growth at the district level over three or more generations of the disease. It has been suggested that behavioral changes or the successful implementation of control measures, or high levels of clustering, or all of them may nave been responsible for polynomial growth. A recent review of mathematical models of past and current EVD outbreaks can be found in [14] and references therein. Authors in [5, 19, 30] attempted to quantify the spread of EDV out of the three Ebola-stricken countries via international flights. For instance, in [19] it was shown hypothetically that, for a short-time period, a reduction of 80 % of international flights from and to these three countries delays the international spread for three week. Similarly, in [30], it is showed that a reduction of 60 % of international flights from and to of the affected area would delay but not prevent the spread of the disease beyond the area. Bogoch et al. [5] estimated about the travelers infected per month for a certain window of reduction of international flights from and to Guinea, Liberia and Sierra Leone, and assessed that exit screening for the departing travelers from the three countries is more efficient in mitigating the risk of Ebola exportation. However, the effects of movement of individuals between two or more neighborhoods or highly connected cities to the best of our knowledge has not been explored. In this paper, we proceed to analyze the effectiveness of forcefully local restrictions in movement on the dynamics of EVD. We study the dynamics of EVD within scenarios that resemble EVD transmission dynamics within locally interconnected communities in West Africa.

3 The Model Derivation

Cordons Sanitaire or "sanitary barriers" are designed to prevent the movement, in and out, of people and goods from particular areas. The effectiveness of the use of *cordons sanitaire* have been controversial. This policy was last implemented nearly one hundred years ago [9]. In desperate attempts to control disease, Ebola-stricken countries enforced public health officials decided to use this medieval control strategy, in the EVD hot-zone, that is, the region of confluence of Guinea, Liberia and Sierra Leone [17]. In this chapter, a framework that allows, in the simplest possible setting, the possibility of assessing the potential impact of the use of a *Cordon Sanitaire* during an EVD outbreak, is introduced and "tested". The population of interest is subdivided into susceptible (S), latent (E), infectious (I), dead (D) and recovered (R). The total population (including the dead) is therefore $N = S + E + I + D + R$. The susceptible population is reduced by the process of infection, which occurs via effective "contacts" between an infectious (I) or a dead body (D) at the rate of $\beta(\frac{I}{N} + \varepsilon\frac{D}{N})$ and susceptible. EVD-induced dead bodies have the highest viral load, that is, more infectious than individuals in the infectious stage (I); and, so, it is assumed that $\varepsilon > 1$. The latent population increases at the rate $\beta S(\frac{I}{N} + \varepsilon\frac{D}{N})$. However since some latent individuals may recover without developing an infection [1, 2, 12, 20, 21, 26], it is assumed that exposed individuals develop symptoms at the rate κ or recover at the rate α. The population of infectious individuals increases at the rate κE and decreases at the rate γI. Further, individuals leaving the infectious stage at rate γ, die at the rate γf_{dead} or recover at the rate $(1 - f_{\text{dead}})\gamma$. The R class includes recovered or the removed individuals from the system (dead and buried). By definition the R-class increases, the arrival of previously infected, grows at the rate $(1 - f_{\text{dead}})\gamma I$.

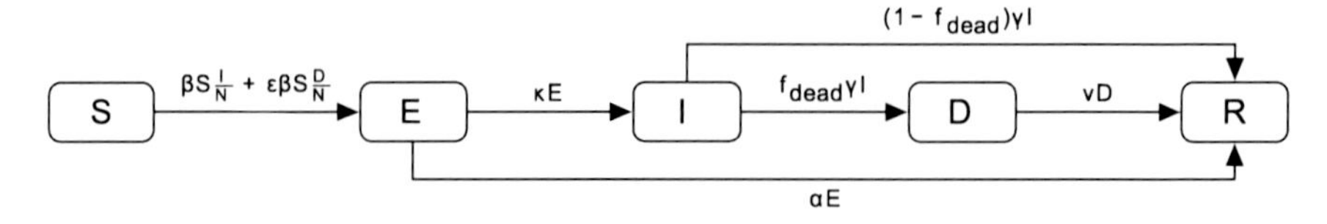

Fig. 1 An SEIDR model for Ebola virus disease

Table 1 Variables and parameters of the contagion model

Parameter	Description	Base model values
α	Rate at which of latent recover without developing symptoms	$0 - 0.458$ [26]
β	Per susceptible infection rate	0.3056 [11, 14, 33]
γ	Rate at which an infected recovers or dies	$\frac{1}{6.5}$ [14]
κ	Per-capita progression rate to **infectious stage**	$\frac{1}{7}$ [11, 33]
ν	Per-capita body disposal rate	$\frac{1}{2}$ [24]
f_{dead}	Proportion of infected who die due to infection	0.708 [14]
ε	Scale: Ebola infectiousness of dead bodies	1.2

A flow diagram of the model is in Fig. 1, The definitions of parameters are collected in Table 1, including the parameter values used in simulations where the mathematical model built from Fig. 1, that models EVD dynamics is given by the following nonlinear systems of differential equations:

$$\begin{cases} N = S + E + I + D + R \\ \dot{S} = -\beta S \frac{I}{N} - \varepsilon \beta S \frac{D}{N} \\ \dot{E} = \beta S \frac{I}{N} + \varepsilon \beta S \frac{D}{N} - (\kappa + \alpha) E \\ \dot{I} = \kappa E - \gamma I \\ \dot{D} = f_{\text{dead}} \gamma I - \nu D \\ \dot{R} = (1 - f_{\text{dead}}) \gamma I + \nu D + \alpha E \end{cases} \tag{1}$$

The total population is constant and the set $\Omega = \{(S, E, I, R) \in \mathbb{R}^4_+ / S + E + I + R \leq N\}$ is a compact positively invariant, that is, solutions behave as expected biologically. Hence Model (1) is well-posed. Following the next generation operator approach [16, 34] (on E, I and D), we find that the basic reproductive number is given by

$$\mathscr{R}_0 = \left(\frac{\beta}{\gamma} + \frac{\varepsilon f_{\text{dead}}\beta}{\nu}\right)\frac{\kappa}{\kappa+\alpha}$$

That is, $\mathscr{R}_0$ is given by the sum of the secondary cases of infection produced by infected and dead individuals during their infection period. The final epidemic size relation that includes dead (to simplify the maths) being given by

$$\log\frac{N}{S^\infty} = \mathscr{R}_0\left(1-\frac{S^\infty}{N}\right).$$

4 EDV Dynamics in Heterogeneous Risk Environments

The work of Eubank et al. [18], Sara de Valle et al. [31], Chowell et al. [4, 13] analyze heterogeneous environments. Castillo-Chavez and Song [10], for example, highlight the importance of epidemiological frameworks that follow a Lagrangian perspective, that is, models that keep track of each individual (or at least its place of residence or group membership) at all times. The Fig. 2 represents a schematic representation of the Lagrangian dispersal between two patches.

Bichara et al. [4] uses a general Susceptible-Infectious-Susceptible (SIS) model involving n-patches given by the following system of nonlinear equations:

$$\begin{cases} \dot{S}_i = b_i - d_i S_i + \gamma_i I_i - \sum_{j=1}^n (S_i \text{ infected in Patch } j) \\ \dot{I}_i = \sum_{j=1}^n (S_i \text{ infected in Patch } j) - \gamma_i I_i - d_i I_i \\ \dot{N}_i = b_i - d_i N_i. \end{cases}$$

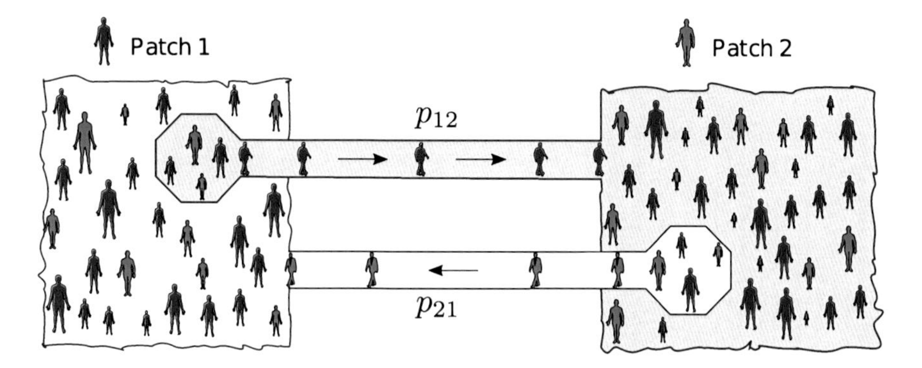

Fig. 2 Dispersal of individuals via a Lagrangian approach where p_{ij} is the proportion of time individual of Patch i spend in Patch j, for $(i, j) \in \{1, 2\}$

where b_i, d_i and γ_i denote the per-capita birth, natural death and recovery rates respectively. Infection is modeled as follows:

$$[S_i \text{ infected in Patch } j] = \underbrace{\beta_j}_{\text{the risk of infection in Patch } j} \times \underbrace{p_{ij} S_i}_{\text{Susceptible from Patch } i \text{ who are currently in Patch } j} \times \underbrace{\frac{\sum_{k=1}^{n} p_{kj} I_k}{\sum_{k=1}^{n} p_{kj} N_k}}_{\text{Proportion of infected in Patch } j}.$$

where the last term accounts for the *effective* infection proportion in Patch j at time. The model reduces to the single n-dimensional system

$$\dot{I}_i = \sum_{j=1}^{n} \left(\beta_j p_{ij} \left(\frac{b_i}{d_i} - I_i \right) \frac{\sum_{k=1}^{n} p_{kj} I_k}{\sum_{k=1}^{n} p_{kj} \frac{b_k}{d_k}} \right) - (\gamma_i + d_i) I_i \quad i = 1, 2, \ldots, n.$$

with a basic reproduction number $\mathcal{R}_0$ that it is a function of the risk vector $\mathcal{B} = (\beta_1, \beta_2, \ldots, \beta_n)^t$ and the residence times matrix $\mathbb{P} = (p_{ij})$, $i, j = 1, \ldots, n$, where $p_{i,j}$ denotes the proportion of the time that an i-resident spends visiting patch j. In [4], it is shown that when $\mathbb{P}$ is irreducible (patches are strongly connected), the disease free state is globally asymptotically stable if $\mathcal{R}_0 \leq 1$ (g.a.s.) while, whenever $\mathcal{R}_0 > 1$ there exists a unique interior equilibrium which is g.a.s.

The Patch-specific basic reproduction number is given by

$$\mathcal{R}_0^i(\mathbb{P}) = \mathcal{R}_0^i \times \sum_{j=1}^{n} \left(\frac{\beta_j}{\beta_i} \right) p_{ij} \left(\frac{\left(p_{ij} \frac{b_i}{d_i} \right)}{\sum_{k=1}^{n} p_{kj} \frac{b_k}{d_k}} \right).$$

where $\mathcal{R}_0^i$ are the *local* basic reproduction number when the patches are isolated. This Patch-specific basic reproduction number gives the dynamics of the disease at Patch level [4], that is, if $\mathcal{R}_0^i(\mathbb{P}) > 1$ the disease persists in Patch i. Moreover, if $p_{kj} = 0$ for all $k = 1, 2, \ldots, n$ and $k \neq i$ whenever $p_{ij>1}$, it has been shown [4] that the disease dies out form Patch i if $\mathcal{R}_0^i(\mathbb{P}) < 1$. The authors in [4] also considered a multi-patch SIR single outbreak model and deduced the final epidemic size. The SIR single outbreak model considered in [4] is the following:

$$\begin{cases} \dot{S}_i = -\left(\frac{\beta_i p_{ii}^2}{p_{ii} N_i + p_{ji} N_j} + \frac{\beta_j p_{1ij}^2}{p_{ij} N_i + p_{jj} N_j} \right) S_i I_i - \left(\frac{\beta_i p_{ii} p_{ji}}{p_{ii} N_i + p_{ji} N_j} + \frac{\beta_j p_{ij} p_{jj}}{p_{ij} N_i + p_{jj} N_j} \right) S_i I_j, \\ \\ \dot{I}_i = \left(\frac{\beta_i p_{ii}^2}{p_{ii} N_i + p_{ji} N_j} + \frac{\beta_j p_{1ij}^2}{p_{ij} N_i + p_{jj} N_j} \right) S_i I_i + \left(\frac{\beta_i p_{ii} p_{ji}}{p_{ii} N_i + p_{ji} N_j} + \frac{\beta_j p_{ij} p_{jj}}{p_{ij} N_i + p_{jj} N_j} \right) S_i I_j - \alpha_i I_i, \\ \\ \dot{R}_i = \alpha_i I_i, \end{cases}$$

where $i, j = 1, 2, i \neq j$, and S_i, I_i and R_i denotes the population of susceptible, infected and recovered immune individuals in Patch i, respectively. The parameter α_i is the recovery rate in Patch i and $N_i \equiv S_i + I_i + R_i$, for $i = 1, 2$.

In this chapter we will be making use of this modeling framework, but with a slightly different formulation, to test under what conditions the movement of individuals from high risk areas to nearby low risk areas due to the use of *cordon sanitaire*, is effective in reducing *overall* transmission by considering two-Patch single outbreak that captures the dynamics of Ebola in a two-patch setting.This Lagrangian approach where dispersal is defined via residence times is useful in describing the movement of commuters between two or more highly connected cities or neighborhoods. The Eulerian approach of metapopulation is useful in describing long distance migration of individuals between cities or countries.

4.1 Formulation of the Model

It is assumed that the community of interest is composed of two adjacent geographic regions facing highly distinct levels of EVD infection. The levels of risk account for differences in population density, availability of medical services and isolation facilities, and the need to travel to a lower risk area to work. So, we let N_1 denote be the population in patch-one (high risk) and N_2 be the population in patch-two (low risk). The classes S_i, E_i, I_i, R_i represent respectively, the susceptible, exposed, infectious and recovered sub-populations in Patch i $(i = 1, 2)$. The class D_i represents the number of disease induced deaths in Patch i. The dispersal of individuals is captured via a Lagrangian approach defined in terms of residence times [3, 4], a concept developed for communicable diseases for n patch setting [4] and applied to vector-borne diseases to an arbitrary number of host groups and vector patches in [3].

We model the new cases of infection per unit of time as follows:

- The density of infected individuals mingling in Patch 1 at time t, who are only capable of infecting susceptible individuals currently in Patch 1 at time t, that is, the *effective* infectious proportion in Patch 1 is given by

$$p_{11}\frac{I_1(t)}{N_1} + p_{21}\frac{I_2(t)}{N_2},$$

  where p_{11} denotes the proportion of time residents from Patch 1 spend in Patch 1 and p_{21} the proportion of time that residents from Patch 2 spend in Patch 1.
- The number of new infections within members of Patch 1, in Patch 1 is therefore given by

$$\beta_1 p_{11} S_1 \left(p_{11}\frac{I_1(t)}{N_1} + p_{21}\frac{I_2(t)}{N_2} \right).$$

- The number of new cases of infection within members of Patch 1, in Patch 2 per unit of time is therefore

$$\beta_2 p_{12} S_1 \left(p_{12} \frac{I_1(t)}{N_1} + p_{22} \frac{I_2(t)}{N_2} \right),$$

where p_{12} denotes the proportion of time that residents from Patch 1 spend in Patch 2 and p_{22} the proportion of time that residents from Patch 2 spend in Patch 2; given by the effective density of infected individuals in Patch 1

$$p_{11} \frac{I_1(t)}{N_1} + p_{21} \frac{I_2(t)}{N_2}, \quad (*)$$

while the *effective* density of infected individuals in Patch 2 is given by

$$p_{12} \frac{I_1(t)}{N_1} + p_{22} \frac{I_2(t)}{N_2}. \quad (**)$$

Further, since, $p_{11} + p_{12} = 1$ and $p_{21} + p_{21} = 1$ then we see that the sum of (*) and (**) gives the density of infected individuals in both patches, namely,

$$\frac{I_1}{N_1} + \frac{I_2}{N_2},$$

as expected. If we further assume that infection by dead bodies occurs only at the local level (bodies are not moved) then, by following the same rationale as in Model (1), we arrive at the following model:

$$\begin{cases} N_1 = S_1 + E_1 + I_1 + D_1 + R_1 \\ N_2 = S_2 + E_2 + I_2 + D_2 + R_2 \\ \dot{S}_1 = -\beta_1 p_{11} S_1 \left(p_{11} \frac{I_1}{N_1} + p_{21} \frac{I_2}{N_2} \right) - \beta_2 p_{12} S_1 \left(p_{12} \frac{I_1}{N_1} + p_{22} \frac{I_2}{N_2} \right) - \varepsilon_1 \beta_1 p_{11} S_1 \frac{D_1}{N_1} \\ \dot{E}_1 = \beta_1 p_{11} S_1 \left(p_{11} \frac{I_1}{N_1} + p_{21} \frac{I_2}{N_2} \right) + \beta_2 p_{12} S_1 \left(p_{12} \frac{I_1}{N_1} + p_{22} \frac{I_2}{N_2} \right) + \varepsilon_1 \beta_1 p_{11} S_1 \frac{D_1}{N_1} - \kappa E_1 - \alpha E_1 \\ \dot{I}_1 = \kappa E_1 - \gamma I_1 \\ \dot{D}_1 = f_{\text{dead}} \gamma I_1 - \nu D_1 \\ \dot{R}_1 = (1 - f_{\text{dead}}) \gamma I_1 + \nu D_1 + \alpha E_1 \\ \dot{S}_2 = -\beta_1 p_{21} S_2 \left(p_{11} \frac{I_1}{N_1} + p_{21} \frac{I_2}{N_2} \right) - \beta_2 p_{22} S_2 \left(p_{12} \frac{I_1}{N_1} + p_{22} \frac{I_2}{N_2} \right) - \varepsilon_2 \beta_2 p_{22} S_2 \frac{D_2}{N_2} \\ \dot{E}_2 = \beta_1 p_{21} S_2 \left(p_{11} \frac{I_1}{N_1} + p_{21} \frac{I_2}{N_2} \right) + \beta_2 p_{22} S_2 \left(p_{12} \frac{I_1}{N_1} + p_{22} \frac{I_2}{N_2} \right) + \varepsilon_2 \beta_2 p_{22} S_2 \frac{D_2}{N_2} - \kappa E_2 - \alpha E_2 \\ \dot{I}_2 = \kappa E_2 - \gamma I_2 \\ \dot{D}_2 = f_{\text{dead}} \gamma I_2 - \nu D_2 \\ \dot{R}_2 = (1 - f_{\text{dead}}) \gamma I_2 + \nu D_2 + \alpha E_2 \end{cases} \quad (2)$$

The difference, in the formulation of the infection term, from the one considered in [4] is the *effective* proportion of infected. Here, the *effective* proportion of infected in Patch 1, for example, is

$$p_{11}\frac{I_1}{N_1} + p_{21}\frac{I_2}{N_2}$$

whereas in [4], it is

$$\frac{p_{11}I_1 + p_{21}I_1}{p_{11}N_1 + p_{21}N_1}.$$

The proportions of infected individuals are taken, in each patch, before the coupling for the former and after the coupling for the latter at the beginning of the infection. Hence, modeling the *effective* proportion of infected as $p_{11}\frac{I_1}{N_1} + p_{21}\frac{I_2}{N_2}$ is well suited for a single outbreak such as the one considered in this paper.

By using the next generation approach [16, 34], we arrive at the basic reproductive number for the entire system, namely,

$$\mathcal{R}_0 = \frac{\kappa}{2(\kappa+\alpha)}\left(\frac{\beta_1 p_{11}^2 + \beta_2 p_{12}^2}{\gamma} + \frac{f_{\text{death}}\varepsilon_1\beta_1 p_{11}}{\nu} + \frac{\beta_1 p_{21}^2 + \beta_2 p_{22}^2}{\gamma} + \frac{f_{\text{death}}\varepsilon_2\beta_2 p_{22}}{\nu}\right.$$

$$+\left.\sqrt{\begin{array}{l}\left(\frac{\beta_1 p_{11}^2 + \beta_2 p_{12}^2}{\gamma} + \frac{f_{\text{death}}\varepsilon_1\beta_1 p_{11}}{\nu}\right)^2 + \left(\frac{\beta_1 p_{21}^2 + \beta_2 p_{22}^2}{\gamma} + \frac{f_{\text{death}}\varepsilon_2\beta_2 p_{22}}{\nu}\right)^2 \\ -2\left(\frac{\beta_1 p_{11}^2 + \beta_2 p_{12}^2}{\gamma} + \frac{f_{\text{death}}\varepsilon_1\beta_1 p_{11}}{\nu}\right)\left(\frac{\beta_1 p_{21}^2 + \beta_2 p_{22}^2}{\gamma} + \frac{f_{\text{death}}\varepsilon_2\beta_2 p_{22}}{\nu}\right) \\ +4\left(\beta_1 p_{11}p_{21}\frac{N_1}{\gamma N_2} + \beta_1 p_{12}p_{22}\frac{N_1}{\gamma N_2}\right)\left(\beta_1 p_{11}p_{21}\frac{N_2}{N_1} + \beta_1 p_{12}p_{22}\frac{N_2}{N_1}\right)\end{array}}\right)$$

We see, for example, that whenever the residents of Patch j $(j = 1, 2)$ live in communities where travel is not possible, that is, when $p_{12} = p_{21} = 0$ or $p_{11} = p_{22} = 1$, then the populations decouple and, consequently, we have that

$$\mathcal{R}_0 = \max\{\mathcal{R}^1, \mathcal{R}^2\}$$

where $\mathcal{R}^i = \left(\frac{\beta_i}{\gamma} + \frac{1}{\nu}f_{\text{death}}\varepsilon_i\beta_i\right)\frac{\kappa}{\kappa+\alpha}$ for $i = 1, 2$; that is, basic reproduction number of Patch i, $i = 1, 2$, if isolated.

4.2 Final Epidemic Size in Heterogeneous Risk Environments

We keep track of the dead to make the mathematics simple. That is, to assuming that the population within each Patch is constant. And so, from the model, we get that

$$
\begin{cases}
\dot{S}_1 = -\beta_1 p_{11} S_1 \left(p_{11}\frac{I_1}{N_1} + p_{21}\frac{I_2}{N_2}\right) - \beta_2 p_{12} S_1 \left(p_{12}\frac{I_1}{N_1} + p_{22}\frac{I_2}{N_2}\right) - \varepsilon_1 \beta_1 p_{11} S_1 \frac{D_1}{N_1} \\
\dot{E}_1 = \beta_1 p_{11} S_1 \left(p_{11}\frac{I_1}{N_1} + p_{21}\frac{I_2}{N_2}\right) + \beta_2 p_{12} S_1 \left(p_{12}\frac{I_1}{N_1} + p_{22}\frac{I_2}{N_2}\right) + \varepsilon_1 \beta_1 p_{11} S_1 \frac{D_1}{N_1} - (\kappa+\alpha) E_1 \\
\dot{I}_1 = \kappa E_1 - \gamma I_1 \\
\dot{D}_1 = f_{\text{dead}} \gamma I_1 - \nu D_1 \\
\dot{S}_2 = -\beta_1 p_{21} S_2 \left(p_{11}\frac{I_1}{N_1} + p_{21}\frac{I_2}{N_2}\right) - \beta_2 p_{22} S_2 \left(p_{12}\frac{I_1}{N_1} + p_{22}\frac{I_2}{N_2}\right) - \varepsilon_2 \beta_2 p_{22} S_2 \frac{D_2}{N_2} \\
\dot{E}_2 = \beta_1 p_{21} S_2 \left(p_{11}\frac{I_1}{N_1} + p_{21}\frac{I_2}{N_2}\right) + \beta_2 p_{22} S_2 \left(p_{12}\frac{I_1}{N_1} + p_{22}\frac{I_2}{N_2}\right) + \varepsilon_2 \beta_2 p_{22} S_2 \frac{D_2}{N_2} - (\kappa+\alpha) E_2 \\
\dot{I}_2 = \kappa E_2 - \gamma I_2 \\
\dot{D}_2 = f_{\text{dead}} \gamma I_2 - \nu D_2,
\end{cases}
\tag{3}
$$

with initial conditions

$$S_1(0) = N_1, \quad E_1(0) = 0, \quad I_1(0) = 0, \quad D_1(0) = 0,$$

$$S_2(0) = N_2, \quad E_2(0) = 0, \quad I_2(0) = 0, \quad D_2(0) = 0,$$

We use the above model to find an "approximate" final size relationship, following the method used in [1, 7–9].

Notation

We make use of the notation $\hat{g}(t)$ for $\int_0^t g(s)ds$ and g^∞ for $\lim_{t\to+\infty} g(t)$. We see that our analysis results guarantee that if $g(t)$ is a positive decreasing function then $g^\infty = 0$.

Since $\dot{S}_1 + \dot{E}_1 = -(\kappa+\alpha)E_1 \leq 0$, then $E_1^\infty = 0$ and since $\dot{S}_1 + \dot{E}_1 + \dot{I}_1 = -\alpha E_1 - \gamma I_1 \leq 0$ then $I_1^\infty = 0$. If we now consider that $\dot{S}_1 + \dot{E}_1 + \dot{I}_1 + \dot{D}_1 = -\alpha E_1 - (1 - f_{\text{dead}})\gamma I_1 - \nu D_1 \leq 0$ then it follows that $D_1^\infty = 0$. Similarly, it can be shown that

$$E_2^\infty = I_2^\infty = D_2^\infty = 0.$$

Focusing on the first two equations of System (3), we arrive at

$$S_1^\infty - N_1 = -(\kappa+\alpha)\hat{E}_1.$$

Consequently, since $\dot{I}_1 = kE_1 - \gamma I_1$, we have that $I_1^\infty = \kappa \hat{E}_1 - \gamma \hat{I}_1$ and therefore

$$\kappa \hat{E}_1 = \gamma \hat{I}.$$

Using the equation for $\dot{D}_1$, we find that

$$\nu \hat{D}_1 = f_{\text{dead}} \gamma \hat{I}_1.$$

Similarly, we can deduce the analogous relationships for Patch 2, namely that,

$$S_2^\infty - N_2 = -(\kappa+\alpha)\hat{E}_2, \quad \kappa \hat{E}_2 = \gamma \hat{I} \quad \text{and} \quad \nu \hat{D}_2 = f_{\text{dead}} \gamma \hat{I}_2$$

From the equation for susceptible populations in Patch 1, we have that

$$\frac{\dot{S}_1}{S_1} = -\beta_1 p_{11}\left(p_{11}\frac{I_1}{N_1} + p_{21}\frac{I_2}{N_2}\right) - \beta_2 p_{12}\left(p_{12}\frac{I_1}{N_1} + p_{22}\frac{I_2}{N_2}\right) - \varepsilon_1\beta_1 p_{11}\frac{D_1}{N_1}$$

and, therefore that,

$$\log\frac{S_1^0}{S_1^\infty} = \beta_1 p_{11}\left(p_{11}\frac{\hat{I}_1}{N_1} + p_{21}\frac{\hat{I}_2}{N_2}\right) + \beta_2 p_{12}\left(p_{12}\frac{\hat{I}_1}{N_1} + p_{22}\frac{\hat{I}_2}{N_2}\right) + \varepsilon_1\beta_1 p_{11}\frac{\hat{D}_1}{N_1}.$$

For the second patch, we have that

$$\log\frac{S_2^0}{S_2^\infty} = \beta_1 p_{21}\left(p_{11}\frac{\hat{I}_1}{N_1} + p_{21}\frac{\hat{I}_2}{N_2}\right) + \beta_2 p_{22}\left(p_{12}\frac{\hat{I}_1}{N_1} + p_{22}\frac{\hat{I}_2}{N_2}\right) + \varepsilon_2\beta_2 p_{22}\frac{\hat{D}_2}{N_2}.$$

Rewriting the expressions of $\hat{I}_i$ and $\hat{D}_i$ in terms of S_i^∞, S_i^0, E_i^0 and I_i^0, we arrive at the following two-patch "approximate" (since we are counting the dead), the final size relation. More precisely, with $N^0 = N$, we have that

$$\begin{aligned}\log\frac{N_1}{S_1^\infty} &= \beta_1 p_{11}\left(\frac{p_{11}\kappa}{\gamma(\kappa+\alpha)}\left(1-\frac{S_1^\infty}{N_1}\right) + \frac{p_{21}\kappa}{\gamma(\kappa+\alpha)}\left(1-\frac{S_2^\infty}{N_2}\right)\right)\\ &+ \beta_2 p_{12}\left(\frac{p_{12}\kappa}{\gamma(\kappa+\alpha)}\left(1-\frac{S_1^\infty}{N_1}\right) + \frac{p_{22}\kappa}{\gamma(\kappa+\alpha)}\left(1-\frac{S_2^\infty}{N_2}\right)\right)\\ &+ \varepsilon_1\beta_1 p_{11}\frac{f_{\text{dead}}}{\nu}\frac{\kappa}{\alpha+\kappa}\left(1-\frac{S_1^\infty}{N_1}\right)\end{aligned}$$

$$\begin{aligned}\log\frac{N_2}{S_2^\infty} &= \beta_1 p_{21}\left(\frac{p_{11}\kappa}{\gamma(\kappa+\alpha)}\left(1-\frac{S_1^\infty}{N_1}\right) + \frac{p_{21}\kappa}{\gamma(\kappa+\alpha)}\left(1-\frac{S_2^\infty}{N_2}\right)\right)\\ &+ \beta_2 p_{22}\left(\frac{p_{12}\kappa}{\gamma(\kappa+\alpha)}\left(1-\frac{S_1^\infty}{N_1}\right) + \frac{p_{22}\kappa}{\gamma(\kappa+\alpha)}\left(1-\frac{S_2^\infty}{N_2}\right)\right)\\ &+ \varepsilon_2\beta_2 p_{22}\frac{f_{\text{dead}}}{\nu}\frac{\kappa}{\alpha+\kappa}\left(1-\frac{S_2^\infty}{N_2}\right)\end{aligned}$$

Or in vectorial notation, we have that

$$\begin{bmatrix}\log\frac{N_1}{S_1^\infty}\\ \\ \log\frac{N_2}{S_2^\infty}\end{bmatrix} = \begin{bmatrix}K_{11} & K_{12}\\ \\ K_{21} & K_{22}\end{bmatrix}\begin{bmatrix}1-\frac{S_1^\infty}{N_1}\\ \\ 1-\frac{S_2^\infty}{N_2}\end{bmatrix} \tag{4}$$

where

$$K_{11} = \left(\frac{\beta_1 p_{11}^2 + \beta_2 p_{12}^2}{\gamma} + \frac{f_{\text{death}} \varepsilon_1 \beta_1 p_{11}}{\nu} \right) \frac{\kappa}{\kappa + \alpha}.$$

Furthermore, we note that $K_{11} = A_1$ also appears in the next generation matrix, used to compute $\mathscr{R}$. Further, we also have that,

$$K_{12} = K_{21} = (\beta_1 p_{11} p_{21} + \beta_2 p_{12} p_{22}) \frac{\kappa}{\gamma(\kappa + \alpha)},$$

$$K_{22} = \left(\frac{\beta_1 p_{21}^2 + \beta_2 p_{22}^2}{\gamma} + \varepsilon_2 \beta_2 p_{22} \frac{f_{\text{dead}}}{\nu} \right) \frac{\kappa}{\alpha + \kappa}$$

Note that the vector in (4) is given by

$$\begin{bmatrix} 1 - \frac{S_1^\infty}{N_1} \\ \\ 1 - \frac{S_2^\infty}{N_2} \end{bmatrix}$$

representing the proportion of people in patches one and two able to transmit Ebola including transmission from handling dead bodies. $K_{12}^2 = K_{12}K_{21} = A_2A_3, K_{22} = A_4$, we conclude that the matrix K and the next generation matrix have the same eigenvalues, a result also found in [4].

5 Simulations

The basic model parameters used in the simulations are taken directly from the literature [11, 14, 24, 26, 33]. We consider two patches and, for simplicity, it is assumed that they house the same number of individuals, namely, $N_1 = N_2 = 1000000$. However, implicitly, it is assumed that the density is considerably higher in the high risk area. We assume that an outbreak starts in the high risk Patch 1 with $\beta_1 = 0.3056$. It propagates into Patch 2, low risk, defined by $\beta_2 = 0.1$. The difference between β_1 and β_2 or $\beta_1 - \beta_2$ provides a rough measure of the capacity to transmit, treat and control Ebola within connected two-patch systems. The initial conditions are set as $S_1(0) = N - 1,\ S_2(0) = N,\ E_{1,2}(0) = 0,\ D_{1,2}(0) = 0,\ R_{1,2}(0) = 0, I_1 = 1, I_2 = 0$. The local basic reproductive numbers for each patch under isolation are $\mathscr{R}_0^1 = 2.41 > 1$ and $\mathscr{R}_0^2 = 1.08 > 1$.

We chose to report on three different mobility scenarios: one way movement, symmetric and asymmetric mobility. For the first case, only residents from Patch 1 travel, that is $p_{12} \geq 0$ and $p_{21} = 0$. Given that Patch 1 is facing an epidemic, it is reasonable to assume that people in Patch 2 prefer to avoid traveling to Patch 1, and so, it is reasonable to assume that $p_{21} = 0$. Mobility is allowed in both directions in a symmetric way, that is, residents of Patch 1 spend the same proportion of time in Patch 2 that individuals from Patch 2 spend in Patch 1; i.e. $p_{21} = p_{12}$. The third scenario assumes that mobility is asymmetric, and so, we make use, in this case, of the relation $p_{21} = 1 - p_{12}$.

5.1 *One Way Mobility*

Simulations show that when only individuals from Patch 1 are allowed to travel, the prevalence and final size are lower that under a cordon sanitaire. Figure 3, shows the levels of Patch prevalence when $p_{12} = 0, 20, 40$ and $60\,\%$. For low p_{12}'s, prevalence decreases in Patch 1 but remains high in both patches, which as expected, has a direct impact in the final size of the outbreak.

In Fig. 4, simulations show that the total final size is only greater than the cordoned case when $p_{12} = 20\,\%$, possibly the result of the assumption that $\gamma_1 = \gamma_2$ and $\nu_1 = \nu_2$. However, we see under the assumption of higher body disposal rates in Patch 2, that the total final size under $p_{12} = 20\,\%$ may turn out to be smaller than in the cordoned case. That is, it is conceivable that a safer Patch 2, may emerge as a result of a better health care infrastructure and efficient protocols in the handling of dead bodies.

Finally, Fig. 4 shows that mobility can produce the opposite effect; that is, reduce the total final epidemic size, given that (for the parameters used) the residence times are greater than $p_{12} = 25\,\%$ but smaller than $p_{12} = 94\,\%$.

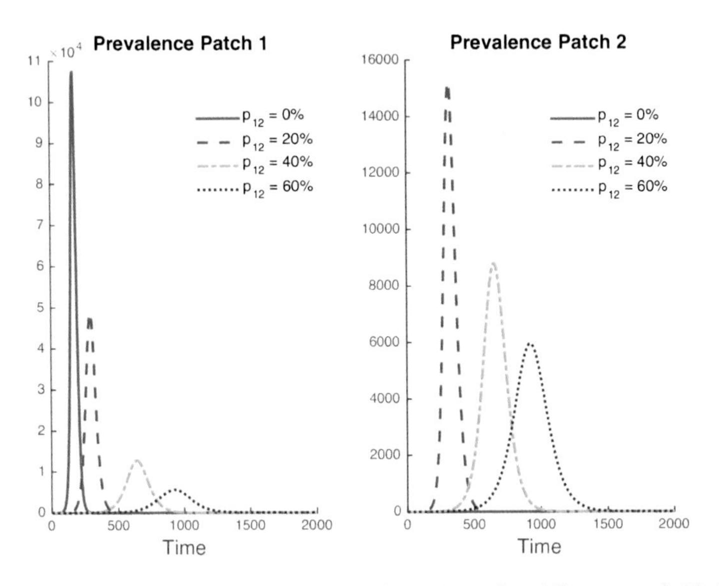

Fig. 3 Dynamics of prevalence in each Patch for values of mobility $p_{12} = 0, 20, 40, 60\,\%$ and $p_{21} = 0$, with parameters: $\varepsilon_{1,2} = 1.2$, $\beta_1 = 0.305$, $\beta_2 = 0.1$, $f_{death} = 0.708$, $k = 1/7$, $\alpha = 0$, $\nu = 1/2$, $\gamma = 1/6.5$

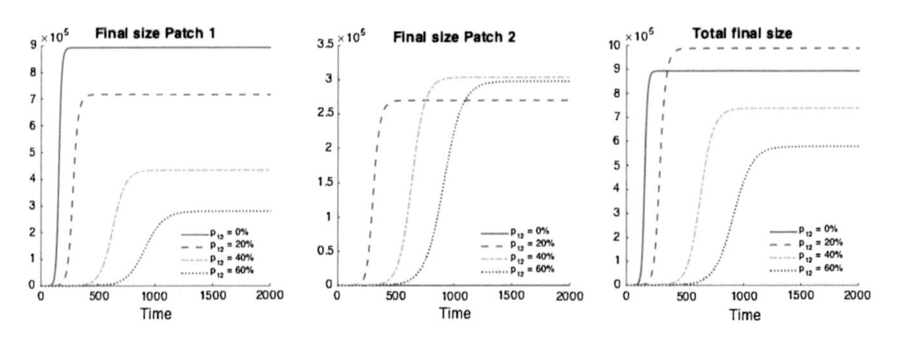

Fig. 4 Dynamics of prevalence in each Patch for values of mobility $p_{12} = 0, 20, 40, 60\,\%$ and $p_{21} = 0$, with parameters: $\varepsilon_{1,2} = 1, \beta_1 = 0.305, \beta_2 = 0.1, f_{death} = 0.708, k = 1/7, \alpha = 0, \nu = 1/2, \gamma = 1/6.5$

5.2 Symmetric Mobility

Simulations under symmetric mobility show that prevalence and final size are severely affected when compared to the cordoned case. Figure 5 shows that the prevalence in Patch 1 exhibits the same behavior as in the one way scenario. However, in this case the prevalence in Patch 1 is decreasing at a slower rate due to the secondary infections produced by individuals traveling from Patch 2. On the other hand, prevalence in Patch 2 is much bigger than in the one way scenario, the result of secondary infections generated by individuals traveling from Patch 2 to Patch 1.

We saw that final size in Patch 1 decreases when residency increases while an increment of the final size in Patch 2. That is, the total final size curve may turn out to be greater than in the cordoned case for almost all residence times. As seen in Fig. 6, allowing symmetric travel would negatively affect the total final size (almost always).

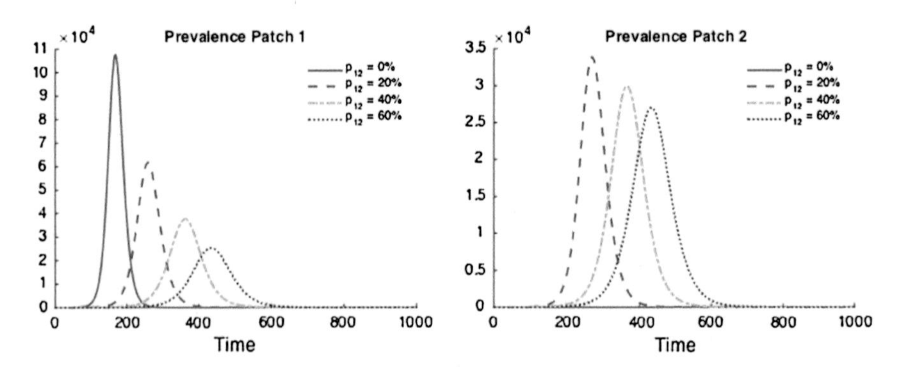

Fig. 5 Dynamics of prevalence in each Patch for values of mobility $p_{12} = 0, 20, 40, 60\,\%$ and $p_{21} = 0$, with parameters: $\varepsilon_{1,2} = 1.2, \beta_1 = 0.305, \beta_2 = 0.1, f_{death} = 0.708, k = 1/7, \alpha = 0, \nu = 1/2, \gamma = 1/6.5$

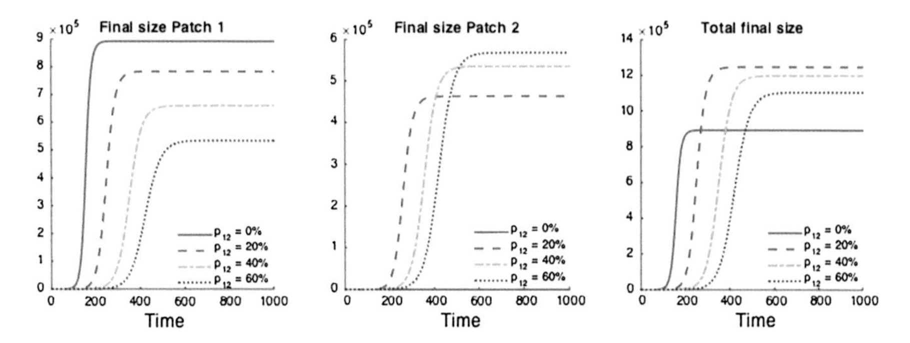

Fig. 6 Dynamics of prevalence in each Patch for values of mobility $p_{12} = 0, 20, 40, 60\,\%$ and $p_{21} = 0$, with parameters: $\varepsilon_{1,2} = 1.2$, $\beta_1 = 0.305$, $\beta_2 = 0.1$, $f_{death} = 0.708$, $k = 1/7$, $\alpha = 0$, $\nu = 1/2$, $\gamma = 1/6.5$

5.3 *Final Size Analysis*

In order to clarify the effects of residence times and mobility on the total final size. We analyze its behavior under one way and symmetric mobility (Fig. 7). Figure 7a shows, one way mobility, the existence of a proportional resident time interval when the total final size is reduced below that generated under the cordoned case. For residence times between 25 and 94 %. In particular, the best case scenario takes place when $p_{12} = 58\,\%$, that is, when the final size reaches its all time minimum.

Figure 7b shows that under symmetric mobility, the total final size increases for almost all resident times. Therefore traveling under these initial conditions has a deleterious effect to the overall population for almost all residence times.

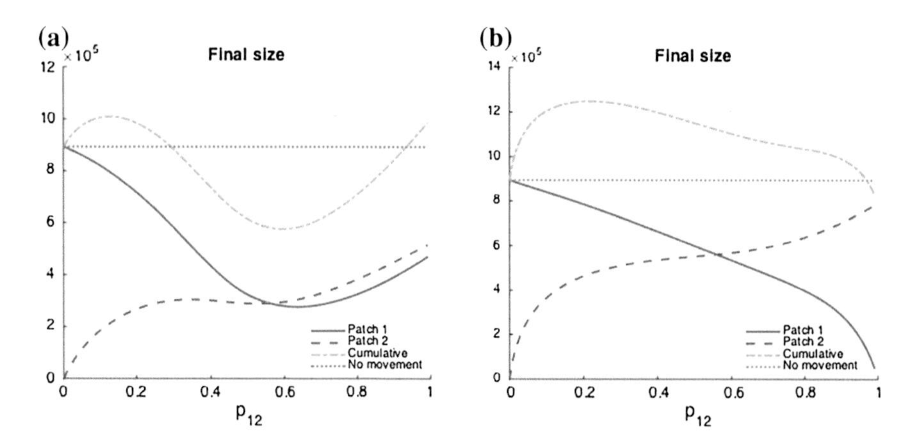

Fig. 7 Dynamics of maximum final size and maximum prevalence in Patch-one with parameters: $\varepsilon_{1,2} = 1.2$, $\beta_1 = 0.305$, $\beta_2 = 0.1$, $f_{death} = 0.708$, $k = 1/7$, $\alpha = 0$, $\nu = 1/2$, $\gamma = 1/6.5$

5.4 Final Size and Basic Reproductive Number Analysis

It is important to notice that reductions in the total final size are related not only to residence times and mobility type but also to the prevailing infection rates. In Fig. 8 simulations show the existence of an interval of residence times for which the total final size is less than the final size under the cordoned case under $\beta_2 < 0.12$.

Simulations (see Fig. 9) show that mobility is always beneficial, that is, it reduces the global $\mathscr{R}_0$. However, mobility on its own is not enough to reduce $\mathscr{R}_0$ below the threshold (less than 1). Bringing $\mathscr{R}_0 < 1$ would require reducing local risk, that is, getting a lower β_2.

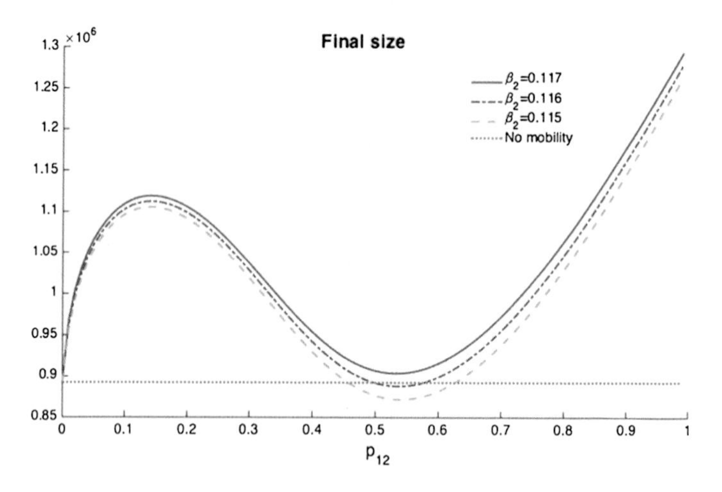

Fig. 8 Dynamics of maximum final size in the one way case with parameters: $\varepsilon_{1,2} = 1.2$, $\beta_1 = 0.305$, $\beta_2 = 0.122, 0.12, 0.118$, $f_{death} = 0.708$, $k = 1/7$, $\alpha = 0$, $\nu = 1/2$, $\gamma = 1/6.5$

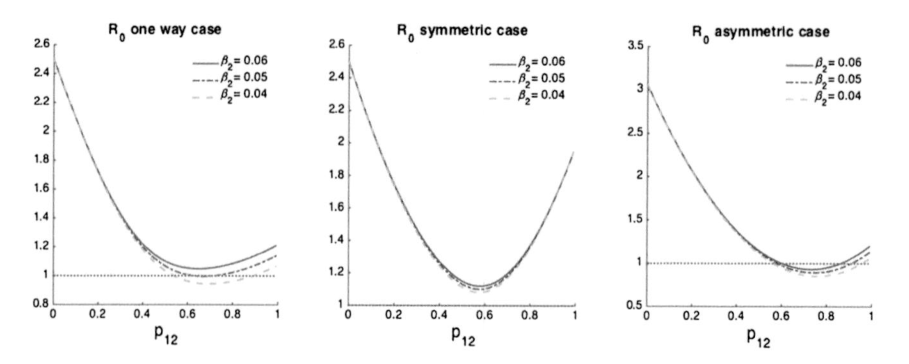

Fig. 9 Dynamics of $\mathscr{R}_0$ with parameters: $\varepsilon_{1,2} = 1.2$, $\beta_1 = 0.305$, $\beta_2 = 0.06, 0.05, 0.04$, $f_{death} = 0.708$, $k = 1/7$, $\alpha = 0$, $\nu = 1/2$, $\gamma = 1/6.5$

6 Conclusion

A West-Africa calibrated two-patch model of the transmission dynamics of EVD is used to show that the use of *cordons sanitaires* not always leads to the best possible global scenario and neither does allowing indiscriminate mobility. Mobility may reduced the total epidemic size as long as the low risk Patch 2 is "safe enough", otherwise mobility would produce a detrimental effect. Having an infection rate $\beta_2 < 0.12$ in Patch 2 guarantees (under our simulations) the existence of non-trivial residence times that reduce the total final size under one way mobility. The global basic reproductive number may be brought bellow one by mobility, whenever a the transmission rate in Patch 2 is low enough. Finally, the choice of non zero α, that is, the recovery rate of asymptomatic that do not develop infection, bring the reproduction number $\mathscr{R}_0$ below one much faster for one way mobility than the case of $\alpha = 0$ for a wide range of residence times.

Acknowledgments We want to thank Kamal Barley for providing us the Fig. 2. These studies were made possible by grant #1R01GM100471-01 from the National Institute of General Medical Sciences (NIGMS) at the National Institutes of Health. The contents of this manuscript are solely the responsibility of the authors and do not necessarily represent the official views of DHS or NIGMS. The funders had no role in study design, data collection and analysis, decision to publish, or preparation of the manuscript.

Appendix 1: Computation of $\mathscr{R}_0$ and Final Epidemic Size

Let us consider the infected compartments, i.e. E, I and D. By following the next generation approach [16, 34], we have that:

$$\mathscr{F} = \begin{pmatrix} \beta S \frac{I}{N} + \varepsilon \beta S \frac{D}{N} \\ 0 \\ 0 \end{pmatrix} \quad \text{and} \quad \mathscr{V} = \begin{pmatrix} -(\kappa + \alpha) E \\ \kappa E - \gamma I \\ f_{\text{dead}} \gamma I - \nu D \end{pmatrix}$$

thus, we have:

$$\mathscr{D}\mathscr{F} = \begin{pmatrix} 0 & \beta \frac{S}{N} & \varepsilon \beta \frac{S}{N} \\ 0 & 0 & 0 \\ 0 & 0 & 0 \end{pmatrix} \quad \text{and} \quad \mathscr{D}V = \begin{pmatrix} -(\kappa + \alpha) & 0 & 0 \\ \kappa & -\gamma & 0 \\ 0 & f_{\text{dead}} \gamma & -\nu \end{pmatrix}.$$

At the DFE, $S = N$, hence

$$F = \begin{pmatrix} 0 & \beta & \varepsilon\beta \\ 0 & 0 & 0 \\ 0 & 0 & 0 \end{pmatrix} \quad \text{and} \quad V = \begin{pmatrix} -(\kappa + \alpha) & 0 & 0 \\ \kappa & -\gamma & 0 \\ 0 & f_{\text{dead}} \gamma & -\nu \end{pmatrix},$$

and the basic reproduction number is the spectral radius of the next generation matrix:

$$-FV^{-1} = \begin{pmatrix} \frac{\kappa\beta}{(\kappa+\alpha)\gamma} + \frac{\varepsilon\kappa f_{\text{dead}}\beta}{(\kappa+\alpha)\nu} & \frac{\beta}{\gamma} + \frac{\varepsilon f_{\text{dead}}\beta}{\nu} & \frac{\varepsilon\beta}{\nu} \\ 0 & 0 & 0 \\ 0 & 0 & 0 \end{pmatrix}.$$

Thus the basic reproduction number is

$$\mathscr{R}_0 = \left(\frac{\beta}{\gamma} + \frac{\varepsilon f_{\text{dead}}\beta}{\nu}\right)\frac{\kappa}{\kappa+\alpha},$$

The total population of system (1) is constant, we can consider only the system

$$\begin{cases} \dot{S} = -\beta S\frac{I}{N} - \varepsilon\beta S\frac{D}{N} \\ \dot{E} = \beta S\frac{I}{N} + \varepsilon_D\beta S\frac{D}{N} - (\kappa+\alpha)E \\ \dot{I} = \kappa E - \gamma I \\ \dot{D} = f_{\text{dead}}\gamma I - \nu D \end{cases} \tag{5}$$

We suppose $S(0) = N$, $E(0) = I(0) = D(0) = 0$. By summing the first two equations of (5), we have: $\dot{S} + \dot{E} = -(\kappa+\alpha)E \leq 0$. This implies that $E^{\infty} = 0$. Similarly by adding the first three and first four equations, we will have $I^{\infty} = 0$ and $D^{\infty} = 0$.

By integrating the first 2 equations, we have $S^{\infty} - N = -(\kappa+\alpha)\hat{E}$. Hence $\hat{E} = \dfrac{N - S^{\infty}}{\kappa+\alpha}$

Similarly, we have $\hat{I} = \dfrac{\kappa}{\gamma(\kappa+\alpha)}(N - S^{\infty})$ and $\hat{D} = \dfrac{f_{\text{dead}}}{\nu}\dfrac{\kappa}{\kappa+\alpha}(N - S^{\infty})$

By using the first equation, we have:

$$\log\frac{N}{S^{\infty}} = \frac{\beta}{\gamma}\frac{\kappa}{\kappa+\alpha}\frac{N-S^{\infty}}{N} + \varepsilon\beta\frac{f_{\text{dead}}}{\nu}\frac{\kappa}{\kappa+\alpha}\frac{N-S^{\infty}}{N}$$

Hence, we have the final epidemic relation:

$$\log\frac{N}{S^{\infty}} = \mathscr{R}_0\left(1 - \frac{S^{\infty}}{N}\right)$$

Appendix 2: Basic Reproduction Number and Final Epidemic Size in Heterogeneous Risk Environments

In heterogeneous risk environments let us consider the infected compartments, i.e. E_1, I_1, D_1, E_2, I_2 and D_2. By following the next generation approach, we have:

$$\mathscr{F} = \begin{pmatrix} \beta_1 p_{11} S_1 \left(p_{11}\frac{I_1}{N_1} + p_{21}\frac{I_2}{N_2}\right) + \beta_2 p_{12} S_1 \left(p_{12}\frac{I_1}{N_1} + p_{22}\frac{I_2}{N_2}\right) + \varepsilon_1 \beta_1 p_{11} S_1 \frac{D_1}{N_1} \\ 0 \\ 0 \\ \beta_1 p_{21} S_2 \left(p_{11}\frac{I_1}{N_1} + p_{21}\frac{I_2}{N_2}\right) + \beta_2 p_{22} S_2 \left(p_{12}\frac{I_1}{N_1} + p_{22}\frac{I_2}{N_2}\right) + \varepsilon_2 \beta_2 p_{22} S_2 \frac{D_2}{N_2} \\ 0 \\ 0 \end{pmatrix}$$

And

$$\mathscr{V} = \begin{pmatrix} -(\kappa+\alpha)E_1 \\ \kappa E_1 - \gamma I_1 \\ f_{\text{dead}}\gamma I_1 - \nu D_1 \\ -(\kappa+\alpha)E_2 \\ \kappa E_2 - \gamma I_2 \\ f_{\text{dead}}\gamma I_2 - \nu D_2 \end{pmatrix}$$

Hence, we have:

$$\mathscr{D}\mathscr{F} = \begin{pmatrix} 0 & \beta_1 p_{11}^2 \frac{S_1}{N_1} + \beta_2 p_{12}^2 \frac{S_1}{N_1} & \beta_1 p_{11} \varepsilon_1 \frac{S_1}{N_1} & 0 & \beta_1 p_{11} p_{21} \frac{S_1}{N_2} + \beta_1 1 p_{12} p_{22} \frac{S_1}{N_2} & 0 \\ 0 & 0 & 0 & 0 & 0 & 0 \\ 0 & 0 & 0 & 0 & 0 & 0 \\ 0 & \beta_1 p_{11} p_{21} \frac{S_2}{N_1} + \beta 1 p_{12} p_{22} \frac{S_2}{N_1} & 0 & 0 & \beta_1 p_{21}^2 \frac{S_2}{N_2} + \beta_2 p_{22}^2 \frac{S_2}{N_2} & \beta_2 p_{22} \varepsilon_2 \frac{S_2}{N_2} \\ 0 & 0 & 0 & 0 & 0 & 0 \\ 0 & 0 & 0 & 0 & 0 & 0 \end{pmatrix}$$

and

$$\mathscr{D}\mathscr{V} = \begin{pmatrix} -(\kappa+\alpha) & 0 & 0 & 0 & 0 & 0 \\ \kappa & -\gamma & 0 & 0 & 0 & 0 \\ 0 & f_{\text{death}}\gamma & -\nu & 0 & 0 & 0 \\ 0 & 0 & 0 & -(\kappa+\alpha) & 0 & 0 \\ 0 & 0 & 0 & \kappa & -\gamma & 0 \\ 0 & 0 & 0 & 0 & f_{\text{death}}\gamma & -\nu \end{pmatrix}$$

At the DFE, $S_1^* = N_1$ and $S_2^* = N_2$, hence

$$F = \begin{pmatrix} 0 & \beta_1 p_{11}^2 + \beta_2 p_{12}^2 & \beta_1 p_{11} \varepsilon_1 & 0 & \beta_1 p_{11} p_{21} \frac{N_1}{N_2} + \beta_1 1 p_{12} p_{22} \frac{N_1}{N_2} & 0 \\ 0 & 0 & 0 & 0 & 0 & 0 \\ 0 & 0 & 0 & 0 & 0 & 0 \\ 0 & \beta_1 p_{11} p_{21} \frac{N_2}{N_1} + \beta 1 p_{12} p_{22} \frac{N_2}{N_1} & 0 & 0 & \beta_1 p_{21}^2 + \beta_2 p_{22}^2 & \beta_2 p_{22} \varepsilon_2 \\ 0 & 0 & 0 & 0 & 0 & 0 \\ 0 & 0 & 0 & 0 & 0 & 0 \end{pmatrix}$$

and

$$V = \begin{pmatrix} -(\kappa+\alpha) & 0 & 0 & 0 & 0 & 0 \\ \kappa & -\gamma & 0 & 0 & 0 & 0 \\ 0 & f_{\text{death}}\gamma & -\nu & 0 & 0 & 0 \\ 0 & 0 & 0 & -(\kappa+\alpha) & 0 & 0 \\ 0 & 0 & 0 & \kappa & -\gamma & 0 \\ 0 & 0 & 0 & 0 & f_{\text{death}}\gamma & -\nu \end{pmatrix}$$

The basic reproduction number is the spectral radius of the next generation matrix:

$$-FV^{-1} = \begin{pmatrix} A_1 & A_2 & \frac{\beta_1 p_{11}\varepsilon_1}{\nu} & A_3 & A_4 & 0 \\ 0 & 0 & 0 & 0 & 0 & 0 \\ 0 & 0 & 0 & 0 & 0 & 0 \\ A_5 & A_6 & 0 & A_7 & A_8 & \frac{\beta_2 p_{22}\varepsilon_2}{\nu} \\ 0 & 0 & 0 & 0 & 0 & 0 \\ 0 & 0 & 0 & 0 & 0 & 0 \end{pmatrix}$$

where

$$A_1 = \left(\frac{\beta_1 p_{11}^2 + \beta_2 p_{12}^2}{\gamma} + \frac{f_{\text{death}}\varepsilon_1 p_{11}\beta_1}{\nu}\right)\frac{\kappa}{\kappa+\alpha},$$

$$A_2 = \frac{\beta_1 p_{11}^2 + \beta_2 p_{12}^2}{\gamma} + \frac{f_{\text{death}}\varepsilon_1\beta_1 p_{11}}{\nu},$$

$$A_3 = (\beta_1 p_{11}p_{21} + \beta_2 p_{12}p_{22})\frac{N_1}{N_2}\frac{\kappa}{\gamma(\kappa+\alpha)},$$

$$A_4 = (\beta_1 p_{11}p_{21} + \beta_2 p_{12}p_{22})\frac{N_1}{\gamma N_2},$$

$$A_5 = (\beta_1 p_{11}p_{21} + \beta_2 p_{12}p_{22})\frac{N_2}{N_1}\frac{\kappa}{\gamma(\kappa+\alpha)} = \left(\frac{N_2}{N_1}\right)^2 A_3,$$

$$A_6 = \frac{1}{\gamma}(\beta_1 p_{11}p_{21} + \beta_2 p_{12}p_{22})\frac{N_2}{N_1},$$

$$A_5 = (\beta_1 p_{11}p_{21} + \beta_2 p_{12}p_{22})\frac{N_2}{N_1}\frac{\kappa}{\gamma(\kappa+\alpha)} = \left(\frac{N_2}{N_1}\right)^2 A_3,$$

$$A_6 = \frac{1}{\gamma}(\beta_1 p_{11}p_{21} + \beta_2 p_{12}p_{22})\frac{N_2}{N_1},$$

$$A_7 = \left(\frac{\beta_1 p_{21}^2 + \beta_2 p_{22}^2}{\gamma} + \frac{f_{\text{death}}\varepsilon_2\beta_2 p_{22}}{\nu}\right)\frac{\kappa}{\kappa+\alpha},$$

$$A_8 = \frac{\beta_1 p_{21}^2 + \beta_2 p_{22}^2}{\gamma} + \frac{f_{\text{death}}\varepsilon_2\beta_2 p_{22}}{\nu}.$$

We can easily see that $-FV^{-1}$ has the same nonzero eigenvalues as the matrix

$$\begin{pmatrix} A_1 & A_3 \\ A_5 & A_7 \end{pmatrix} = \begin{pmatrix} \tilde{A}_1 & \tilde{A}_2 \\ \tilde{A}_3 & \tilde{A}_4 \end{pmatrix}$$

$$\begin{aligned}
\mathscr{R}_0 &= \frac{1}{2}\left(\tilde{A}_1 + \tilde{A}_4 + \sqrt{(\tilde{A}_1 + \tilde{A}_4)^2 - 4(\tilde{A}_1\tilde{A}_4 - \tilde{A}_2\tilde{A}_3)}\right)\frac{\kappa}{\kappa+\alpha} \\
&= \frac{1}{2}\left(\tilde{A}_1 + \tilde{A}_4 + \sqrt{\tilde{A}_1^2 + \tilde{A}_4^2 + 2\tilde{A}_1\tilde{A}_4 - 4(\tilde{A}_1\tilde{A}_4 - \tilde{A}_2\tilde{A}_3)}\right) \\
&= \frac{1}{2}\left(\tilde{A}_1 + \tilde{A}_4 + \sqrt{\tilde{A}_1^2 + \tilde{A}_4^2 - 2\tilde{A}_1\tilde{A}_4 + 4\tilde{A}_2\tilde{A}_3}\right)
\end{aligned}$$

More precisely, we have:

$$\mathscr{R}_0 = \frac{\kappa}{2(\kappa+\alpha)}\left(\frac{\beta_1 p_{11}^2 + \beta_2 p_{12}^2}{\gamma} + \frac{f_{\text{death}}\varepsilon_1\beta_1 p_{11}}{\nu} + \frac{\beta_1 p_{21}^2 + \beta_2 p_{22}^2}{\gamma} + \frac{f_{\text{death}}\varepsilon_2\beta_2 p_{22}}{\nu}\right.$$

$$\left. + \sqrt{\begin{array}{l} \left(\frac{\beta_1 p_{11}^2 + \beta_2 p_{12}^2}{\gamma} + \frac{f_{\text{death}}\varepsilon_1\beta_1 p_{11}}{\nu}\right)^2 + \left(\frac{\beta_1 p_{21}^2 + \beta_2 p_{22}^2}{\gamma} + \frac{f_{\text{death}}\varepsilon_2\beta_2 p_{22}}{\nu}\right)^2 \\ -2\left(\frac{\beta_1 p_{11}^2 + \beta_2 p_{12}^2}{\gamma} + \frac{f_{\text{death}}\varepsilon_1\beta_1 p_{11}}{\nu}\right)\left(\frac{\beta_1 p_{21}^2 + \beta_2 p_{22}^2}{\gamma} + \frac{f_{\text{death}}\varepsilon_2\beta_2 p_{22}}{\nu}\right) \\ +4\left(\beta_1 p_{11} p_{21}\frac{N_1}{\gamma N_2} + \beta_1 p_{12} p_{22}\frac{N_1}{\gamma N_2}\right)\left(\beta_1 p_{11} p_{21}\frac{N_2}{N_1} + \beta_1 p_{12} p_{22}\frac{N_2}{N_1}\right) \end{array}}\right)$$

References

1. Baxter, A.G.: Symptomless infection with Ebola virus. Lancet **355**, 2178–2179 (2000)
2. Bellan, S.E., Pulliam, J.R.C.: Ebola control: effect of asymptomatic infection and acquired immunity. Lancet **384**(9953), 1499–1500 (2014)
3. Bichara, D., Castillo-Chavez, C.: Vector-borne diseases models with residence times - a Lagrangian perspective. arXiv preprint arXiv:1509.08894 (2015)
4. Bichara, D., Kang, Y., Castillo-Chavez, C., Horan, R., Perrings, C.: SIS and SIR epidemic models under virtual dispersal. Bull. Math. Biol. (2015). doi:10.1007/s11538-015-0113-5
5. Bogoch, I.I., Creatore, M.I., Cetron, M.S., Brownstein, J.S., Pesik, N., Miniota, J., Tam, T., Hu, W., Nicolucci, A., Ahmed, S., et al.: Assessment of the potential for international dissemination of Ebola virus via commercial air travel during the: West African outbreak. Lancet **385**(2015), 29–35 (2014)
6. Brauer, F.: Some simple epidemic models. Math. Biosci. Eng. **3**, 1–45 (2006)
7. Brauer, F.: Age of infection and final epidemic size. Math. Biosci. Eng. **5**, 681–690 (2008)
8. Brauer, F., Watmough, J.: Age of infection epidemic models with heterogeneous mixing. J. Biol. Dyn. **3**, 324–330 (2009)

9. Byrne, J.P.: Encyclopedia of Pestilence, Pandemics, and Plagues: AM, vol. 1. ABC-CLIO, Santa Barbara (2008)
10. Castillo-Chavez, C., Song, B., Zhangi, J.: An epidemic model with virtual mass transportation: the case of smallpox. Bioterrorism Math. Model. Appl. Homel. Secur. **28**, 173 (2003)
11. Chowell, D., Castillo-Chavez, C., Krishna, S., Qiu, X., Anderson, K.S.: Modelling the effect of early detection of Ebola. Lancet Infect. Dis. **15**, 148–149 (2015)
12. Chowell, G., Hengartner, N., Castillo-Chavez, C., Fenimore, P., Hyman, J.: The basic reproductive number of Ebola and the effects of public health measures: the cases of Congo and Uganda. J. Theor. Biol. **229**, 119–126 (2004)
13. Chowell, G., Hyman, J.M., Eubank, S., Castillo-Chavez, C.: Scaling laws for the movement of people between locations in a large city. Phys. Rev. E **68**, 066102 (2003)
14. Chowell, G., Nishiura, H.: Transmission dynamics and control of Ebola virus disease (EVD): a review. BMC Med. **12**, 196 (2014)
15. Chowell, G., Viboud, C., Hyman, J.M., Simonsen, L.: The Western Africa Ebola virus disease epidemic exhibits both global exponential and local polynomial growth rates. PLoS Curr. **7** (2014)
16. Diekmann, O., Heesterbeek, J.A.P., Metz, J.A.J.: On the definition and the computation of the basic reproduction ratio R_0 in models for infectious diseases in heterogeneous populations. J. Math. Biol. **28**, 365–382 (1990)
17. Donald, G., McNeil, Jr.: NYT: Using a Tactic Unseen in a Century, Countries Cordon Off Ebola-Racked Areas, 12 Aug 2014
18. Eubank, S., Guclu, H., Kumar, V.A., Marathe, M.V., Srinivasan, A., Toroczkai, Z., Wang, N.: Modelling disease outbreaks in realistic urban social networks. Nature **429**, 180–184 (2004)
19. Gomes, M.F., y Piontti, A.P., Rossi, L., Chao, D., Longini, I., Halloran, M.E., Vespignani, A.: Assessing the international spreading risk associated with the West African Ebola outbreak. PLoS Curr. **6** (2014)
20. Hawryluck, L., Gold, W.L., Robinson, S., Pogorski, S., Galea, S., Styra, R., et al.: Sars control and psychological effects of quarantine, Toronto, Canada. Emerg. Infect. Dis. **10**, 1206–1212 (2004)
21. Heffern, R.T., Pambo, B., Hatchett, R.J., Leman, P.A., Swanepoel, R., Ryder, R.W.: Low seroprevalence of IgG antibodies to Ebola virus in an epidemic zone: Ogooué-Ivindo region, Northeastern Gabon. J. Infect. Dis. **191**(2005), 964–968 (1995)
22. Hethcote, H.W.: The mathematics of infectious diseases. SIAM Rev. **42**, 599–653 (2000) (electronic)
23. House, T.: Epidemiological dynamics of Ebola outbreaks. Elife **3**, e03908 (2014)
24. Legrand, J., Grais, R.F., Boelle, P.Y., Valleron, A.J., Flahault, A.: Understanding the dynamics of Ebola epidemics. Epidemiol. Infect. **135**, 610–621 (2007)
25. Lekone, P.E., Finkenstädt, B.F.: Statistical inference in a stochastic epidemic SEIR model with control intervention: Ebola as a case study. Biometrics **62**, 1170–1177 (2006)
26. Leroy, E., Blaise, S., Volchkov, V.: Human asymptomatic Ebola infection and strong inflammatory response. Lancet **355**, 2210–2215 (2000)
27. Nishiura, H., Chowell, G.: Early transmission dynamics of Ebola virus disease (EVD), West Africa, March to August 2014. Eur. Surveill. **19**(36) (2014)
28. Pandey, A., Atkins, K.E., Medlock, J., Wenzel, N., Townsend, J.P., Childs, J.E., Nyenswah, T.G., Ndeffo-Mbah, M.L., Galvani, A.P.: Strategies for containing Ebola in West Africa. Science **346**, 991–995 (2014)
29. Peters, C.J., LeDuc, J.W., An introduction to Ebola: the virus and the disease. J. Infect. Dis. **179**(Suppl 1), ix–xvi (1999)
30. Poletto, C., Gomes, M.F., y Piontti, A.P., Rossi, L., Bioglio, L., Chao, D.L., Longini, I.M., Halloran, M.E., Colizza, V., Vespignani, A.: Assessing the impact of travel restrictions on international spread of the 2014 West African Ebola epidemic, Euro surveillance: bulletin Europeen sur les maladies transmissibles = European communicable disease bulletin **19** (2014)
31. Stroud, P., Del Valle, S., Sydoriak, S., Riese, J., Mniszewski, S.: Spatial dynamics of pandemic influenza in a massive artificial society. J. Artif. Soc. Soc. Simul. **10**, 9 (2007)

32. Towers, S., Patterson-Lomba, O., Castillo-Chavez, C.: Emerging disease dynamics: the case of Ebola, April 2014
33. Towers, S., Patterson-Lomba, O., Castillo-Chavez, C.: Temporal variations in the effective reproduction number of the 2014 West Africa Ebola outbreak. PloS Curr. Outbreaks **1** (2014)
34. van den Driessche, P., Watmough, J.: Reproduction numbers and sub-threshold endemic equilibria for compartmental models of disease transmission. Math. Biosci. **180**, 29–48 (2002)
35. World Health Organization: Ebola virus disease, April 2015

Patch Models of EVD Transmission Dynamics

Bruce Pell, Javier Baez, Tin Phan, Daozhou Gao, Gerardo Chowell and Yang Kuang

Abstract Mathematical models have the potential to be useful to forecast the course of epidemics. In this chapter, a family of logistic patch models are preliminarily evaluated for use in disease modeling and forecasting. Here we also derive the logistic equation in an infectious disease transmission context based on population behavior and used it for forecasting the trajectories of the 2013–2015 Ebola epidemic in West Africa. The logistic model is then extended to include spatial population heterogeneity by using multi-patch models that incorporate migration between patches and logistic growth within each patch. Each model's ability to forecast epidemic data was assessed by comparing model forecasting error, parameter distributions and parameter confidence intervals as functions of the number of data points used to calibrate the models. The patch models show an improvement over the logistic model in short-term forecasting, but naturally require the estimation of more parameters from limited data.

Keywords Logistic equation · Infectious disease forecasting · Patch model · Ebola · Behavior change · Bootstrap

1 Introduction

The 2013–2015 Ebola epidemic in West Africa has become the most severe Ebola virus disease (EVD0) outbreak in history, with a case fatality rate of 70–71 % and

B. Pell · J. Baez · T. Phan · Y. Kuang (✉)
Arizona State, Tempe, USA
e-mail: kuang@asu.edu

B. Pell
e-mail: bepell@asu.edu

D. Gao
Mathematics and Science College, Shanghai Normal University, Shanghai 200234, China

G. Chowell
School of Public Health, Georgia State University, Atlanta, GA 30302, USA

G. Chowell and J.M. Hyman (eds.), *Mathematical and Statistical Modeling for Emerging and Re-emerging Infectious Diseases*,
DOI 10.1007/978-3-319-40413-4_10

a hospitalized fatality rate of 57–59 % [7, 23, 24]. This epidemic is significantly different in both size and duration compared to previously reported EVD epidemics. As of August 30, 2015, over 28,000 cases have been reported, of which over 11,000 patients have succumbed to the disease, making it the deadliest Ebola epidemic in history [24]. This latest outbreak far surpasses the number of reported cases and deaths from ten major previous ebola outbreaks combined with an estimated 1,531 cases and 1,002 deaths [6].

Although, EVD was first discovered in 1976, the virus had not triggered a major regional epidemic until Dec. 2013. Standard practices to prevent the outbreak in these countries were not as effective partly due to their poor health infrastructure, including the lack of public health surveillance systems to rapidly detect emerging outbreaks [11]. In addition, no licensed vaccine against EVD was available during the 2013–2015 epidemic [1, 26]. Instead, quarantine, isolation and education programs were used to mitigate the spread of the disease.

Measuring the effect that control interventions have on epidemics can be achieved by measuring shifts in R_0 and $R_e(t)$, the basic and effective reproduction numbers, respectively. R_0 is defined as the average number of secondary infections generated by one infectious agent in a completely susceptible population. Nevertheless, R_0 assumes the epidemic first occurs in a fully susceptible population and thus does not account for time-dependent variations. $R_e(t)$ is defined as the actual average number of new infections by one infectious agent in a population with both infected and uninfected individuals at time t. $R_e(t)$ shows time-dependent variation due to the implementation of control strategies and the decline in susceptible individuals.

Several studies have used mathematical models to quantify the effect that control interventions and behavior changes have on managing the epidemic. In [3], Althaus, employs an SEIR (susceptible-exposed-infectious-removed, [4]) model and the estimated effective reproduction number to gain insights into the real-time intervention effects for the 2013–2015 EVD epidemic. They suggest that the effective reproduction numbers in Guinea and Sierra Leone decreased to around unity by the end of May and July 2014 due to sufficient control measures. However, that was not the case in Liberia where efforts needed to be improved. In a similar spirit, Chowell et al. [8], employed the logistic model to capture early signs of intervention and behavior changes in the population. Furthermore, they showed that phenomenological models are useful for understanding early epidemic dynamics, specifically because of the small number of parameters that need to be estimated. With more complexity, Agusto et al. [2], used a mathematical model to explore the effects of traditional belief systems and customs on the transmission process, concluding that the 2014 outbreaks may be controllable by using a moderately-effective basic public health intervention plan.

Other studies have used mathematical models to investigate the affects of spatial structure on disease dynamics. For instance, Valdez et al. [22], embeds a compartmental model into a 15-patch spatial framework (representing 15 counties of Liberia) and shows that reducing mobility only delays the overall control of the epidemic. Their findings suggest that safe burials and hospitalizations are key to controlling EVD. In particular, if safe burials and hospitalizations were established in mid-July 2014, their model predicts that the epidemic would have been three months shorter and infected individuals would have been 80 % less than if the controls were implemented in mid-August. Gomes et al., employs the Global Epidemic and Mobility Model that incorporates mobility and demographic data at a worldwide scale coupled to a stochastic epidemic model [13]. They concluded that the probability of the disease spreading outside of Africa was highly unlikely. Merler et al., employs a spatial agent-based model to examine the effectiveness of safe burials, household protection kits and to estimate Ebola virus transmission parameters [18]. They suggest that the majority of infections occur within hospitals and households. Their findings indicate that the decline in disease incidence is due in part by the increased number of Ebola treatment units, safe burials and household protection kits. Using a discrete, stochastic SEIR model that is embedded within a three-scale community network model, Kiskowski, shows that effects from community mixing along with stochasticity can explain the different growth rates of reported cases observed in Sierra Leone, Liberia and Guinea [15].

Multiple studies have used mathematical models for forecasting the potential number of future cases and estimating transmission parameters for the 2013–2015 Ebola epidemic. Meltzer et al., constructs the EbolaResponse modeling tool that tracks patients through multiple stages of infection and categorizes patient infectiousness depending on whether they are in a hospital, a low-risk community setting or at home with no isolation [17]. The EbolaResponse model was used to estimate how control and prevention measures could stop the epidemic and to forecast future cases. Meltzer et al., suggest that policy makers rapidly increase the number of Ebola treatment units. In another study by Shaman et al., a stochastic compartmental model is coupled with the Ensemble Adjusted Kalman Filter (EAKF) to forecast state variables and parameters six weeks into the future [21]. The EAKF adjusts the parameters and ensemble state variables as more data becomes available. Parameter estimations provided some evidence that the epidemic growth was slowing down in Liberia.

We present a simple approach that phenomenologically connects the effects of behavior changes to mitigate transmission rates and population spatial structure. Our method derives the logistic equation from an assumption about the effect of population behavior and introduces spatial heterogeneity via logistic patch models. In particular, we contribute the following:

- The logistic model is derived from a susceptible-infected compartmental model in Sect. 2.1, justifying its use in [8].
- Formulas for the basic and effective reproduction numbers are presented in Sect. 2.2.
- We build upon the work done in [8], by incorporating spatial heterogeneity via logistic patch models.
- Models are validated by comparing their fits to total reported case data in Sect. 4.1.
- As seen in Fig. 4, we show that these models improve upon the short term forecasting error in Sect. 4.2. Furthermore we perform Kruskal–Wallis tests to analyze the variation across the different models.
- Further model validation and comparison is presented in Sect. 4.3, via parameter estimations and confidence intervals. This section shows that patch models are not well constrained due to limited data.

- We provide estimates and 95 % confidence intervals of R_0 for Liberia, Sierra Leone and Guinea respectively in Sect. 4.4.

2 Modeling Methods

2.1 *Logistic Equation as an Ebola Cumulative Infections Case Model*

From a basic SI compartmental model and an assumption about population behavior we can derive the logistic equation. Assuming there are no births, natural deaths or immigration of susceptible individuals and that infected individuals do not return to the susceptible class, the classical Kermack and McKendrick infectious disease model can be adapted to obtain the following:

$$\begin{aligned} S(t)' &= -\frac{\beta S(t)I(t)}{S(t)+I(t)}, \\ I(t)' &= \frac{\beta S(t)I(t)}{S(t)+I(t)} - \mu I(t), \end{aligned} \tag{1}$$

where β is the infection rate and μ is the disease induced death rate. From system (1) the cumulative number of infections at time t, denoted by $x(t)$, has derivative $x'(t) = \beta \frac{SI}{S+I} \approx \beta I$, (assuming $\frac{S}{S+I} \approx 1$). Below we assume that $x'(t) = \beta I$.

As an increasing number of cases are reported during an outbreak, the behavior of the individuals in the affected region may change due to disease education programs, an increase in care or quarantine facilities and help from health care workers.

As an example, dead bodies infected with Ebola virus remain infectious, causing participants to unknowingly contract the infection during funeral burials. In the beginning stage of the outbreak, unsuspecting mourners would carry the infection back to other parts of the community and would infect more individuals. By having specific handling guidelines of human remains, communities were able to decrease exposure to the Ebola virus [27]. In general, this is the notion of a positive behavioral change in the community. Based on these observations we make what we call the behavior assumption:

- **(Behavior assumption)**: During an epidemic, a change in behavior in the community that mitigates the transmission rates is expected as an epidemic unfolds. This response is modeled by a function of the total reported cases and has a decreasing effect on per-capita infection rate. That is,

$$\frac{I'(t)}{I(t)} = f(x(t)) \tag{2}$$

is a decreasing function of the total number of reported cases $x(t)$.

In the following, we assume that $f(x(t)) = r(1 - ax(t))$ for some positive constants $r := \beta - \mu$ and a. Hence

$$I'(t) = rI(t)(1 - ax(t)) = \frac{r}{\beta}x'(t)(1 - ax(t)).$$

Therefore,

$$I(t) - I(0) = \frac{r}{\beta}\left(x(t) - \frac{a}{2}[x(t)]^2\right) - \frac{r}{\beta}\left(x(0) - \frac{a}{2}[x(0)]^2\right).$$

Since $I(0) = x(0) \approx 0$, we see that $I(t)$ can be approximated by $\frac{r}{\beta}\left(x(t) - \frac{a}{2}[x(t)]^2\right)$. Therefore

$$x'(t) = \beta I(t) = r\left(x(t) - \frac{a}{2}[x(t)]^2\right) = rx(t)\left(1 - \frac{x(t)}{K}\right), \tag{3}$$

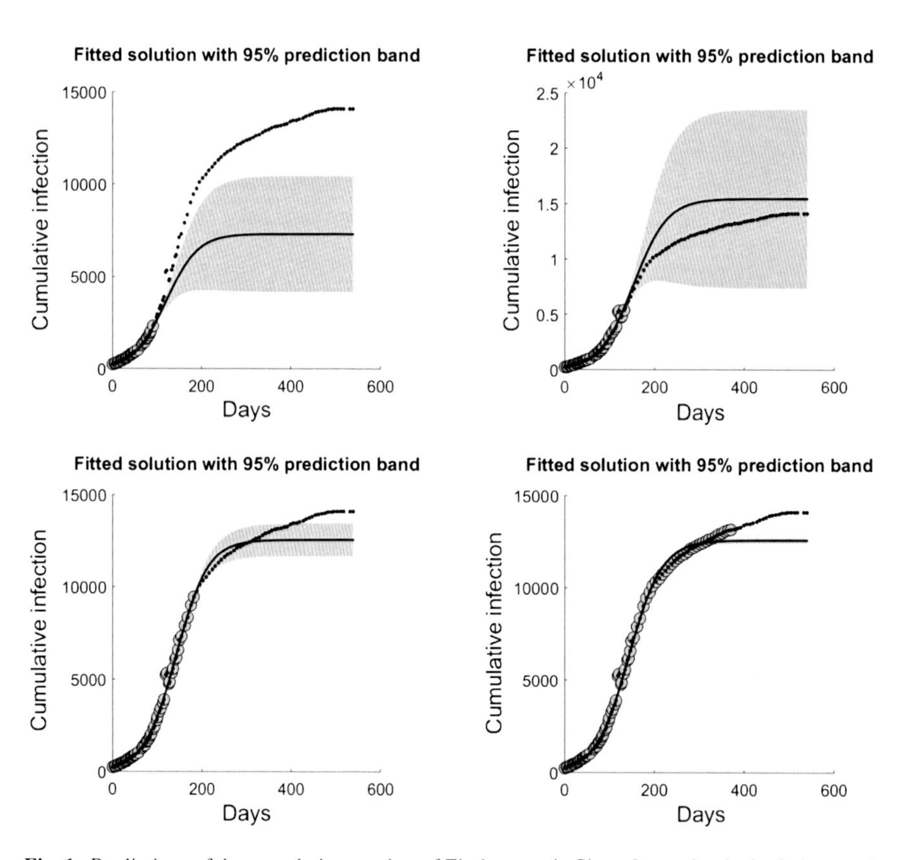

Fig. 1 Predictions of the cumulative number of Ebola cases in Sierra Leone by the logistic growth Eq. (3). Data points start on June 2, 2014 and end December 23, 2015. 95 % prediction bands are superimposed. *Gray disks* are data points for model calibration, while *black dots* are forecasting data points

where $K = 2/a$. Here we interpret r as the *intrinsic infection rate*, a is a proportionality constant that corresponds to strength and effectiveness of disease interventions and preventive strategies and K is the *final epidemic size*.

In [8], the saturation effect of the logistic equation was used to implicitly account for the behavior change in the population. The above derivation provides a rigorous framework of this modeling effort and emphasizes the role behavior plays in the saturation effect. Figure 1 shows the change in the 95 % prediction band using the delta method as more data points are incorporated when fitting the logistic model to epidemic data [5].

2.2 Derivation of R_0 and R_e

During an outbreak, there may not be enough data to calibrate mechanistic models of the exact transmission processes, thus the logistic model can provide useful insights into the early outbreak dynamics. To derive R_0 and R_e first observe that,

$$I(t+T) = R_e(t)\, I(t), \tag{4}$$

where T is the mean generation interval and is defined as the time between infection in an index case patient and infection in a patient infected by that index case patient [23]. From Eq. (2), we have that $I'(t) = f(x(t))\, I(t)$, integrating both sides from t to $t+T$ yields

$$\ln(I(t+T)) - \ln(I(t)) = \int_t^{t+T} f(x(s))\, ds.$$

Solving for $I(t+T)$ and dividing by $I(t)$ yields $\frac{I(t+T)}{I(t)} = e^{\int_t^{t+T} f(x(s))ds}$, which from Eq. (4) yields

$$R_e(t) = e^{\int_t^{t+T} f(x(s))ds}. \tag{5}$$

Lastly, define $R_0 := e^{rT}$ which is approximately equal to the usual definition of the basic reproduction number, $\frac{\beta}{\mu}$, of model 1 when $\frac{\beta}{\mu}$ is close to 1.

2.3 Incorporating Population Heterogeneity: Multi-patch Models

District geography, topology, health care centers and quarantined regions can influence population movement. This motivates the need for incorporating spatial structure in transmission models. We do this by partitioning a district into a network of two or more sub-districts (patches). In each sub-district, cumulative infections obey logistic growth individually.

Let x_i be the **cumulative infections** in patch i and let m_{ij} be the rate of cumulative infections that travel from patch i to patch j, where $i, j = 1, 2, i \neq j$.

The equations for the two-patch model are:

$$x_1' = r_1 x_1 \left(1 - \frac{x_1}{K_1}\right) - m_{12}x_1 + m_{21}x_2,$$

$$x_2' = r_2 x_2 \left(1 - \frac{x_2}{K_2}\right) - m_{21}x_2 + m_{12}x_1.$$

Similarly, the three-patch model is given by:

$$x_1' = r_1 x_1 \left(1 - \frac{x_1}{K_1}\right) - (m_{12} + m_{13})\, x_1 + m_{21}x_2 + m_{31}x_3,$$

$$x_2' = r_2 x_2 \left(1 - \frac{x_2}{K_2}\right) - (m_{21} + m_{23})\, x_2 + m_{12}x_1 + m_{32}x_3,$$

$$x_3' = r_3 x_3 \left(1 - \frac{x_3}{K_3}\right) - (m_{31} + m_{32})\, x_3 + m_{13}x_1 + m_{23}x_2.$$

In addition, we will consider two special cases of each model: symmetric migration (S) with $m_{ij} = m_{ji}$ and homogeneous migration (H) with, $m_{ij} = m$ for all i, j and $i \neq j$.

Assume that r_i and K_i are positive in the above models. It is easy to see that these patch models are cooperative in nature which generate a strictly monotone semiflow. It is shown that the positive solutions of the above models tend to a unique positive steady state (see Lemma 3.1 in [12]).

Let $x = \sum_{i=1}^{N} x_i$. As with the derivation of R_e and R_0 for the logistic model above, define the basic reproduction number for an N-patch model as

$$R_e(t) = \exp\left(\hat{r} \int_t^{t+T} 1 - \frac{2}{\hat{K}} x(s)\, ds\right),$$

where $\hat{r} = \frac{\sum_{i=1}^{N} r_i K_i}{\hat{K}}$, $\hat{K} = \sum_{i=1}^{N} K_i$ are weighted averages and for simplicity we assume $T = 2$ weeks, instead of 2.18 [1]. Similarly to above, we define $R_0 := R_e(0) \approx e^{rT}$.

3 Comparison Methods

We use district data from the World Health Organization (WHO) patient database, which contains weekly reported confirmed, suspected and probable infections from Liberia, Sierra Leone and Guinea [24]. Data ranges from Mar. 1, 2014 to Aug. 5, 2015.

Table 1 Number of parameters for each model

	Logistic	Two-patch (H)	Two-patch	Three-patch (H)	Three-patch (S)	Three-patch
Number of parameters	2	5	6	7	9	12

Table 1 lists the number of parameters of each model. By studying the special cases of the patch models we reduce the number of parameters that need to be estimated, which constrains model fits and reduces the likelihood of over-fitting the data.

We use Matlab's built-in function, fminsearch, to help locate optimized parameter values for data fitting. fminsearch is a derivative-free method that is based on the Nelder-Mead Simplex [16] and searches for minimums, but does not guarantee global minimums. We are searching for a biologically reasonable parameter set that minimizes the error between the simulations and the observed data. To this end, we define the weighted error function:

$$E_w = \frac{1}{N-P}\sum_{i=1}^{N} \left| y_i - \hat{y}_i \right| e^{-0.1(t_f - t_i)}, \tag{6}$$

where t_f is the final date that we have an observation for, P is the number of parameters and N is the number of observations. $\hat{y}_i$ denotes the observation at time t_i and y_i the value of our model at the ith observation. We make the assumption that recent data has higher significance for forecasting future cases, as reflected by the exponential factor. The value of 0.1 in the exponential term is used because it gave a reasonable temporal-weight to the data points.

3.1 *Ranking Models by Fitting and Forecasting Errors*

To compare the models, we use absolute and relative errors that penalize models that have more parameters. The absolute error is calculated using the following equation,

$$E_{abs} = \frac{1}{\sqrt{N-P}}\sqrt{\sum_{i=1}^{N} \left(y_i - \hat{y}_i\right)^2} \tag{7}$$

and the relative error is given by,

$$E_{rel} = \frac{1}{\sqrt{N-P}}\sqrt{\sum_{i=1}^{N} \left(\frac{y_i - \hat{y}_i}{\hat{y}_i}\right)^2}. \tag{8}$$

Since we are interested in assessing and ranking the forecasting performance of all models, we define the *forecasting error* as follows:

$$E_{fcst} = \frac{1}{\sqrt{N - \hat{N} - P}} \sqrt{\sum_{i=i^*}^{N} \left[y(t_i) - \hat{y}(t_i)\right]^2}, \tag{9}$$

where i^* corresponds to the temporal index at which we start forecasting our models, N is the total number of observations and $\hat{N}$ is the total number of observations used for model calibration and P is the number of parameters. If i^* was not an integer value, we took its floor value.

3.2 Parameters and Confidence Interval Assessment

To further compare and assess the models we compute 95 % confidence intervals for the logistic, two-patch (H) and three-patch (H) models. Only these models were considered, because they have the least number of parameters which reduces the likelihood of overfitting the models to data. Bootstrapping can be used as a way to estimate standard errors of parameter estimates in statistical models. The basic idea is to fit the model to data, find the residuals and add them to the data. Next, randomly sample with replacement B times, where B is large and fit the model to each of these newly created data sets to obtain B different parameter sets from the fitted model. This allows one to obtain a distribution of the parameters without assuming anything prior about them. For further details see [9, 10, 20].

Recall a statistical model, with $y = (y_1, \ldots, y_n)$ being explained by k explanatory variables $\boldsymbol{x} = (x_1, \ldots, x_k)$ using p parameters $\boldsymbol{\theta} = (\theta_1, \ldots, \theta_p)$:

$$y_i = g(\boldsymbol{x}_i|\boldsymbol{\theta}) + \varepsilon_i$$

for $i = 1, \ldots, n$. Where g is a mathematical model such as an ordinary differential equation model, partial differential equation model, algebraic model, etc. ε is the error and is a random variable and y is another random variable. Let G be the partial derivative matrix with respect to θ and the leverages, $h_1, \ldots, h_n$ be the diagonal elements of the $G(G^{\dagger}G)^{-1}G^{\dagger}$ matrix, where $\dagger$ denotes matrix transpose.

The bootstrapping method is described below.

1. Fit the model to the original data with an initial parameter set, $\hat{\boldsymbol{\theta}}$, and for each x_i, compute the corresponding residual $\hat{\varepsilon}_i = y_i - \hat{y}_i$ for $i = 1, 2, \ldots n$, where n is the total number of data points and $\hat{y}_i = g(x_i, \hat{\boldsymbol{\theta}})$.
2. Correct for the potential heteroscedasticity in the residual variances by computing the **modified residuals**: $\hat{r}_i = \frac{\hat{\varepsilon}_i}{\sqrt{1-h_i}}$ and compute the centered residuals $r_i^* = \hat{\varepsilon}_i - \hat{r}_i$, where h_i are the leverages.
3. Sample with replacement from the n modified and centered residuals.

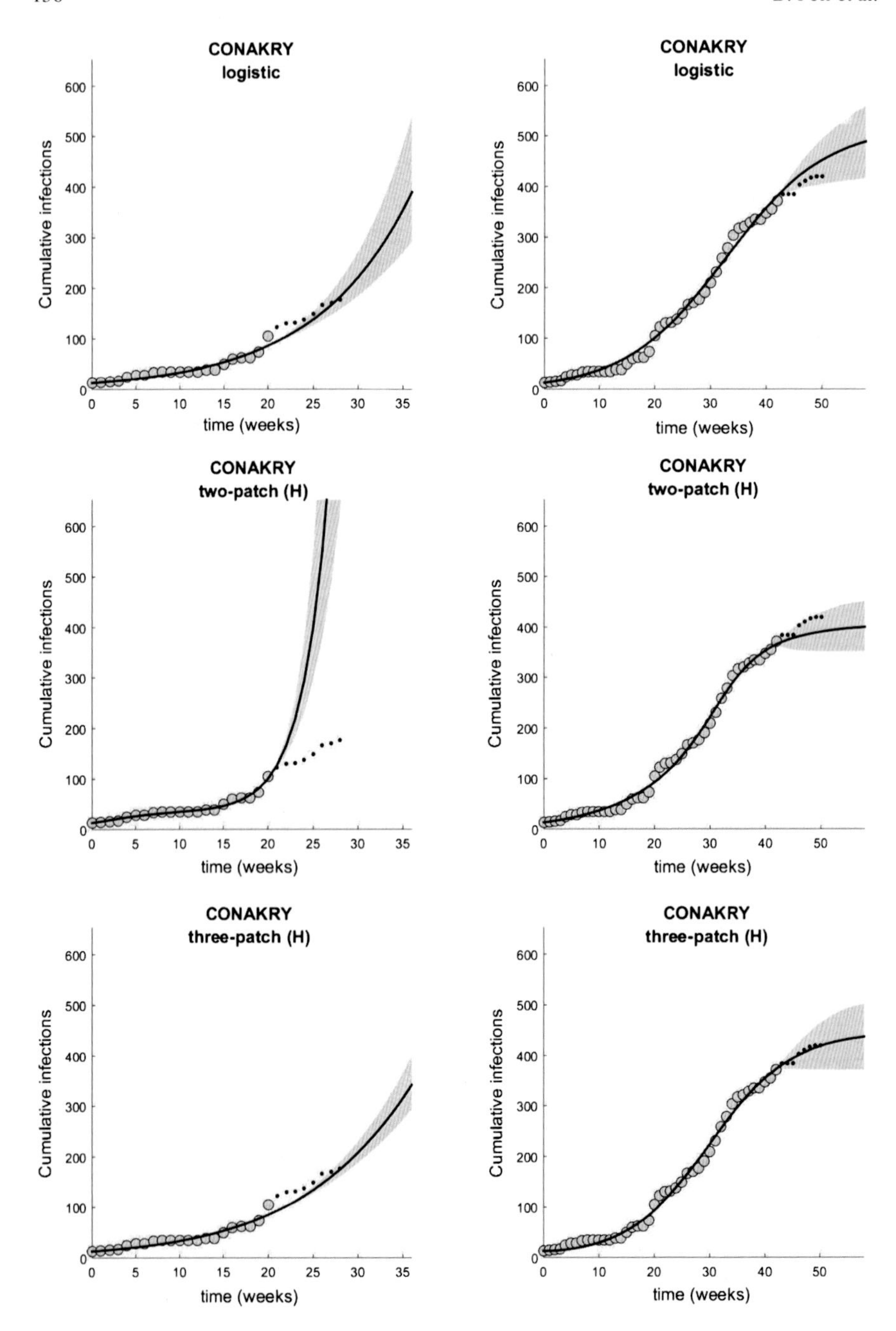

Fig. 2 Illustration of the model fitting and forecasting for Conakry, the capital and largest city of Guinea. *Left column* models trained on the first one-third data. *Right column* models trained on the first two-thirds of data. *Gray shaded region* represents 95 % prediction bands

4. Generate bootstrap sample, $\bar{y}_i := \hat{y}_i + r_j^*$, for all i and where j is random.
5. Fit the model to these new $\bar{y}_i$ values and obtain a new set of parameter values, $\bar{\boldsymbol{\theta}}$.
6. Repeat steps 3, 4 and 5 a large number of times[1] of times (say 2,000). This generates 2,000 bootstrap samples and corresponding sets of parameter estimations.
7. Use the 2,000 parameter estimates to generate distributions to find confidence intervals.

3.3 Challenges

Whenever fitting a mathematical model to time series data that ranges from small values to very large values, deciding at what time to initiate the model can seriously influence its forecasting ability. For example, training a model on a large set of data that is relatively near zero except for the last couple of points will force the fitting to be heavily biased by the large amount of initial points near zero, thus not providing a good forecast. We remedied this by starting the models after there were no three consecutive weeks that had no infections and by using the weighted error (Eq. 6) for fitting. This was done due to the fact that smaller outbreak waves happened before the main wave of infections appeared.

Forecasting an ongoing disease outbreak in real-time brings many challenges. New data being available means that computer programs must be designed to process and incorporate new data sets with ease and in a timely fashion. In our case, fitting six models (including special cases) to forty-one data sets requires a significant amount of computing resources.

4 Results

4.1 Data Based Model Validation

To validate the patch models for epidemic modeling, we fit all models to all data sets and compare model fits and errors. To illustrate this fitting process, Fig. 2 shows model fits of the logistic, two-patch and three-patch models with homogenous migration to cumulative reported case data from Conakry, Guinea.

We report the means for the weighted, relative and absolute error (respectively Eqs. 6, 7 and 8) for all 39 data sets in Table 2. Observe that the patch models show an improvement over the logistic model when fitting the data. Additionally, we see that the homogeneous migration models perform better than their free migration versions.

---

[1] Results from Efron and Tibshirani [10] suggest that accurate results for confidence intervals can be obtained from 1000 bootstrap samples. For standard errors this number is reduced to 200.

Table 2 Mean error statistics

Model	Weighted error	Relative error	Absolute
Logistic	82.2822	1.3387	102.198
2-Patch (H)	53.6764	1.1271	63.1193
2-Patch	58.6311	1.2124	72.7197
3-Patch (H)	48.709	1.1256	59.3391
3-Patch (S)	55.0951	1.1515	65.1694
3-Patch	54.215	1.1727	66.0885

In what follows, we summarize the different fitting and forecasting cases. Let FTG be the fitting error from Eq. 6 and FCST be the forecasting error from Eq. 9. We use the following convention to denote the different errors: FTG-Δ and FCST-Δ-Ω, where Δ is the fraction of data used for fitting and Ω is the number of weeks forecasted ahead (Table 5).

Fitting errors were calculated using Eq. 6 and the first one-third and the first two-thirds of each data set. All fitting errors are provided in Table 5 given in the appendix. From Fig. 3, most of the patch models had smaller mean fitting error than the logistic model.

Four and eight week forecasts were made after training all models to the first one-third and first two-thirds of the data set. Figure 3 shows that in all cases, the patch models had smaller mean forecasting errors. This supports the hypothesis that modeling spatial structure within the district improved forecasting error. Additionally, all models perform better when forecasting the short-term rather than long-term epidemic trajectory. Forecasting error variance was lowest with FCST-2/3-4. In contrast, the variance was the largest with FCST-1/3-8.

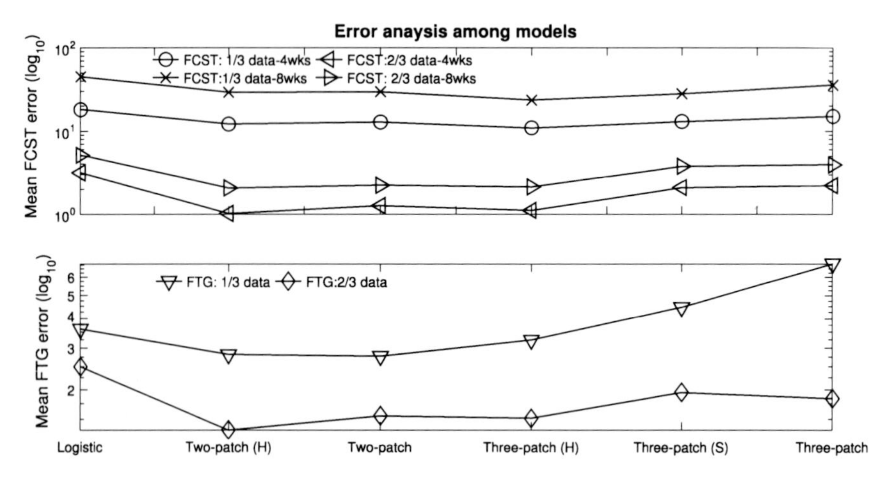

Fig. 3 Mean forecasting and fitting errors. Models are along the x-axis and variance is along the y-axis. We connect points for aesthetic purposes

Table 3 p-values of the Kruskal–Wallis test show forecasting errors do not significantly differ across models

Case	p-value
FCST-3-4	0.9806
FCST-3-8	0.9872
FCST-23-4	0.9933
FCST-23-8	0.9894

Results of Kruskal-Wallis tests were not significant for FCST-1/3-4, FCST-1/3-8, FCST-2/3-4 and FCST-2/3-8; the mean ranks for all forecasting cases did not significantly differ. We include the p-values (95 %) in Table 3 for this test.

4.2 Forecasting Error as a Function of Forecasting Points

Forecasting error for Port Loko, Guinea, Liberia and Sierra Leone was calculated for varying amounts of forecasting points.

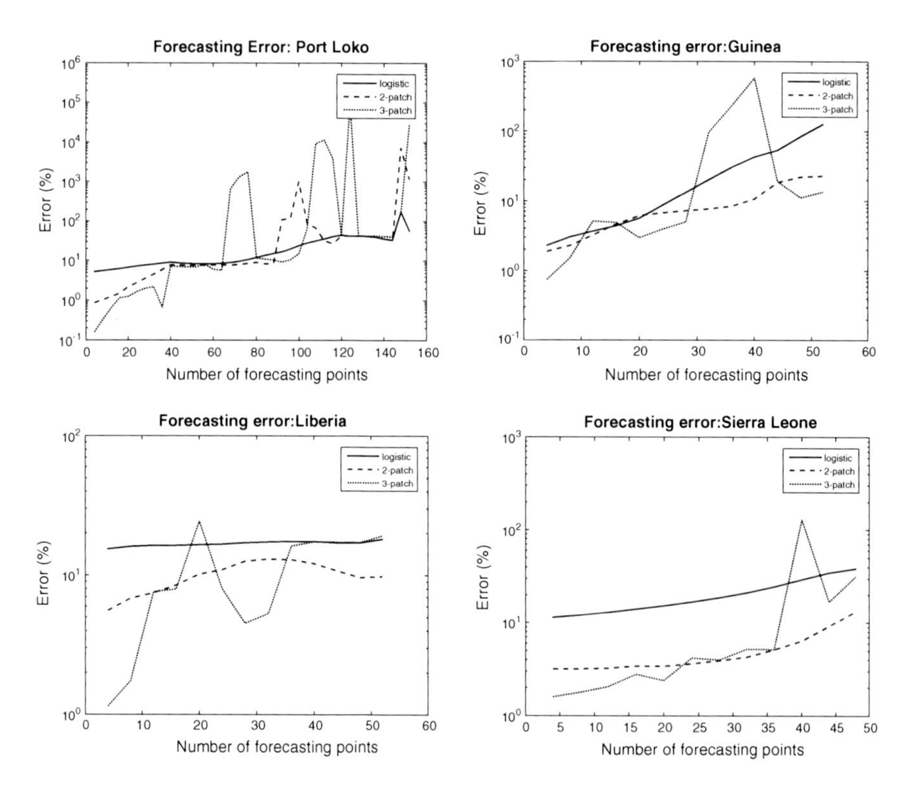

Fig. 4 Relative error of forecasting points for the logistic, two and three patch models with homogeneous migration rate: Port Loko, Guinea, Liberia and Sierra Leone

The forecasting error for Port Loko in Fig. 4, suggests that the patch models have smaller forecasting errors than the logistic equation for short-term forecasts (4–70 days). Additionally, it shows erratic long-term forecasting of the patch models for Port Loko, because they are not well constrained due to the limited data. Figure 4 further shows lower short-term error for Sierra Leone and Liberia by the two-patch model. We note that the three-patch model yielded the smallest error when forecasting ten prediction points or less (4–10 days).

4.3 *Confidence Interval Assessment*

Parameter confidence intervals for the logistic equation decrease in length as we decrease the number of prediction points (Fig. 5) for Port Loko. Similar assessments were done using data from Sierra Leone, Liberia and Guinea at the country level. Results were similar as the Port Loko case except for Liberia, where confidence interval lengths begin to increase when we forecast less data points. In summary, the logistic model shows well behaved parameter values when we fit to an increasing number of data points for three out of four data sets used.

The patch models tell a different story. The confidence intervals are larger and show erratic behavior when forecasting a large number of points. Indeed for the two-patch model (Fig. 6), the confidence intervals for r_1 actually increase when we are predicting a small number of data points from Port Loko. This variability is seen to be worse in the confidence intervals for the final epidemic sizes (K_i's) for both two and three patch models, but they are so erratic that they cannot be shown in a reasonable way and therefore are not included. The fact that the patch models have more parameters allows for different parameter sets that produce a well fit curve, but allow for large variability in the parameter sets. The same is seen in the confidence

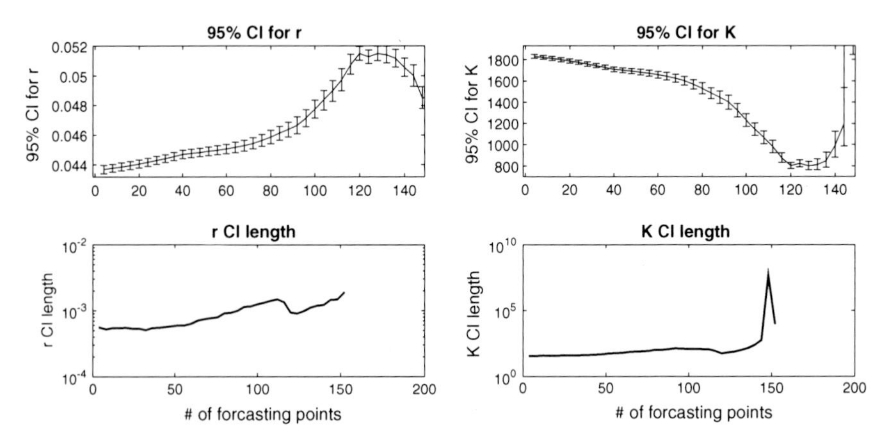

Fig. 5 95 % CI for r and K from (3). (*Bottom*) Plot of the length of the CI for r and K as a function of the number of forecasting points. District: Port Loko

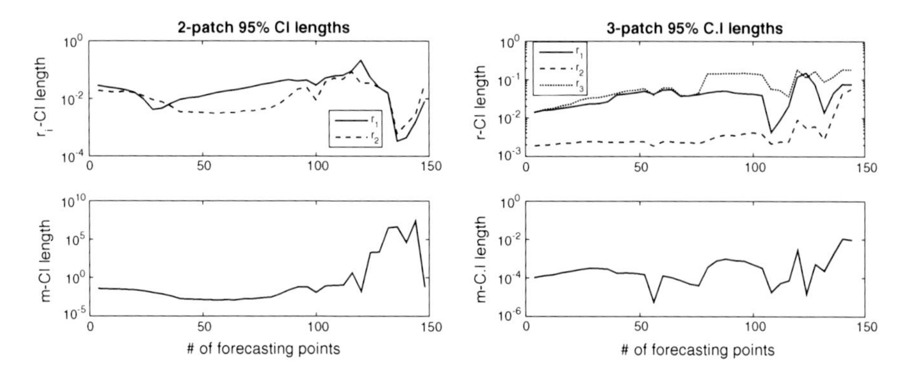

Fig. 6 95 % CI for r_i and m for $i = 1, 2, 3$ from (6) for Port Loko. (*Left*) two-patch confidence interval lengths for intrinsic infection rate and migration parameter. (*Right*) Three-patch 95 % confidence interval lengths for intrinsic infection rate and migration rate. Note the variability for high numbers of prediction points for both models and the high variability in r_1 for the two-patch model for low numbers of prediction points

interval assessment using data from Sierra Leone, Guinea and Liberia, (not shown here).

4.4 Implications for Liberia, Sierra Leone and Guinea: R_0

From the bootstrapping method, we calculated 95 % confidence intervals for R_0 in Guinea, Liberia and Sierra Leone (see Table 4).

5 Discussion

In this chapter, a family of logistic patch models were preliminarily evaluated for use in disease modeling and forecasting. An explicit formula for the cumulative number of infectious individuals was derived from a SI compartmental model which takes the form of the well known logistic model. This derivation follows from the behavior change assumption, Eq. (2). We then extended the logistic model to include spatial population heterogeneity by using multi-patch models that incorporate migration between patches and logistic growth within each patch. Each model's ability to forecast epidemic data was assessed by comparing model forecasting error, parameter distributions and parameter confidence intervals as functions of the number of data points used to calibrate the models. The patch models show an improvement over the logistic model in short-term forecasting, but naturally require the estimation of more parameters from limited data.

The models were tested by fitting them to the total reported case data from 39 districts in West Africa. In particular, the means of the weighted, relative and absolute errors of the patch models are less than the logistic model's, suggesting that spatial structure improved the data fitting. Next, models were compared by their forecasting capabilities in two ways: comparing forecasting error and comparing parameter confidence intervals. These latter efforts were restricted to the logistic, two-patch and three-patch models with homogeneous migration. The forecasting errors from Fig. 3 show that the patch models forecast better than the logistic model. However, Fig. 4 shows long-term forecasting variability from the patch models, because of the limited data. In contrast to these results, the Kruskal-Wallis test showed no significant difference in the forecasting errors across the models.

The value of R_0 during the outbreak in Liberia, Guinea and Sierra Leone were estimated to be in the same range as previous studies that were based on compartmental models [3, 13, 14, 28]. In particular, from Table 4 the estimates from the two and three patch models for R_0 are similar with Althaus et al., but our confidence intervals are not as small [3]. This agreement further supports the reliability of the logistic and patch models with homogeneous migration.

In reality, early in the Ebola 2013–2015 epidemic, the public's behavior in Liberia, Sierra Leone and Guinea did not swiftly change in a manner that mediated disease transmission nor has there been any evidence supporting that the per-capita infection rate decreased linearly. Actually, the public's misunderstanding of the disease, lack of resources and fear fostered high-risk behaviors and resulted in an increased disease transmission in West Africa during the epidemic [19, 25]. However, health-care workers supplied valuable public awareness programs and medical resources that helped manage the spread. Our modeling assumptions approximate these notions and provide immediate behavior change in the spirit of Eq. (2), but this is modeled simultaneously everywhere in space and is one reason why the logistic model does not fit the data well. The patch-models overcome this issue by modeling behavior changes at different times, rates and locations, but require more data to be constrained. Indeed, an issue with the patch models is that the number of parameters increase quickly as more patches are introduced.

Table 4 R_0 and 95 % confidence intervals for R_0

	Althaus [3]	Team et al. [23]	Logistic	2-Patch (H)	3-Patch (H)
Guinea	1.51 (1.50–1.52)	1.71 (1.44–2.01)	1.252 (1.249, 1.255)	1.52 (1.42, 1.92)	1.45 (1.39, 1.51)
Liberia	1.59 (1.57–1.60)	1.83 (1.72–1.94)	2.11 (2.07, 2.15)	1.45 (1.12, 1.94)	1.43 (1.06, 2.199)
Sierra Leone	2.53 (2.41–2.67)	2.02 (1.79–2.26)	2.28 (2.25, 2.32)	2.27 (2, 2.62)	2.12 (1.87, 2.26)

Further work can be done with between-country and between-district scales. The latter would allow for more parameter constraint, but would have to be restricted to a small number of patches that represent a small number of neighboring districts. The problem with incorporating all districts is that it ultimately requires a high-dimensional patch model with many parameters on a complicated network. This may be remedied with a partial differential equation model or by using mobility data to constrain the migration parameters. In addition, exploring different behavior functions would be another direction to expand this work.

Although the logistic model is phenomenological, it is capable of fitting the sigmoid curves that usually result from plotting the cumulative reported cases of disease outbreaks. The logistic and the patch models provide a general framework for disease modeling, because they do not model specific disease transmission processes. Specifically, they are based on two fundamental mechanisms that influence disease outbreaks: behavior change in the community and movement of individuals within that community. We find that incorporating the latter mechanism decreased forecasting errors with respect to the logistic model, but also require more data for model calibration.

Acknowledgments This work is partially supported by NSF grant DMS-1518529.

Appendix

Forecast and Fitting Error Tables

See Table 5.

Table 5 Fitting errors for all models

District	Logistic		Two-patch (H)		Two-patch		Three-patch (H)		Three-patch (S)		Three-patch	
	One-third	Two-thirds	One-third	Two-thirds	One-third	Two-thirds	One-third	Two-thirds	One-third	Two-thirds	One-third	Two-thirds
BOMI	3.6147	1.198	1.7439	0.39968	2.23	0.49683	1.9891	0.4395	3.1711	0.52022	3.9724	0.47549
BONG	1.4365	0.54448	1.5116	0.42227	1.6447	0.46937	1.6753	0.5351	2.1265	0.49347	2.9081	0.58443
GBARPOLU	0.71881	0.078303	0.6592	0.087046	1.001	0.0887	1.1162	0.095164	1.1436	0.077254	2.5221	0.11758
GRAND BASSA	1.8093	0.68238	1.1774	0.29884	1.8118	0.41695	1.7176	0.38735	2.2839	0.44523	3.2918	0.58292
GRANDAPE MOUNT	3.333	0.5762	3.7319	0.63049	3.8035	0.65232	3.3711	0.67542	5.0092	0.73396	8.0373	0.83729
GRAND KRU	0.61518	0.17033	0.80231	0.099753	0.84577	0.17673	0.64961	0.12372	1.0854	0.1753	2.3581	0.2528
LOFA	5.2755	0.36486	5.6001	0.26833	6.9035	0.36263	7.9303	0.34862	6.4173	0.27562	11.1918	0.47298
MARGIBI	3.4293	0.73833	4.4185	0.67457	4.3363	0.72399	4.5471	0.72418	5.619	0.79608	7.7291	0.89117
MONTSERRADO	4.2503	8.3487	4.922	2.2296	5.2784	1.8897	5.6934	2.3507	6.7871	1.5	9.1043	2.424
NIMBA	1.2104	0.12813	1.351	0.13701	1.4561	0.14135	1.5792	0.1464	1.9673	0.15578	2.7993	0.17449
RIVER GEE	0.15977	0.01381	0.1785	0.015599	0.17445	0.015513	0.18504	0.014329	0.23398	0.019005	0.3597	0.019446
RIVERCESS	0.68386	0.077873	0.51155	0.093633	0.54034	0.027355	1.1207	0.1403	1.6564	0.10546	3.84	0.20521
SINOE	0.71361	0.074711	0.76264	0.069135	0.92105	0.089601	1.1015	0.095067	1.5029	0.099703	2.8564	0.13226
CONAKRY	2.4851	2.2749	2.4127	2.428	3.1721	2.443	3.4615	2.5474	4.0175	2.6153	7.2811	2.9771
COYAH	2.9429	3.1608	1.6338	3.4047	2.0082	2.9153	3.1834	3.1261	5.2135	3.2436	5.4088	4.6479
DUBREKA	1.8975	1.0283	0.84368	1.0297	2.5879	0.70316	5.2154	1.0243	3.0884	1.0003	5.7692	1.1607
FARANAH	2.1281	0.37701	2.1799	0.42643	2.4097	0.41307	3.8266	0.50515	5.0919	0.53024	25.1464	0.24839
FORECARIAH	1.6364	3.1111	2.0821	2.8257	2.2314	3.3816	1.6743	13.7987	2.9266	3.4089	5.3969	3.8571
KANKAN	1.1965	0.14143	2.3918	0.1566	1.4882	0.1561	3.15	0.49163	3.0055	0.16257	3.7905	0.23459
KINDIA	2.0281	1.136	1.1496	0.91487	1.6464	1.071	1.5116	0.38334	2.5737	1.0592	5.3894	1.2542
KISSIDOUGOU	2.9894	0.40939	2.3094	0.47537	3.0904	0.53037	2.3511	1.1683	5.3364	0.39528	21.0685	0.77644

(continued)

Table 5 (continued)

District	Logistic		Two-patch (H)		Two-patch		Three-patch (H)		Three-patch (S)		Three-patch	
	One-third	Two-thirds	One-third	Two-thirds	One-third	Two-thirds	One-third	Two-thirds	One-third	Two-thirds	One-third	Two-thirds
MACENTA	0.4115	5.2217	1.6022	5.5868	1.8795	5.3856	2.0131	0.62805	4.0898	5.9809	6.7702	6.1607
NZEREKORE	2.5579	0.38891	0.44257	0.40024	0.42032	0.41519	1.0254	5.7162	1.3283	0.49414	0.68875	0.53331
SIGUIRI	0.44141	0.30196	3.1856	0.32252	3.5061	0.25171	3.8516	0.4314	5.0128	0.35819	8.8683	0.41559
TELIMELE	0.10555	0.55761	0.42019	0.593	0.4517	0.62469	0.65173	0.34477	0.75666	0.6742	1.8585	0.72794
BO	5.0701	2.2253	0.12915	2.4011	0.13449	2.0631	0.175	0.61298	0.15866	2.4455	0.24843	2.6633
BOMBALI	8.8538	9.0596	1.9431	3.2113	1.7743	4.476	4.0898	2.2312	5.8781	3.8964	6.1361	4.9203
KAILAHUN	13.4441	2.3216	3.0016	0.67132	3.8811	0.66044	4.9654	3.3201	7.8443	2.2252	8.5021	1.2032
KAMBIA	3.0924	2.8205	5.1435	1.6991	3.718	1.1592	7.6597	1.0176	11.6425	1.4946	13.382	1.5634
KENEMA	10.8483	2.4777	1.3423	1.2226	2.1451	0.83164	3.4772	1.4973	4.8896	0.85422	4.7483	1.0399
KOINADUGU	2.18	0.38465	8.1016	0.25254	4.9844	0.44878	6.3207	1.2681	15.0373	0.35363	6.2745	0.40977
KONO	5.3272	3.2919	2.7568	3.3897	3.1007	3.3525	1.7213	0.4554	4.7125	3.2659	7.5391	3.6874
MOYAMBA	2.18	0.38465	6.7662	0.25254	6.8282	0.44878	7.4665	3.6681	9.9778	0.35363	15.8279	0.40977
PORT LOKO	15.4465	15.1163	2.7568	2.2217	3.1007	6.4625	1.7213	0.4554	4.7125	14.2096	7.5391	2.7181
PUJEHUN	0.22985	0.02164	16.4268	0.017028	11.313	0.017084	13.17	3.6144	12.6916	0.017823	17.257	0.048621
TONKOLILI	11.6003	3.3944	0.18359	1.598	0.29053	1.9964	0.2574	0.016134	0.42985	4.0286	0.62986	1.8315
PUJEHUN	0.22985	0.02164	7.3516	0.017028	4.5375	0.017084	4.5832	1.6187	6.898	0.017823	10.2676	0.048621
WESTERN AREA RURAL	8.5967	11.4656	0.18359	3.0142	0.29053	5.9014	0.2574	0.016134	0.42985	7.0712	0.62986	4.0112
WESTERN AREA URBAN	5.639	13.5544	5.7848	8.6758	6.0817	8.771	6.0987	3.1066	7.3591	10.3357	8.545	16.817

Models were trained on one-third and two-thirds of each district data set

References

1. Agnandji, S.T., Huttner, A., Zinser, M.E., Njuguna, P., Dahlke, C., Fernandes, J.F., Yerly, S., Dayer, J.A., Kraehling, V., Kasonta, R., et al.: Phase 1 trials of rVSV Ebola vaccine in Africa and Europe–preliminary report. N. Engl. J. Med. (2015)
2. Agusto, F.B., Teboh-Ewungkem, M.I., Gumel, A.B.: Mathematical assessment of the effect of traditional beliefs and customs on the transmission dynamics of the 2014 Ebola outbreaks. BMC Med. **13**(1), 96 (2015)
3. Althaus, C.L.: Estimating the reproduction number of Ebola virus (EBOV) during the 2014 outbreak in West Africa. PLoS currents **6** (2014)
4. Anderson, R.M., May, R.M.: Infectious Diseases of Humans, vol. 1. Oxford University Press, Oxford (1991)
5. Bickel, P.J., Doksum, K.A.: Mathematical Statistics: Basic Ideas and Selected Topics, Volume I, vol. 117. CRC Press, Boca Raton (2015)
6. Center for Disease Control: Outbreaks Chronology: Ebola Virus Disease. Website (2015). http://www.cdc.gov/vhf/ebola/outbreaks/history/chronology.html
7. Chowell, G., Nishiura, H.: Transmission dynamics and control of Ebola virus disease (EVD): a review. BMC Med. **12**(1), 196 (2014)
8. Chowell, G., Simonsen, L., Viboud, C., Kuang, Y.: Is West Africa approaching a catastrophic phase or is the 2014 Ebola epidemic slowing down? Different models yield different answers for Liberia. PLoS currents **6** (2014)
9. Davison, A.C., Hinkley, D.V.: Bootstrap Methods and Their Application, vol. 1. Cambridge university press, Cambridge (1997)
10. Efron, B., Tibshirani, R.J.: An Introduction to the Bootstrap. CRC press, Boca Raton (1994)
11. Frieden, T.R., Damon, I., Bell, B.P., Kenyon, T., Nichol, S.: Ebola 2014 – new challenges, new global response and responsibility. N. Engl. J. Med. **371**(13), 1177–1180 (2014)
12. Gao, D., Ruan, S.: A multipatch malaria model with logistic growth populations. SIAM J. Appl. Math. **72**(3), 819–841 (2012)
13. Gomes, M.F., y Piontti, A.P., Rossi, L., Chao, D., Longini, I., Halloran, M.E., Vespignani, A.: Assessing the international spreading risk associated with the 2014 West African Ebola outbreak. PLOS Curr. Outbreaks **1** (2014)
14. Khan, A., Naveed, M., Dur-e Ahmad, M., Imran, M.: Estimating the basic reproductive ratio for the Ebola outbreak in Liberia and Sierra Leone. Infect. Dis. Poverty **4**(1), 13 (2015)
15. Kiskowski, M.A.: A three-scale network model for the early growth dynamics of 2014 West Africa Ebola epidemic. PLoS Curr. **6** (2014)
16. Lagarias, J.C., Reeds, J.A., Wright, M.H., Wright, P.E.: Convergence properties of the Nelder-Mead simplex method in low dimensions. SIAM J. Optim. **9**(1), 112–147 (1998)
17. Meltzer, M.I., Atkins, C.Y., Santibanez, S., Knust, B., Petersen, B.W., Ervin, E.D., Nichol, S.T., Damon, I.K., Washington, M.L.: Estimating the future number of cases in the Ebola epidemic–Liberia and Sierra Leone, 2014–2015. MMWR Surveill Summ **63**(suppl 3), 1–14 (2014)
18. Merler, S., Ajelli, M., Fumanelli, L., Gomes, M.F., y Piontti, A.P., Rossi, L., Chao, D.L., Longini, I.M., Halloran, M.E., Vespignani, A.: Spatiotemporal spread of the 2014 outbreak of Ebola virus disease in Liberia and the effectiveness of non-pharmaceutical interventions: a computational modelling analysis. Lancet Infect. Dis. **15**(2), 204–211 (2015)
19. Nielsen, C.F., Kidd, S., Sillah, A., Davis, E., Mermin, J., Kilmarx, P.H.: Improving burial practices and cemetery management during an ebola virus disease epidemic-Sierra Leone, 2014. MMWR Surveill Summ **64**, 1–8 (2015)
20. Pardoe, I., Weisberg, S.: An Introduction to bootstrap methods using Arc. Unpublished Report available at www.stat.umn.edu/arc/bootmethREV.pdf (2001)
21. Shaman, J., Yang, W., Kandula, S.: Inference and forecast of the current West African Ebola outbreak in Guinea, Sierra Leone and Liberia. PLoS Curr. **6** (2014)
22. Valdez, L., Rêgo, H.H.A., Stanley, H., Braunstein, L.: Predicting the extinction of Ebola spreading in Liberia due to mitigation strategies. Scientific Reports **5**, Article no. 12172

23. WHO Ebola virus disease in West Africa–the first 9 months of the epidemic and forward projections. N. Engl. J. Med. **371**(16), 1481–1495 (2014)
24. World Health Organization: Ebola Response Roadmap Situation report 03-05-2015 (2015). http://www.who.int/csr/disease/ebola/situation-reports/en/
25. World Health Organization: Ebola response: What needs to happen in 2015 (2015). http://www.who.int/csr/disease/ebola/one-year-report/response-in-2015/en/
26. World Health Organization: Ebola vaccines, therapies, and diagnostics (2015). http://www.who.int/medicines/emp_ebola_q_as/en
27. World Health Organization: Guidance for Safe Handling of Human Remains of Ebola Patients in U.S. Hospitals and Mortuaries (2015). http://www.cdc.gov/vhf/ebola/healthcare-us/hospitals/handling-human-remains.html
28. Yamin, D., Gertler, S., Ndeffo-Mbah, M.L., Skrip, L.A., Fallah, M., Nyenswah, T.G., Altice, F.L., Galvani, A.P.: Effect of Ebola progression on transmission and control in Liberia. Ann. Intern. Med. **162**(1), 11–17 (2015)

From Bee Species Aggregation to Models of Disease Avoidance: The *Ben-Hur* effect

K.E. Yong, E. Díaz Herrera and C. Castillo-Chavez

Abstract The movie *Ben-Hur* highlights the dynamics of contagion associated with leprosy, a pattern of forced aggregation driven by the emergence of symptoms and the fear of contagion. The 2014 Ebola outbreaks reaffirmed the dynamics of redistribution among symptomatic and asymptomatic or non-infected individuals as a way to avoid contagion. In this manuscript, we explore the establishment of clusters of infection via density-dependence avoidance (diffusive instability). We illustrate this possibility in two ways: using a phenomenological driven model where disease incidence is assumed to be a decreasing function of the size of the symptomatic population and with a model that accounts for the deliberate movement of individuals in response to a gradient of symptomatic infectious individuals. The results in this manuscript are preliminary but indicative of the role that behavior, here modeled in crude simplistic ways, may have on disease dynamics, particularly on the spatial redistribution of epidemiological classes.

Keywords Ebola · Leprosy · Behavior epidemics · Behavioral ecology · Infection clusters · Diffusive instability

---

K.E. Yong (✉)
Mathematics/Science Subdivision, University of Hawai'i - West O'ahu,
Kapolei, HI 96707, USA
e-mail: kamuela.yong@hawaii.edu

E. Díaz Herrera
Instituto Nacional De Salud Pública, Universidad 655, Santa María Ahuacatitlán,
62100 Cuernavaca, Morelos, Mexico
e-mail: edgar.diaz@insp.mx

C. Castillo-Chavez (✉)
Simon A. Levin Mathematical, Computational and Modeling Science Center,
Arizona State University, Tempe, AZ 85287, USA
e-mail: ccchavez@asu.edu

G. Chowell and J.M. Hyman (eds.), *Mathematical and Statistical Modeling for Emerging and Re-emerging Infectious Diseases*,
DOI 10.1007/978-3-319-40413-4_11

1 Introduction

The effect that aggregation of susceptible and infected populations of individuals has on the basic reproduction number, $\mathscr{R}_0$, and the *final size* has been studied by various researchers (see [1–3, 6, 7, 16, 25]). The effect of aggregation on $\mathscr{R}_0$ and the final outbreak size is not necessarily the same as a small core group with a high activity level can substantially contribute to $\mathscr{R}_0$ while having little impact on the final outbreak size [15]. O. Diekmann et al. [14] showed that aggregation of susceptible and infective individuals reduces the number of groups required to capture the dynamics of a large system provided that one assumes identical levels of infectivity for all groups. These researchers also observed that increased levels of aggregation may lead to lower values of $\mathscr{R}_0$ [7, 14].

Spatial transmission of diseases has been studied by various researchers [21, 26, 27, 31, 38], often using reaction diffusion equations (see [5, 8, 10, 11, 24, 28, 37, 40]). In this paper, two novel reaction-diffusion models are introduced that model the spread of a communicable disease when the presence of symptoms reduces contacts among all types and, in the process, ameliorates disease spread (Model (1)). We also examine the impact that the movement of individuals, in response to gradients of symptomatic infectious individuals modeled via cross-diffusion (Model (18)), has on disease dynamics. This paper is organized as follows: Sect. 2 introduces a phenomenological model and identifies conditions for clustering via diffusive instability; Sect. 3 examines the role of cross-diffusion on epidemiological spatial aggregation; Sect. 4 collects thoughts and conclusions.

2 Phenomenological Model

Epidemics are capable of generating shifts on population level interactions possibly as a function of the presence of growing levels of severe infection as reflected by the impact of symptomatic populations [9, 17, 18] on the contacts between individuals and survival. A simple epidemiological model that accounts for reductions in transmission as the size of the symptomatic population increases is described below motivated by observed disease patterns in leprosy [4, 33, 34], Ebola [12, 22, 30, 39], and influenza [32]. We let $S(x, y, t)$ denote the susceptible population at time t and position (x, y), and divide the infected population in two groups, a group that exhibits symptoms and a group that does not, the "asymptomatic" infectious group. Specifically, we let $I_1(x, y, t)$ denote the symptomless infectious population, assumed to be infectious, and let $I_2(x, y, t)$ denote the infected population with visible symptoms. The incidence term in a susceptible-infectious-susceptible (SIS) type model is modified by the addition of spatial diffusion to each class under the assumption that the symptomatic class, that is, I_2-members are in principle, to be avoided. The model equations are given by the following phenomenologically derived reaction-diffusion epidemiological model:

$$\begin{aligned} \frac{\partial S}{\partial t} &= -\frac{\beta}{1+I_2} S I_1 + \alpha I_2 + D_S \nabla^2 S, \\ \frac{\partial I_1}{\partial t} &= \frac{\beta}{1+I_2} S I_1 - \delta I_1 + D_{I_1} \nabla^2 I_, \\ \frac{\partial I_2}{\partial t} &= \delta I_1 - \alpha I_2 + D_{I_2} \nabla^2 I_2, \end{aligned} \tag{1}$$

where $\nabla^2 = \Delta = \partial^2/\partial x^2 + \partial^2/\partial y^2$, the Laplace operator. Setting $I_2 = 0$ leads to the "standard" SIS system with diffusion [21]. The incidence term gets altered by assuming that all contacts decrease with the size of the I_2-population, that is, the incidence is modeled as follows:

$$\frac{\beta}{1 + I_2} S I_1. \tag{2}$$

The question posed in [13] is whether or not System (1) can support non-uniform distributions via diffusive instability. The assumption of constant population size implies, without loss of generality, that we can take $S \equiv 1 - I_1 - I_2$, a substitution that allows us to focus on the equations for I_1 and I_2. We observe that System (1) supports the following positive steady states in the absence of diffusion ($D_S = D_{I_1} = D_{I_2} = 0$):

$$(I_1^*, I_2^*) = \left(\frac{\alpha(\beta - \delta)}{\beta\alpha + \beta\delta + \delta^2}, \frac{\delta(\beta - \delta)}{\beta\alpha + \beta\delta + \delta^2} \right),$$

from where we identify the basic reproductive number as

$$\mathscr{R}_0 = \frac{\beta}{\delta}.$$

The effects of small perturbations of the (I_1^*, I_2^*)-equilibrium are introduced via the following variables:

$$\ell_i(x, y, t) = I_i(x, y, t) - I_i^*, \qquad i = 1, 2. \tag{3}$$

Substituting (3) into the last two equations of System (1) leads, after ignoring higher order terms, to the following linearized system

$$\begin{aligned} \frac{\partial \ell_1}{\partial t} &= J_{11}\ell_1 + J_{12}\ell_2 + D_{I_1} \nabla^2 \ell_1, \\ \frac{\partial \ell_2}{\partial t} &= J_{21}\ell_1 + J_{22}\ell_2 + D_{I_2} \nabla^2 \ell_2, \end{aligned} \tag{4}$$

where the matrix (J_{ij}) is the Jacobian of System (1) in the absence of diffusion evaluated at the equilibrium (I_1^*, I_2^*), namely

$$J = (J_{ij}) = \begin{pmatrix} \frac{\alpha(\delta-\beta)}{\alpha+2\delta} & \frac{\alpha(\alpha^2-\beta^2)}{\beta(\alpha+2\delta)} \\ \delta & -\alpha \end{pmatrix}. \tag{5}$$

The three conditions that guarantee diffusive instability [35] are given by the following inequalities:

$$J_{11} + J_{22} < 0, \tag{6}$$
$$J_{11}J_{22} - J_{12}J_{21} > 0, \tag{7}$$
$$J_{11}D_{I_2} + J_{22}D_{I_1} > 2\sqrt{D_{I_1}D_{I_2}(J_{11}J_{22} - J_{12}J_{21})}. \tag{8}$$

Condition (6) always holds, since

$$J_{11} + J_{22} = -\alpha\left(\frac{\delta + \beta + \alpha}{\alpha + 2\delta}\right) < 0.$$

Condition (7) is satisfied provided that

$$J_{11}J_{22} - J_{12}J_{21} = \frac{\beta\alpha^2(\beta - \delta) + \delta\alpha(\alpha^2 - \beta^2)}{\beta(\alpha + 2\delta)}$$

is positive, which is true as long as

$$\beta^2(\alpha + \beta) > \alpha\delta(\beta + \alpha),$$

or, equivalently as long as $\mathscr{R}_0 = \frac{\beta}{\delta} > 1$ and $\frac{\beta}{\alpha} > 1$. Now, we make use of the fact that Condition (8) is equivalent to the inequality

$$J_{11}J_{22} - J_{12}J_{21} - \frac{1}{4D_{I_1}D_{I_2}}\left(J_{11}D_{I_2} + J_{22}D_{I_1}\right)^2 < 0. \tag{9}$$

After substituting the corresponding values from Eq. (5) we see that whenever the following inequality

$$2D_{I_1}D_{I_2}\frac{\alpha + 2\delta}{\alpha\beta}\left[\beta^2(\alpha + 2\delta) - \alpha\delta(\beta + 2\alpha)\right] - D_{I_1}^2(\delta - \beta) - D_{I_2}^2(\alpha + 2\delta)^2 < 0, \tag{10}$$

is satisfied, Condition (9) is satisfied. Using $\mathscr{R}_0 > 1$ leads to

$$\frac{\delta}{\beta}(\beta + 2\alpha) < \beta + 2\delta; \tag{11}$$

while $\alpha < \beta$ leads to

$$-\frac{\beta}{\alpha}(\alpha + 2\delta) < -(\alpha + 2\delta). \tag{12}$$

The addition of Conditions (11) and (12) leads to the inequality

$$\frac{\delta}{\beta}(\beta + 2\alpha) - \frac{\beta}{\alpha}(\alpha + 2\delta) < \beta - \alpha. \tag{13}$$

Thus, we conclude that Condition (8) (Inequality (10)) holds as long as

$$\mathscr{R}_0 = \frac{\beta}{\delta} > 1 \quad \text{and} \quad \frac{\beta}{\alpha} > 1 \tag{14}$$

The main conclusion of this section can be stated as follows:

Theorem 1 *The linear System (4) satisfies necessary and sufficient conditions for diffusive instability whenever $\mathscr{R}_0 > 1$ and $\frac{\beta}{\alpha} > 1$. In other words, diffusive instability takes place when the endemic state exists ($\mathscr{R}_0 > 1$) and I_2 individuals are not infectious for too long.*

The steady state non-uniform distribution of infected individuals (symptomatic and asymptomatic) loses stability due small perturbations of the form

$$\ell_i(x,t) = \alpha_i \cos(qx) e^{\sigma t}, \qquad i = 1, 2. \tag{15}$$

The present analysis works as long as the perturbations are sufficiently small to make the linear approximation (Model (4)) a valid representation of the truly nonlinear representation of Model (1). When the perturbations have been amplified beyond a small size, the analysis is no longer adequate. As a result of the above analysis, we expect that an initial spatially distributed population, will begin to "break up" and aggregate according to the presence or absence of symptoms. See Figs. 1, 2 and 3 generated via the simulations carried out under Condition (14). We see that aggregation occurs faster if the difference in diffusion rates is large for both the linear Model (4) (see Figs. 1 and 2) and nonlinear Model (1) (see Fig. 3).

3 Cross-Diffusion Models

The dynamics of solitary and honey bees and their role in enhancing cross-pollination in California almond tree farms was studied via a cross-diffusion model in [41]. The model for the interaction of honey bees, $u_1(x, y, t)$, and solitary bees, $u_2(x, y, t)$ at time t and position $(x, y) \in \Omega$, proposed in [41], is given by the system:

$$\begin{aligned}
\frac{\partial}{\partial t} u_i &= \nabla^2 (\alpha_i + \beta_{i1} u_1 + \beta_{i2} u_2) u_i + \gamma_i \nabla \cdot (u_i \nabla W) && \text{in } \Omega \times (0, T), \\
u_i(x, y, 0) &= \xi_i(x, y) && \text{on } \Omega \times \{t = 0\}, \\
\frac{\partial u_i}{\partial \nu} &= 0 && \text{on } \partial\Omega \times (0, T),
\end{aligned} \tag{16}$$

where $\alpha_i \geq 0$ represents the intrinsic diffusion, $\beta_{ij} \geq 0$ represents the self-diffusion for $i = j$ and cross-diffusion for $i \neq j$, $W = W(x, y, t)$ represents the environmental potential, and $\gamma_i \in \mathbb{R}$ is the coefficient associated with W. The dynamics of avoidance between honey and solitary bees was captured by the addition of cross- and self-diffusion terms to the model in [36]. Numerical simulations were used to show

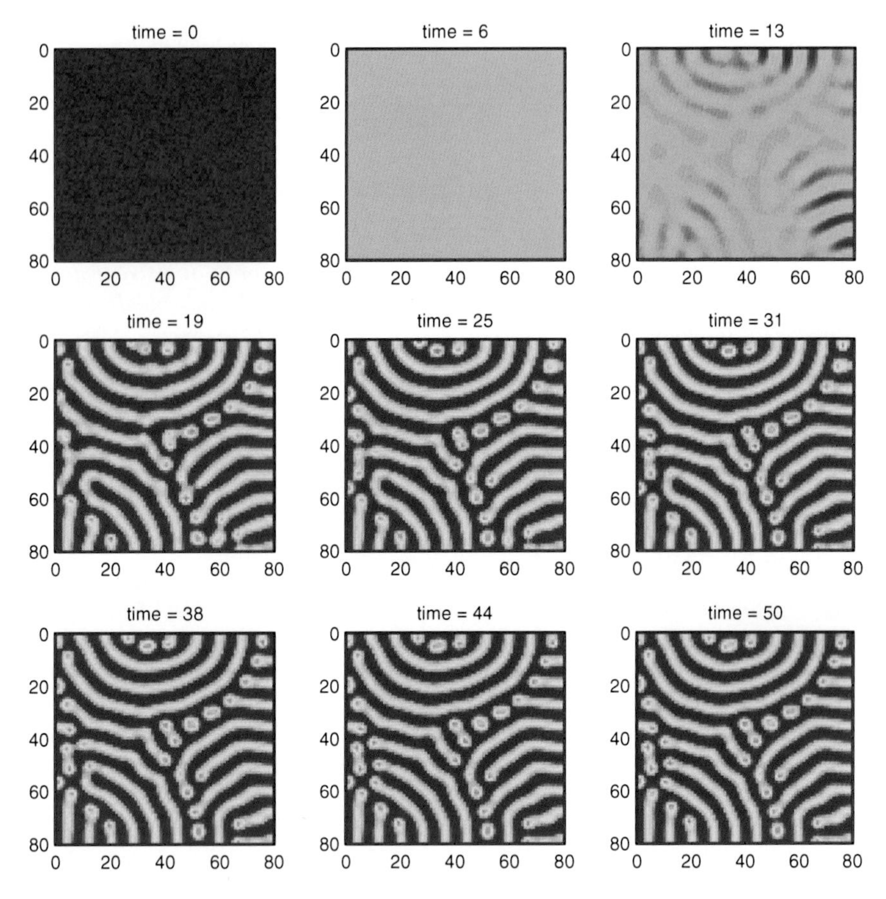

Fig. 1 Spatial aggregation for Model (4) occurs quickly when the difference between diffusion rates is large. ($D_{I_1} = 10$ and $D_{I_2} = 80$. $\alpha = 0.05$, $\beta = 0.13$ and $\delta = 1.3$, chosen so that Condition (14) is satisfied)

that cross-diffusion was indeed capable of capturing the observed spatial aggregation of individuals by species. The resulting spatial aggregating of bees by species, as a result of a strong cross-diffusion (β_{12}), is illustrated in Fig. 4. This figure shows that in areas of high solitary bee density (u_2) result in low honey bee density (u_1) and in areas of low solitary bee densities result in honey bees aggregating in high densities.

The use of cross-diffusion to model spatially explicit epidemics has been studied in the past (see [24, 28, 37, 40]). Most recently, the role of density-dependent cross-diffusion in epidemiology has been explored numerically by Berres and Ruiz-Baier [5] via the model

$$
\begin{aligned}
\frac{\partial S}{\partial t} &= rS\left(1 - \frac{S}{K}\right) - \beta\frac{SI}{S+I} + D_S\nabla^2 S + c\nabla\cdot(S\nabla I)\\
\frac{\partial I}{\partial t} &= \beta\frac{SI}{S+I} - \gamma I + D_I\nabla^2 I
\end{aligned}
\tag{17}
$$

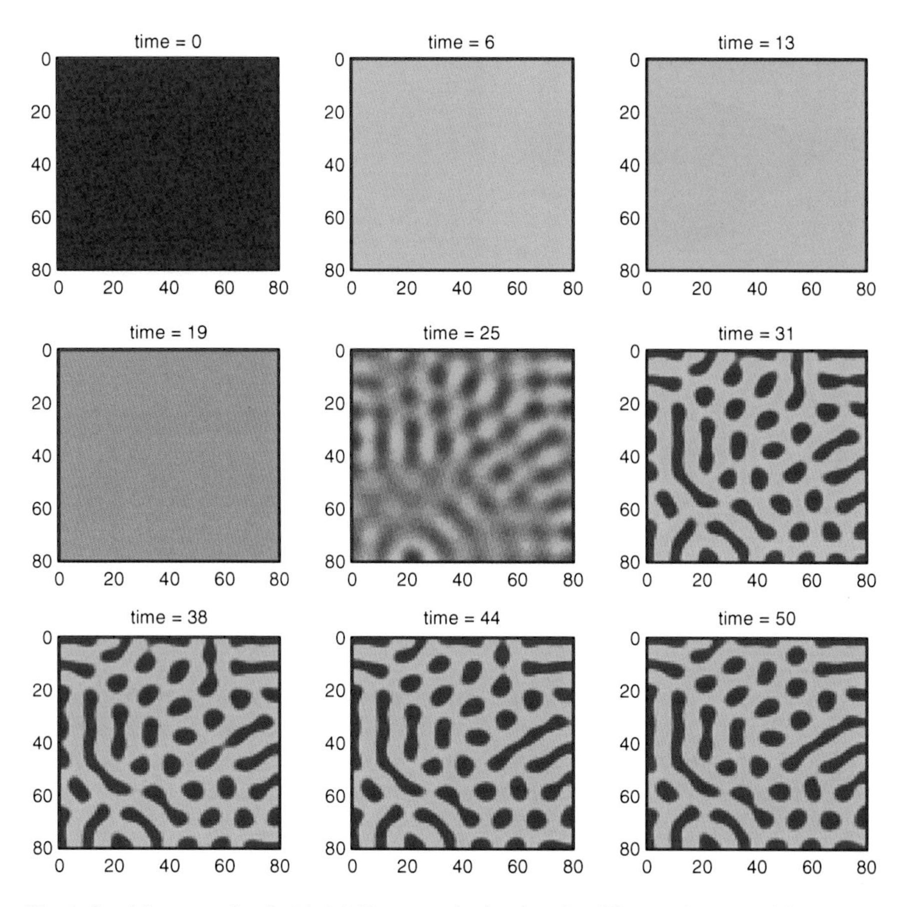

Fig. 2 Spatial aggregation for Model (4) occurs slowly when the difference between diffusion rates is small. ($D_{I_1} = 10$ and $D_{I_2} = 20$. $\alpha = 0.05$, $\beta = 0.13$ and $\delta = 1.3$, chosen so that (14) is satisfied)

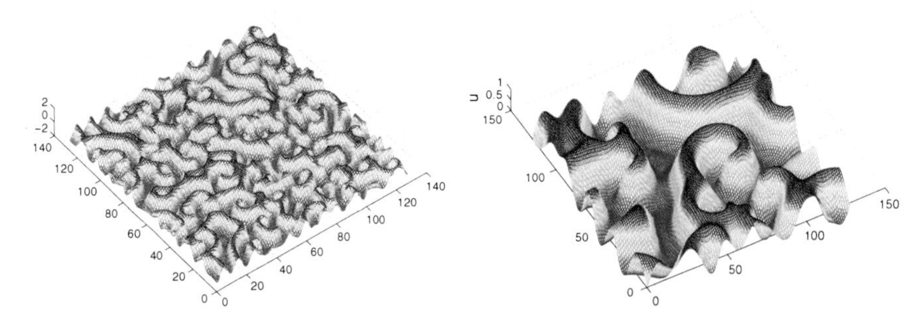

Fig. 3 When the difference between diffusion rates, D_{I_1} and D_{I_2} from Model (1) is large (*left*) aggregation occurs faster than when the difference between diffusion rates is small (*right*). Not linear model, we use the same parameters from model (4), except for a bigger β ($\alpha = 0.05$, $\beta = 1$ and $\delta = 1.3$, chosen so that (14) is satisfied)

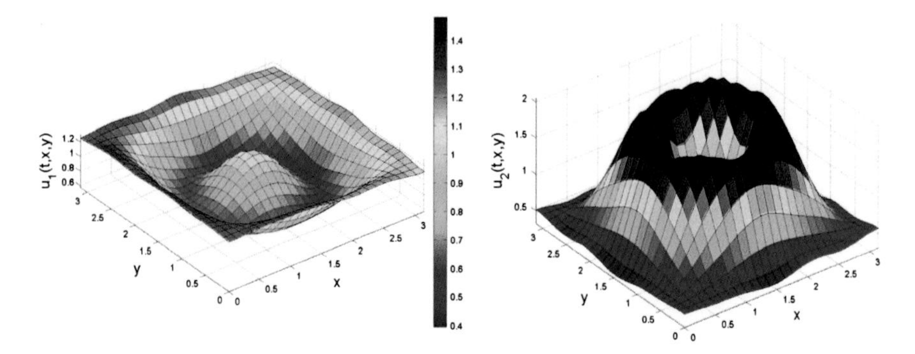

Fig. 4 The effects of a high cross-diffusion effect of solitary bees on honey bees ($\alpha_1 = \alpha_2 = \beta_{11} = \beta_{21} = \beta_{22} = 1, \gamma_1 = \gamma_2 = 5, \beta_{12} = 10$). Honey bees ($u_1$) are in low densities in areas where solitary bees (u_2) are in high densities and honey bees are found in high densities in areas where solitary bees are in low densities, thus demonstrating the avoidance effects of cross-diffusion [41]

where K is the carrying capacity, r is the intrinsic birth rate, β is the transmission rate, γ is the recovery rate, D_S and D_I are the susceptible and infective diffusion coefficients, respectively, and c is the cross-diffusion coefficient.

Following the approach in [41], the role of density-dependent cross-diffusion in the aggregation of individuals according to epidemiological states during a nefarious disease outbreak is carried out below. We expand on the type of cross-diffusion model in [6] via the use only of a population of S-individuals (susceptible) and I-individuals (infectives), that is, symptomatic infectious individuals. The model below assumes that symptoms generate avoidance.

3.1 *SI Model with Diffusion*

Let the densities for populations susceptible to a disease and infective with a disease, at time t and position $(x, y) \in \Omega$ be $S(x, y, t)$ and $I(x, y, t)$, respectively. We use the following SI epidemiological system

$$\begin{aligned} \frac{\partial S}{\partial t} &= rS^{\alpha_1}\left(1 - \frac{S^{\alpha_1}}{K}\right) - \beta\frac{SI}{(S+I)^{\alpha_2}} + D_S\nabla^2 S + c\nabla\cdot(S\nabla I) \\ \frac{\partial I}{\partial t} &= \beta\frac{SI}{(S+I)^{\alpha_2}} - \gamma I + D_I\nabla^2 I. \end{aligned} \tag{18}$$

Finally, it is further assumed that we have a closed system involving no external input; thus the use of Neumann boundary conditions

$$\frac{\partial}{\partial \nu} S = \frac{\partial}{\partial \nu} I = 0, \tag{19}$$

is acceptable. The initial conditions are as follows

$$S(x, y, 0) = S_0(x, y) \quad \text{and} \quad I(x, y, 0) = I_0(x, y). \tag{20}$$

Whenever D_S and D_I are the dominant coefficients, System (18) reduces essentially to the heat equation, which under Neumann boundary conditions will go to the average of the initial data as $t \to \infty$ [29].

3.2 *Effects of Recruitment*

Next we examine System (18) with $\alpha_2 = 1$, that is, we focus on the study of the effects of recruitment. When $\alpha_1 = 1$, logistic recruitment, System (18) reduces to System (17).

Lemma 1 *System* (17) *will support Turing's diffusive instability if*

$$\mathcal{R}_0 := \frac{\beta}{\gamma} < \frac{r}{\gamma} + 1, \tag{21}$$

$$Z := -D_S \frac{(\beta - \gamma)}{\mathcal{R}_0} - D_I r + D_I \beta - D_I \frac{\gamma}{\mathcal{R}_0} - \frac{(\beta - \gamma)^2}{\beta} c \frac{K(r - (\beta - \gamma))}{r} > 0, \tag{22}$$

and

$$Z^2 \geq D_S D_I \gamma (\beta - \gamma)(r - \beta + \gamma). \tag{23}$$

Proof To show Turing's diffusive instability, we first examine System (17) without diffusion terms ($D_S = D_I = c = 0$). The corresponding endemic equilibrium point is

$$(S^*, I^*) = \left(\frac{K(r - \beta + \gamma)}{r}, \frac{K(r - \beta + \gamma)(\beta - \gamma)}{r\gamma} \right), \tag{24}$$

the basic reproduction number is

$$\mathcal{R}_0 = \frac{\beta}{\gamma}, \tag{25}$$

and the Jacobian of System (17) without diffusion evaluated at the endemic equilibrium is

$$J = \begin{pmatrix} -r + \beta - \frac{\gamma^2}{\beta} & -\frac{\gamma^2}{\beta} \\ \frac{(\beta-\gamma)^2}{\beta} & -\frac{\gamma(\beta-\gamma)}{\beta} \end{pmatrix}. \tag{26}$$

By [23, 42], Turing's diffusive instability occurs if the following four conditions are satisfied

$$\mathrm{tr} J = J_{11} + J_{22} < 0 \tag{27}$$
$$\det J = J_{11}J_{22} - J_{12}J_{21} > 0 \tag{28}$$
$$\det \hat{D} = \hat{D}_{11}\hat{D}_{22} - \hat{D}_{12}\hat{D}_{21} > 0 \tag{29}$$
$$(\hat{D}_{11} - \hat{D}_{22})^2 + 4\hat{D}_{12}\hat{D}_{21} \geq 0 \tag{30}$$
$$\hat{D}_{11}J_{22} + \hat{D}_{22}J_{11} - \hat{D}_{12}J_{21} - \hat{D}_{21}J_{12} > 0 \tag{31}$$
$$(\hat{D}_{11}J_{22} + \hat{D}_{22}J_{11} - \hat{D}_{12}J_{21} - \hat{D}_{21}J_{12})^2 - 4 \det \hat{D} \det J \geq 0 \tag{32}$$

where the diffusion matrix is given by

$$\hat{D} = \begin{pmatrix} \hat{D}_{11} & \hat{D}_{12} \\ \hat{D}_{21} & \hat{D}_{22} \end{pmatrix} = \begin{pmatrix} D_S & c\frac{K(r-(\beta-\gamma))}{r} \\ 0 & D_I \end{pmatrix}.$$

Notice that in the absence of cross-diffusion, $D_{12} = D_{21} = 0$, Conditions (27), (28), and (32) become Conditions (6)–(8) from Model (1).

Conditions (27) and (28) hold if

$$\beta < r + \gamma, \tag{33}$$

which is equivalent to

$$\mathscr{R}_0 < \frac{r}{\gamma} + 1. \tag{34}$$

thus we must have that

$$1 < \mathscr{R}_0 < \frac{r}{\gamma} + 1. \tag{35}$$

It can be shown that Conditions (29) and (30) hold if $D_S, D_I \neq 0$, while Condition (31) holds if

$$Z := -D_S\frac{(\beta-\gamma)}{\mathscr{R}_0} - D_I r + D_I\beta - D_I\frac{\gamma}{\mathscr{R}_0} - \frac{(\beta-\gamma)^2}{\beta}c\frac{K(r-(\beta-\gamma))}{r} > 0 \tag{36}$$

and Condition (32) holds if

$$Z^2 \geq D_S D_I \gamma(\beta-\gamma)(r-\beta+\gamma) \tag{37}$$

□

When $\alpha_1 = 0$, constant recruitment, System (18) becomes

$$\begin{aligned}\frac{\partial S}{\partial t} &= \Lambda - \beta\frac{SI}{S+I} + D_S\nabla^2 S + c\nabla\cdot(S\nabla I)\\ \frac{\partial I}{\partial t} &= \beta\frac{SI}{S+I} - \gamma I + D_I\nabla^2 I\end{aligned} \tag{38}$$

where $\Lambda = r\left(1 - \frac{1}{K}\right)$.

Lemma 2 *Model* (38) *does not support Turing's diffusive instability.*

Proof The endemic equilibrium is

$$(S^*, I^*) = \left(\frac{\Lambda}{\beta-\gamma}, \frac{\Lambda}{\gamma}\right). \tag{39}$$

The basic reproductive number is

$$\mathscr{R}_0 = \frac{\beta}{\gamma}. \tag{40}$$

and we assume $\beta > \gamma$ so that $\mathscr{R}_0 > 1$.

The Jacobian is

$$J = \begin{pmatrix} -\frac{(\beta-\gamma)^2}{\beta} & -\frac{\gamma^2}{\beta} \\ \frac{(\beta-\gamma)^2}{\beta} & -\frac{\gamma(\beta-\gamma)}{\beta}\end{pmatrix}, \tag{41}$$

and the diffusion matrix is

$$\hat{D} = \begin{pmatrix} D_S & c\frac{\Lambda}{\beta-\gamma} \\ 0 & D_I\end{pmatrix}.$$

Note that Condition (31) fails due to the assumption that $\beta > \gamma$, and thus from [23, 42] we know that Turing diffusive instability is not possible. □

In short, logistic recruitment seems critical for supporting Turing's diffusive instability in the proposed cross-diffusion model.

3.3 *Effects of Incidence Functions*

The literature has often focused on modeling epidemics using the so called "mass-action" law ($\alpha_2 = 0$) or "standard" incidence ($\alpha_2 = 1$). In this section, we explore the role of this assumption in support of diffusive instability in our setting.

When $\alpha_2 = 0$, the mass action law comes into play and System (18) becomes

$$\begin{aligned}\frac{\partial S}{\partial t} &= rS\left(1 - \frac{S}{K}\right) - \beta SI + D_S \nabla^2 S + c\nabla \cdot (S\nabla I) \\ \frac{\partial I}{\partial t} &= \beta SI - \gamma I + D_I \nabla^2 I\end{aligned} \tag{42}$$

Lemma 3 *System* (42) *will not support Turing's diffusive instability.*

Proof The endemic equilibrium is

$$(S^*, I^*) = \left(\frac{\gamma}{\beta}, \frac{r(K\beta - \gamma)}{K\beta^2}\right), \tag{43}$$

where the basic reproductive number is

$$\mathscr{R}_0 = \frac{\beta K}{\gamma}. \tag{44}$$

The Jacobian evaluated at the endemic equilibrium is

$$J = \begin{pmatrix} -\frac{r}{\mathscr{R}_0} & -\gamma \\ r\left(1 - \frac{1}{\mathscr{R}_0}\right) & 0 \end{pmatrix}. \tag{45}$$

The diffusion matrix is

$$\hat{D} = \begin{pmatrix} D_S & c\frac{\gamma}{\beta} \\ 0 & D_I \end{pmatrix}.$$

Notice that Condition (31) fails if $\mathscr{R}_0 > 1$ is imposed. Thus (42) will not result in Turing's diffusive instability. □

The case $\alpha_2 = 1$, standard incidence, corresponds to the case when System (18) becomes System (17), and so, Turing's diffusive instability is possible. The use of standard incidence seems critical to the support of Turing's diffusive instability in our setting.

3.4 Necessary and Sufficient Conditions

Theorem 2 *For a density dependent cross-diffusion SI model of the form System* (18), *logistic recruitment and standard incidence functions are necessary for Turing's diffusive instability.*

Proof The proof is a direct result of the preceding lemmas. □

See Fig. 5 for simulations for Model (17) carried out under Conditions (21)–(23).

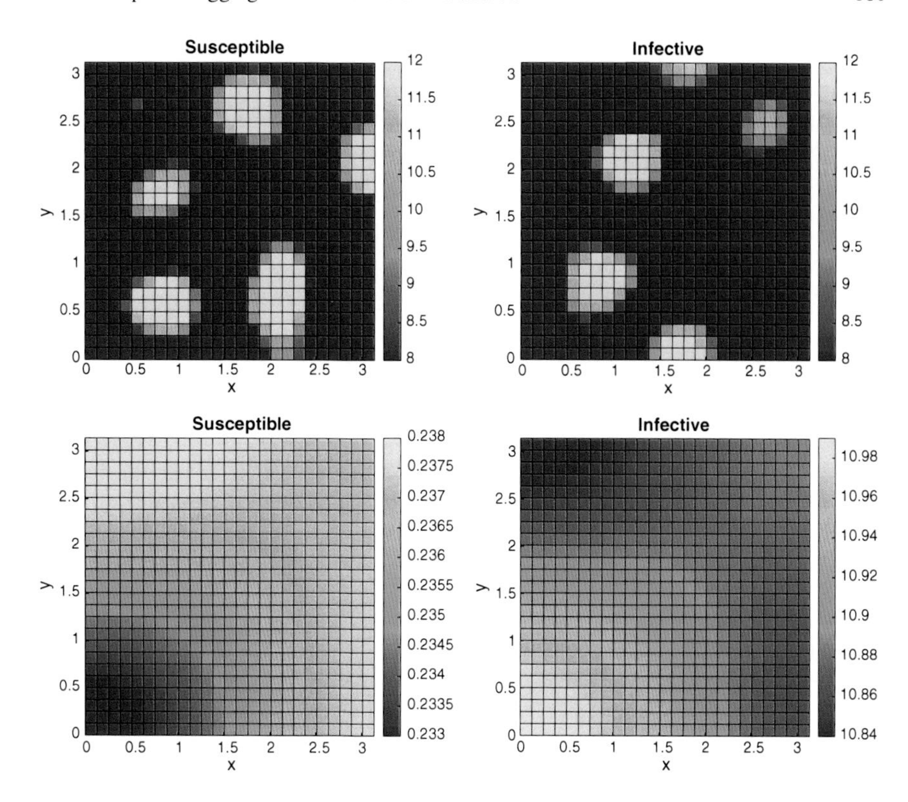

Fig. 5 The distribution for Model (18) under constant recruitment ($\alpha_1 = 0$) and mass action incidence function ($\alpha_2 = 0$) under the conditions $D_S = 0.1$, $D_I = 2$, $c = 0.02$, $r = 0.4$, $K = 100$, $\beta = 0.5$, chosen so that Conditions (21)–(23) are satisfied for $t = 0$ (*top*), $t = 500$ (*bottom*). As time increases the distributions of both susceptible and infective populations have a homogeneous distribution, with no patches

4 Discussion and Conclusion

We have proposed two models: a phenomenological model that examined the effects of an "unusual" incidence function and a cross-diffusion model. Model (1) can be applied to the study of sexually transmitted diseases such as *chlamydia* and *gonorrhea* as well as to communicable diseases like *leprosy* or possibly Ebola. In all three examples some form of *social distancing* is assumed to be generated in response to the presence of symptoms. Model (1) predicts that changes in behavior will result in spatial aggregation (via diffusive instability) and that such natural responses help, in fact, to reduce the population's levels of infection.

An SI model with density dependent cross-diffusion, where susceptible individuals avoid increasing gradients of infective individuals is also considered. Indeed if the sign of the diffusion coefficient is negated, individuals would be attracted to increasing gradients of infective populations, as shown in the Keller–Segel model

[19, 20], rather than repelled from infective populations. Using Model (18) as a starting point, we examine the effects of the choice of recruitment and incidence functions and conclude that a logistic recruitment and standard incidence functions are necessary to have pattern formations, Turing's diffusive instability. Mass action incidence function, a popular choice, does not result in diffusive instability.

Appendix: Derivation of the SI Model with Diffusion

As a starting point, let the densities for populations susceptible to a disease and infective with a disease, at time t and position $(x, y) \in \Omega$ be $S(x, y, t)$ and $I(x, y, t)$, respectively. We assume the model takes the form of the following reaction-diffusion model

$$\begin{aligned} \frac{\partial S}{\partial t} &= -\nabla \cdot \mathbf{J}_1 + f_1(S, I) \quad \text{in } \Omega \times (0, T), \\ \frac{\partial I}{\partial t} &= -\nabla \cdot \mathbf{J}_2 + f_2(S, I) \quad \text{in } \Omega \times (0, T), \end{aligned} \tag{46}$$

where f_1, f_2 and $\mathbf{J}_1$, $\mathbf{J}_2$ are the reaction and flux terms for the susceptible and infective populations, respectively. The reaction terms are modeled as follows:

$$f_1(S, I) = rS^{\alpha_1}\left(1 - \frac{S^{\alpha_1}}{K}\right) - \beta\frac{SI}{(S+I)^{\alpha_2}}, \qquad f_2(S, I) = \beta\frac{SI}{(S+I)^{\alpha_2}} - \gamma I,$$

where K is the carrying capacity, r is the intrinsic birth rate, β is the transmission rate, γ is the recovery rate, $\alpha_1 \in \{0, 1\}$, $\alpha_2 \in \{0, 1\}$; $\alpha_1 = 1$ corresponding to logistic growth and $\alpha_1 = 0$ to constant recruitment; $\alpha_2 = 0$ accounts for mass-action transmission while $\alpha_2 = 1$ models standard incidence.

It is assumed that each population is influenced by increasing gradients of infectious individuals that result in the "directional"s dispersive migrations of each population towards its own type. Let D_S and D_I be the intrinsic-diffusion constants of the susceptible and infective populations, respectively, then the intrinsic dispersal forces of S and I in the flux are given by the gradient of the densities, $D_S\nabla S$, $D_I\nabla I$, respectively [28]. The assumption that $D_S, D_I \geq 0$ means that the dispersal is in directions away from high densities, the last assumption justified by the tendency of susceptible to avoid increasing gradient populations of symptomatic infectious individuals, that is, it is assumed that they tend to move towards decreasing gradients of symptomatic individuals. The cross-diffusion coefficient measuring the impact of the infective population on the susceptible population is denoted by the constant $c \geq 0$. Therefore, the cross-diffusion force of infective on susceptible populations in the flux is given by $cS\nabla I$. We further assume that there are no other cross-diffusion forces. Thus the flux for S and I are modeled as

$$\mathbf{J}_1 = -D_S \nabla S - cS\nabla I$$
$$\mathbf{J}_2 = -D_I \nabla I,$$

which takes the form of the celebrated Keller–Segel model [19, 20].

Incorporating the reaction and diffusion terms leads to the following SI epidemiological system

$$\begin{aligned} \frac{\partial S}{\partial t} &= rS^{\alpha_1}\left(1 - \frac{S^{\alpha_1}}{K}\right) - \beta \frac{SI}{(S+I)^{\alpha_2}} + D_S \nabla^2 S + c\nabla \cdot (S\nabla I) \\ \frac{\partial I}{\partial t} &= \beta \frac{SI}{(S+I)^{\alpha_2}} - \gamma I + D_I \nabla^2 I. \end{aligned} \tag{47}$$

Finally, it is further assumed that we have a closed system involving no external input; thus the use of Neumann boundary conditions

$$\frac{\partial}{\partial \nu} S = \frac{\partial}{\partial \nu} I = 0, \tag{48}$$

is acceptable. The initial conditions are as follows

$$S(x, y, 0) = S_0(x, y) \quad \text{and} \quad I(x, y, 0) = I_0(x, y). \tag{49}$$

Whenever D_S and D_I are the dominant coefficients, System (18) reduces essentially to the heat equation, which under Neumann boundary conditions will go to the average of the initial data as $t \to \infty$ [29].

References

1. Adler, F.R.: The effects of averaging on the basic reproduction ratio. Math. Bioscie. **111**(1), 89–98 (1992)
2. Adler, F.R., Kretzschmar, M.: Aggregation and stability in parasitehost models. Parasitology **104**(02), 199–205 (1992)
3. Andersson, H., Britton, T., et al.: Heterogeneity in epidemic models and its effect on the spread of infection. J. Appl. Probab. **35**(3), 651–661 (1998)
4. Balina, L.M., Valdez, R.P.: Reflections on the international leprosy congresses and other events in research, epidemiology, and elimination of leprosy. Int. J. Lepr. **62**, 412–427 (1994)
5. Berres, S., Ruiz-Baier, R.: A fully adaptive numerical approximation for a two-dimensional epidemic model with nonlinear cross-diffusion. Nonlinear Anal. Real World Appl. **12**(5), 2888–2903 (2011)
6. Bichara, D., Kang, Y., Castillo-Chavez, C., Horan, R., Perrings, C:. Sis and sir epidemic models under virtual dispersal. B. Math. Biol. **77**, 2004–2034 (2015)
7. Brauer, F., Van den Driessche, P., Wu, J.: Mathematical Epidemiology, vol. 1945. Springer, Berlin (2008)
8. Carrero, G., Lizana, M.: Pattern formation in a SIS epidemiological model. Can. Appl. Math. Q. **11**(1), 1–22 (2003)
9. Castillo-Chavez, C., Li, B.: Spatial spread of sexually transmitted diseases within susceptible populations at demographic steady state. Math. Biosci. Eng. **5**(4), 713–727 (2008)

10. Castillo-Chavez, C., Huang, W., Li, J.: Competitive exclusion in gonorrhea models and other sexually transmitted diseases. SIAM J. Appl. Math. **56**(2), 494–508 (1996)
11. Castillo-Chavez, C., Blower, S., Driessche, P., Kirschner, D., Yakubu, A.-A.: Mathematical Approaches for Emerging and Reemerging Infectious Diseases: Models, Methods, and Theory, vol. 126. Springer, Berlin (2002)
12. Chowell, G., Hengartner, N.W., Castillo-Chavez, C., Fenimore, P.W., Hyman, J.M.: The basic reproductive number of ebola and the effects of public health measures: the cases of congo and uganda. J. Theor. Biol. **229**(1), 119–126 (2004)
13. Herrera, E.D.: Diffusive instability and aggregation in epidemics. Ph.D. thesis, Arizona State University (2010)
14. Diekmann, O., Dietz, K., Heesterbeek, V.: The basic reproduction ratio for sexually transmitted diseases: I. theoretical considerations. Math. Biosci. **107**(2), 325–339 (1991)
15. Diekmann, O., Heesterbeek, H., Britton, T.: Mathematical Tools for Understanding Infectious Disease Dynamics. Princeton University Press, Princeton (2012)
16. Fenichel, E.P., Carlos Castillo-Chavez, M.G., Ceddia, G.C., Gonzalez, P.A., Parra, G.J., Hickling, G.H., Horan, R., Morin, B., Perrings, C., et al.: Adaptive human behavior in epidemiological models. Proc. Natl. Acad. Sci. **108**(15), 6306–6311 (2011)
17. Hadeler, K.P., Castillo-Chávez, C.: A core group model for disease transmission. Math. Biosci. **128**(1), 41–55 (1995)
18. Heiderich, K.R., Huang, W., Castillo-Chavez, C.: Nonlocal response in a simple epidemiological model. Mathematical Approaches for Emerging and Reemerging Infectious Diseases: an Introduction (Minneapolis, MN, 1999), vol. 125, IMA vol. Math. Appl., pp. 129–151. Springer, New York (2002)
19. Keller, F.E., Segel, L.A.: Initiation of slime mold aggregation viewed as an instability. J. Theor. Biol. **26**(3), 399–415 (1970)
20. Keller, E.F., Segel, L.A.: Model for chemotaxis. J. Theor. Biol. **30**(2), 225–234 (1971)
21. Kermack, W.O., McKendrick, A.G.: Contributions to the mathematical theory of epidemics. ii. the problem of endemicity. Proc. R. Soc. Lond. Ser. A **138**(834), 55–83 (1932)
22. Kiskowski, M.A.: A three-scale network model for the early growth dynamics of 2014 west africa ebola epidemic. PloS Curr. Outbreaks (2014)
23. Kumar, N., Horsthemke, W.: Effects of cross diffusion on turing bifurcations in two-species reaction-transport systems. Phys. Rev. E **83**(3), 036105 (2011)
24. Li, L., Zhen, J., Gui-Quan, S.: Spatial pattern of an epidemic model with cross-diffusion. Chin. Phys. Lett. **25**(9), 3500 (2008)
25. Morin, B.R., Fenichel, E.P., Castillo-Chavez, C.: Sir dynamics with economically driven contact rates. Nat. Resour. Model. **26**(4), 505–525 (2013)
26. Murray, J.D.: Mathematical Biology I: An Introduction, vol. 17. Springer, New York (2002)
27. Murray, J.D.: Mathematical Biology II: Spatial Models and Biomedical Applications, vol. 17. Springer, New York (2002)
28. Nallaswamy, R., Shukla, B.: Effects of dispersal on the stability. Math. Biosci. **72**, 63–72 (1982)
29. Ni, W.M.: Diffusion, cross-diffusion, and their spike-layer steady states. Not. AMS, pp. 9–18 (1998)
30. Nishiura, H., Chowell, G.: Early transmission dynamics of ebola virus disease (evd), west africa, march to august 2014. Euro Surveill **19**(36), 20894 (2014)
31. Riley, S.: Large-scale spatial-transmission models of infectious disease. Science **316**(5829), 1298–1301 (2007)
32. Rıos-Soto, K.R., Song, B., Castillo-Chavez, C.: Epidemic spread of influenza viruses: the impact of transient populations on disease dynamics. Math. Biosci. Eng. **8**(1), 199–222 (2011)
33. Robbins, G., Mushrif Tripathy, V., Misra, V.N., Mohanty, R.K., Shinde, V.S., Gray, K.M., Schug, M.D.: Ancient skeletal evidence for leprosy in india (2000 bc). PloS One **4**(5), e5669 (2009)
34. Rodrigues, L.C., Lockwood, D.N.J.: Leprosy now: epidemiology, progress, challenges, and research gaps. Lancet Infect. Dis. **11**(6), 464–470 (2011)

35. Segel, L.A., Jackson, J.L.: Dissipative structure: an explanation and an ecological example. J. Theor. Biol. **37**(3), 545–559 (1972)
36. Shigesada, N., Kawasaki, K., Teramoto, E.: Spatial segregation of interacting species. J. Theor. Biol. **79**(1), 83–99 (1979)
37. Sun, G.-Q., Jin, Z., Liu, Q.-X., Li, L.: Spatial pattern in an epidemic system with cross-diffusion of the susceptible. J. Biol. Syst. **17**(01), 141–152 (2009)
38. Thieme, H.R.: Mathematics in Population Biology. Princeton University Press, Princeton (2003)
39. Towers, S., Patterson-Lomba, O., Castillo-Chavez, C.: Temporal variations in the effective reproduction number of the 2014 west africa ebola outbreak. PLOS Curr. Outbreaks (2014)
40. Wang, Y., Wang, J., Zhang, L.: Cross diffusion-induced pattern in an si model. Appl. Math. Comput. **217**(5), 1965–1970 (2010)
41. Yong, K.E., Li, Y., Hendrix, S.D.: Of multiple pollinators in almond trees and its potential effect on pollen movement and productivity: A theoretical approach using the Shigesada-Kawasaki-Teramoto model. J. Theor. Biol. **305**, 103–109 (2012)
42. Zemskov, E.P., Kassner, K., Hauser, M.J.B., Horsthemke, W.: Turing space in reaction-diffusion systems with density-dependent cross diffusion. Phys. Rev. E **87**(3), 032906 (2013)

Designing Public Health Policies to Mitigate the Adverse Consequences of Rural-Urban Migration via Meta-Population Modeling

Zhilan Feng, Yiqiang Zheng, Nancy Hernandez-Ceron and Henry Zhao

Abstract This study extends the model considered in [3] (Chap. 8 in this volume) by incorporating spatially explicit migration of individuals. A three-patch meta-population model is used to explore vaccination strategies for a vaccine-preventable disease. Spatial movements of individuals between patches are mainly migration from rural to urban and peri-urban for greater economic opportunities. Stochastic simulations evaluate the effects of alternative vaccination strategies on preventing disease outbreaks, examine the distribution of possible outcomes, and compare the likelihood of outbreak mitigation and prevention across immunization policies. Two types of vaccine coverage are compared. One is homogeneous coverage, in which relevant sub-populations receive vaccination with equal probability; and the other is heterogeneous coverage, in which sub-populations can receive vaccination with different probabilities. Results suggest that when sub-populations differ in density (which may affect contact rates), heterogeneous vaccination coverage among migrants is most effective according to measures such as final epidemic size, peak size, number of vaccine doses needed to prevent outbreaks, and likelihood of containing an outbreak. This suggests that public health efforts to mitigate vaccine-preventable diseases must consider migration.

Keywords Epidemic model · Migration · Meta-population model · Infectious disease · Public health policy · Vaccination

---

Z. Feng (✉) · Y. Zheng · H. Zhao
Purdue University, West Lafayette, IN 47907, USA
e-mail: zfeng@math.purdue.edu

Y. Zheng
e-mail: zheng30@purdue.edu

H. Zhao
e-mail: zhao137@purdue.edu

N. Hernandez-Ceron
University of Michigan, 48109 Ann Arbor, MI, USA
e-mail: nhceron@umich.edu

G. Chowell and J.M. Hyman (eds.), *Mathematical and Statistical Modeling for Emerging and Re-emerging Infectious Diseases*,
DOI 10.1007/978-3-319-40413-4_12

1 Introduction

Rural people migrate to urban areas largely because economic opportunities are greater there, even absent education or special skills. Such migrations may be seasonal, to sell goods produced or harvested locally where potential consumers are more concentrated. Migration may also be motivated by the need for medical or other services available only in densely populated areas. Depending on sojourn duration, immigrants may stay with friends or relatives in peri-urban shanty towns. Those wishing to remain permanently and are able to sustain themselves in urban environments may move from peri-urban to urban areas while others return to the rural areas from whence they came.

By virtue of the difference in population density, infectious diseases against which immunity is long-lasting may be epidemic in rural, but endemic in urban areas. If so, immigrants are less likely to be immune than urban people the same age. Together with births, rural-urban migration thus increases the proportions of urban or peri-urban populations that are susceptible to infection by the pathogens causing these diseases. In the preceding chapter, Jos Cassio de Moraes et al. argue that–insofar as the coverage required to prevent outbreaks is lower in rural than urban areas—rural-urban migration motivates regional versus local design of optimal vaccination programs.

Here we consider a model with three sub-populations consisting of urban, peri-urban, and rural populations. One of the main differences between these sub-populations is their density (and immunity, naturally acquired or vaccine-induced). The model is constructed to include not only the usual mixing between the three sub-populations (deterministic) but also seasonally-driven migrations of individuals from rural to urban areas (stochastic). In addition to routine vaccination within each patch, supplementary vaccination may be used to mitigate the consequences of the migration.

While deterministic models provide the expected effects of various immunization policies, policymakers must consider the inherent randomness of contact between susceptible and infectious people. Stochastic models allow us to examine the distribution of possible outcomes and compare the likelihood of certain results across immunization policies. When the threat of a disease outbreak cannot be eliminated entirely, it may be possible to limit those exceeding specific levels, whatever those might be. Stochastic simulations can be used to analyze the likelihood of containing outbreaks to any prescribed final or peak size. Perhaps the goal is a below 5 % risk of the disease spreading to more than that threshold level, because the policies necessary to eliminate that final 5 % are prohibitively expensive or unrealistic to implement. Stochastic models are more suitable for obtaining such insights than deterministic ones. Detailed examples are presented in the following sections.

Effects of spatial movement of humans on the spread and control of infectious diseases have been studied using mathematical models in other settings, particularly for the 2014 West Africa Ebola outbreak (see, for example, [1, 5, 9]). These studies focus on international spread of Ebola virus via air travel, and the efficacy of control measures including travel restrictions or exit and entry screening of travelers. They provide important quantitative information about the benefits and associated costs of screening and restriction of travel, which can be very helpful for policy-making. The study presented in the current paper aims at assessing the role of vaccinating migrants from a rural area at their entry to urban and peri-urban areas, where disease transmission rates can be much higher due to greater population densities. Results in this work suggest that such a difference in population densities can have important implications for disease outbreaks and vaccination strategies.

2 Models and Analysis

Because the objective of this study is to identify the best short-term vaccination policy to mitigate outbreaks, we focus on an epidemic model (neither births nor deaths) and stochastic simulations over a short period. On the other hand, population immunity is influenced by the routine vaccination policy over a longer period. Thus, we use a deterministic endemic model for each sub-population to compute the steady-state distribution of the epidemiological classes, which is then used as initial conditions for short-term stochastic simulations. Following the approach of Lloyd et al. [8], we use discrete-time models here.

2.1 *The Long-Term Endemic Model*

Consider three sub-populations representing urban, peri-urban, and rural populations, each of which consists of six epidemiological classes: individuals with maternal immunity (M_i); individuals with temporary immunity due to vaccination (V_i); susceptible individuals (S_i); exposed or latent (L); infectious (I); and those who have recovered from infection (and are immune) (R_i), where the subscripts $i = 1, 2, 3$ correspond to urban, peri-urban, and rural populations, respectively. Individuals in both V and M classes can lose their immunity. Birth and death rates within each patch are assumed to be equal so that the total population remains constant. A transition diagram is shown in Fig. 1

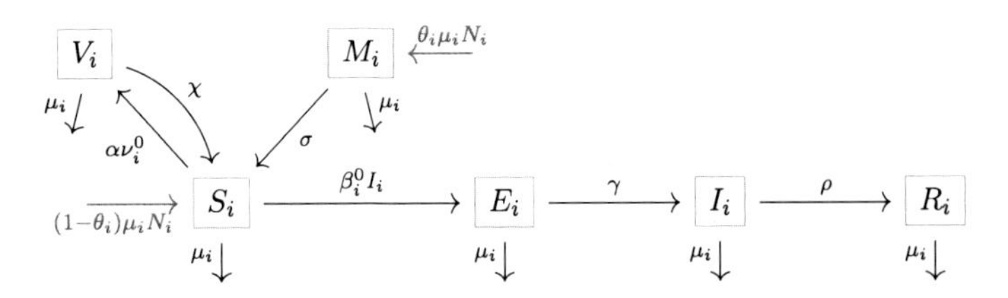

Fig. 1 Transition diagram for the long-term model

The model reads

$$
\begin{aligned}
M_i(n+1) &= \theta_i \mu_i N_i + (1-\mu_i)(1-\sigma)M_i(n) \\
V_i(n+1) &= \alpha \nu_i^0 (1-\mu_i) e^{-\beta_i^0 \frac{I_i(n)}{N_i}} S_i(n) + (1-\mu_i)(1-\chi)V_i(n) \\
S_i(n+1) &= (1-\theta_i)\mu_i N_i + (1-\mu_i)(1-\alpha \nu_i^0) e^{-\beta_i^0 \frac{I_i(n)}{N_i}} S_i(n) \\
&\quad + \sigma(1-\mu_i)M_i(n) + \chi(1-\mu_i)V_i(n) \\
E_i(n+1) &= (1-\mu_i)(1-e^{-\beta_i^0 \frac{I_i(n)}{N_i}})S_i(n) + (1-\mu_i)(1-\gamma)E_i(n) \\
I_i(n+1) &= (1-\mu_i)\gamma E_i(n) + (1-\mu_i)(1-\rho)I_i(n) \\
R_i(n+1) &= (1-\mu_i)\rho I_i(n) + (1-\mu_i)R_i(n), \quad i = 1, 2, 3,
\end{aligned}
\tag{1}
$$

where $N_i = M_i + V_i + S_i + E_i + I_i + R_i$. For patch i, θ_i is the proportion of newborns with maternal immunity; μ_i is the daily per-capita birth and death probability ($1/\mu_i$ is the average lifespan) in patch i; σ is the daily probability of immunity loss due to maternal antibodies ($1/\sigma$ is the average period of maternal immunity); α is the vaccine efficacy; ν_i^0 is the daily probability of being vaccinated; β_i^0 is the daily transmission rate; $1/\chi$ is the duration of immunity due to vaccination; $1/\gamma$ and $1/\rho$ are the average periods of latency and infection, respectively. The probability of infection for a susceptible individual in patch i, $e^{-\beta_i^0 \frac{I_i}{N_i}}$, has the same form as in [2, 6–8]. All parameters and their meanings are listed in Table 1.

The parameter values listed in Table 1 are based on measles, and the three subpopulations have a similar spatial structure to the urban, peri-urban and rural populations in São Paulo, Brazil. Some parameter values are selected from the literature while others are calculated or estimated from available data. For example, given the

Table 1 Parameters in the long-term model (1) for patch i ($i = 1, 2, 3$)

Symbol	Description	Value (patch 1, 2, 3)
θ_i	Fraction of newborns with maternal immunity	(0.7, 0.7, 0.7)
$1/\mu_i$	Lifespan	(70, 70, 68) years
$1/\sigma$	Duration of maternal immunity	6 months
$1/\chi$	Duration of vaccine-induced immunity	60 years
α	Vaccine efficacy	92–95 %
ν_i^0	Daily probability of being vaccinated	determined by p_i
β_i^0	Daily transmission rate	(1.4, 1.1, 0.85)
$\mathcal{R}_{vi}$	Effective reproduction number (long-term)	(1.25, 1.16, 1.03)
$\mathcal{R}_{0i}$	Basic reproduction number (long-term)	(9.79, 7.70, 5.95)
$1/\gamma$	Latent period	7 days
$1/\rho$	Infectious period	7 days
N	Total population size $= N_1 + N_2 + N_3$	$(0.125N, 0.2N, 0.675N)$

The subscripts $i = 1, 2, 3$ correspond to urban, peri-urban, rural patches, respectively long-term vaccination policy of vaccinating $p_i = 0.9$ of susceptibles within 10 years, the daily probability ν_i^0 of being vaccinated can be determined from using the relationship $1 - p_i = (1 - \nu_i^0)^{10\times 360}$. Also, knowing the basic reproduction number $\mathscr{R}_{0i}$ and all other parameter values except β_i, we can estimate β_i. Using these parameter values, we can numerically compute the steady-state values of each epidemiological class, which then can be used in stochastic simulations of the short-term model.

Because the long-term model is used to determine the local population immunity within each patch under the routine vaccination policy, no interactions between patches are modeled. Even though the interactions between patches are ignored, it is difficult to obtain an explicit expression for the non-trivial steady state of the system for sub-population i. Numerical computations of these steady states will be used for short-term simulations. Nevertheless, the effective reproduction number for sub-population i, denoted by $\mathscr{R}_{vi}$, can be computed (see Appendix) and is given by

$$\mathscr{R}_{vi} = \left(\frac{(1-\mu_i)\gamma}{1-(1-\mu_i)(1-\gamma)}\right)\left(\frac{\beta_i^0(1-\mu_i)}{1-(1-\mu_i)(1-\rho)}\right)\frac{S_i^0}{N_i}, \tag{2}$$

in which the first factor is the probability that a newly infected individual survives the latent period, the second factor is the number of new infections that a typical infectious individual produces during the entire infectious period in a completely susceptible population, and the third factor is the fraction of the population i that is susceptible at the disease-free equilibrium. Note that, under the routine vaccination policy represented by vaccination at rate ν_i^0, the fraction of susceptibles (see Appendix) at the disease-free equilibrium is

$$\frac{S_i^0}{N_i} = \frac{\left[(1-\theta_i) + \theta_i \frac{\sigma(1-\mu_i)}{1-(1-\mu_i)(1-\sigma)}\right]\mu_i}{1-(1-\mu_i)(1-\alpha\nu_i^0) - \frac{\chi(1-\mu_i)\alpha\nu_i^0(1-\mu_i)}{1-(1-\mu_i)(1-\chi)}}, \quad \frac{V_i^0}{N_i} = \frac{\alpha\nu_i^0(1-\mu_i)S_i^0/N_i}{1-(1-\mu_i)(1-\chi)}. \tag{3}$$

The expressions in (2) and (3) illustrate how the population susceptibility S_i^0/N_i and level of immunity V_i^0/N_i depend on vaccination at rate ν_i^0, which may differ among the three sub-populations. Similarly, it is clear that the endemic equilibrium of patch i,

$$\hat{E}_i = (\hat{M}_i, \hat{V}_i, \hat{E}_i, \hat{I}_i, \hat{R}_i), \quad i = 1, 2, 3, \tag{4}$$

depends on both vaccination rate ν_i^0 and transmission rate β_i^0. For example, susceptibility of the rural population might be much higher than that of the urban population due to vaccination coverage and population density (which affects the values of β_i^0 through contact rates). Consequently, migrants from rural to urban or peri-urban might have a significant impact on the potential for an outbreak (see Chap. 8).

Although it is difficult to obtain analytic expressions for $\hat{E}_i$, it can be solved for numerically (see Fig. 2). The long-term steady state values of the components in $\hat{E}_i$ will be used as initial conditions for simulations of the short-term model, and the effects of various vaccination policies on controlling disease outbreaks will be compared in Sect. 3.

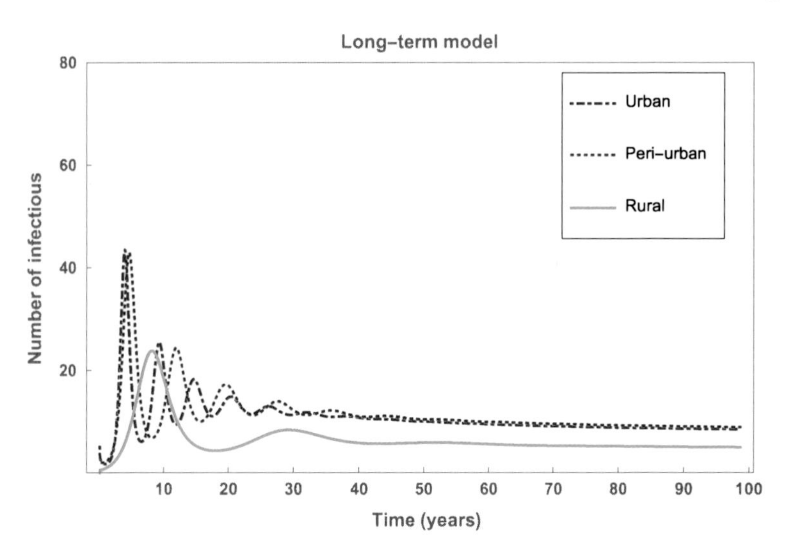

Fig. 2 Long-term dynamics of the model (1) for each of the three patches when rural-urban migration is ignored

2.2 The Short-Term Model

The short-term stochastic model focuses on mitigating a single outbreak during one season. It ignores the birth and death processes, as well as the vaccination/immunity loss considered in the long-term model. In this case, the individuals in the V, M, and R classes are all considered immune so can be combined in the same compartment, denoted by R. Disease transmission and migration for the short-term model are depicted in Fig. 3.

The stochasticity is modeled following the approach used in [8]. The model equations are given by:

$$
\begin{aligned}
S_i(n+1) &= \sum_{j=1}^{3} m_{ji}(n) S_j(n) e^{-\lambda_j(n)}(1-\eta_{ji}(n)) \\
E_i(n+1) &= \sum_{j=1}^{3} m_{ji}(n) S_j(n) \left[1 - e^{-\lambda_j(n)}\right] + \sum_{j=1}^{3} (1-\gamma) m_{ji}(n) E_j(n) \\
I_i(n+1) &= \sum_{j=1}^{3} \gamma m_{ji}(n) E_j(n) + (1-\rho) I_i(n) \\
R_i(n+1) &= \rho I_i(n) + \sum_{j=1}^{3} m_{ji}(n) R_j(n) \\
V_i^s(n+1) &= \sum_{j=1}^{3} m_{ji}(n) S_j(n) e^{\lambda_j(n)} \eta_{ji}(n) + \sum_{j=1}^{3} m_{ji}(n) V_j^s(n), \quad i = 1, 2, 3,
\end{aligned}
\tag{5}
$$

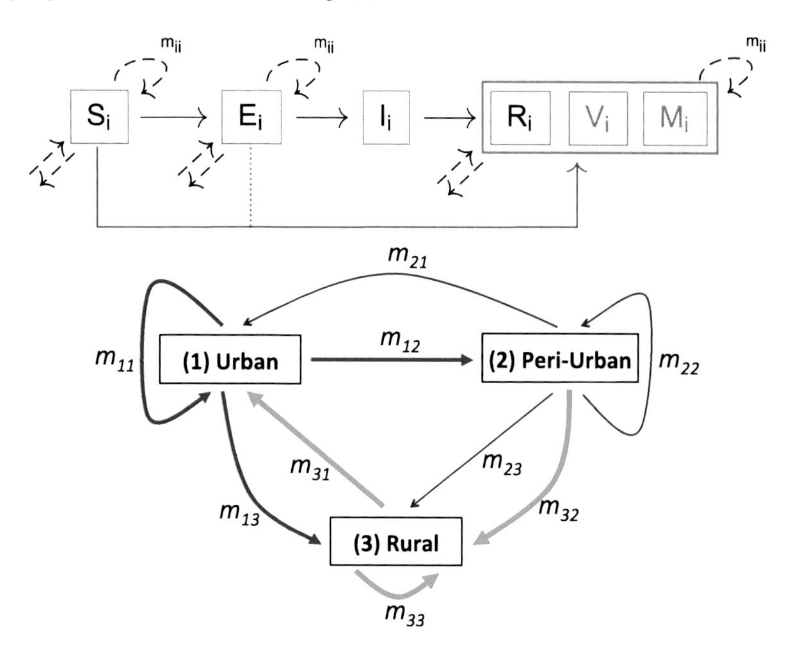

Fig. 3 A disease transmission diagram for the short-term model (*top*) and a depiction of the movement between the three patches (*bottom*). The dashed arrows in the top diagram represent migration. The parameter m_{ij} represents the daily per capita migration probability from patch i to patch j

where V_i^s denotes the individuals in patch i who are vaccinated due to supplemental efforts (in addition to the routine vaccination program); $m_{ij}(n)$ is the time-dependent exiting probability from patch i to patch j at time step n (see the migration diagram in Fig. 3); η_{ij} represents the combined routine and supplementary vaccination; γ and ρ have the same meanings as in the long-term model (1). The force of infection, λ_i is given by

$$\lambda_i(n) = \beta a_i \sum_{j=1}^{3} c_{ij} \frac{I_j(n)}{N_j(n)}, \quad i = 1, 2, 3. \tag{6}$$

Here, the c_{ij} represent casual mixing between patches i and j, which we consider to be preferential and are given by

$$c_{ij} = \varepsilon_i \delta_{ij} + (1 - \varepsilon_i) f_j, \quad f_j = \frac{(1 - \varepsilon_j) a_j N_j}{\sum_k (1 - \varepsilon_k) a_k N_k}, \tag{7}$$

where a_i denotes the number of contacts per day in patch i, and $N_i(n) = S_i(n) + E_i(n) + I_i(n) + R_i(n) + V_i^s(n)$ is the total population in patch i at time n. Note that the M_i and V_i classes are included in the R_i class in the short-term model.

We remark that, although vaccinations are also given to individuals in the E_i class (assuming that no testing will be done before vaccinating), these individuals will remain in the E_i class, which is why this process need not be explicitly modeled. However, the wasted vaccines are included in determining the number of doses used. The parameter ε_i denotes the proportion of contacts of patch i that is reserved for others in the same patch. The rest $1 - \varepsilon_i$ of contacts are distributed proportionately among all patches including i. The parameter a_i denotes the per-capita number of contacts in population i, and the balance equation $a_i N_i c_{ij} = a_j N_j c_{ji}$ must be satisfied. That is, the total number of contacts from individuals in patch i with individuals in patch j must equal to the total contacts of individuals in patch j with those in patch i. We remark that, although $N_i(n)$ may change with time n when migration rates are not zero, the balance equation will always hold as long as c_{ij} are defined as in (7).

To evaluate the effect of various short-term vaccination programs, particularly those involving migrants, it is important to get reasonable parameter values for the migration probabilities m_{ij}. Although these parameters are chosen to be constant in many patch models, it is not appropriate here as the migration that we are considering is driven by seasonally-available job opportunities, and migrants will return to their home patch within one year. To capture this seasonally varying pattern, we consider piecewise-constant m_{ij} values as described below.

For demonstration purposes, consider the case in which a proportion of rural individuals will move to urban and peri-urban for jobs during a fixed period of time in a year and return to their rural homes afterwards; there is no migration between patches during the rest of the year. Let $M = (m_{ij})$ denote the 3×3 migration matrix. Denote by M_{ru}, M_{ur}, and M_0 the matrices for the migration from rural to urban/peri-urban, the migration from urban/peri-urban back to rural, and no migration, respectively, during the corresponding periods of a year.

To determine the elements in M_{ru}, assume that the migration season lasts for d days, and that a fraction l_3 of the rural population move to the urban/peri-urban patches, of which a fraction q_1 go to the urban patch and fraction q_2 go to the peri-urban patch. Then $1 - l_3 = m_{33}^d$ or

$$m_{33} = (1 - l_3)^{\frac{1}{d}}. \tag{8}$$

Note that $m_{31} + m_{32} + m_{33} = 1$ and that

$$q_1 = \frac{m_{31}}{m_{31} + m_{32}}, \quad q_2 = \frac{m_{32}}{m_{31} + m_{32}}.$$

It follows that

$$m_{31} = q_1(1 - m_{33}), \quad m_{32} = q_2(1 - m_{33}). \tag{9}$$

Thus, the matrix M_{ru} is given by

$$M_{ru} = \begin{bmatrix} 1 & 0 & 0 \\ 0 & 1 & 0 \\ q_1[1-(1-l_3)^{\frac{1}{d}}] & q_2[1-(1-l_3)^{\frac{1}{d}}] & (1-l_3)^{\frac{1}{d}} \end{bmatrix}. \tag{10}$$

For the matrix M_{ur} for migrants returning from urban/peri-urban to rural, let $n_i = N_i/(N_1 + N_2 + N_3)$ denote the ratio of sub-population N_i of patch i to the total population N. Let l_i $(i = 1, 2)$ denote the ratios of rural migrants in patch i to the total population in patches i ($i = 1, 2$ for urban and peri-urban, respectively). Then

$$l_i = \frac{n_3 l_3 q_i}{n_i + n_3 l_3 q_i} = 1 - m_{ii}^d, \quad i = 1, 2, \tag{11}$$

and thus,

$$m_{11} = (1-l_1)^{\frac{1}{d}}, \quad m_{22} = (1-l_2)^{\frac{1}{d}}.$$

Noticing that $m_{21} = m_{31} = m_{12} = m_{32} = 0$, $m_{33} = 1$, and $\sum_{j=1}^{3} m_{ij} = 1$ ($i = 1$, 2, 3), we have

$$M_{ur} = \begin{bmatrix} (1-l_1)^{\frac{1}{d}} & 0 & 1-(1-l_1)^{\frac{1}{d}} \\ 0 & (1-l_2)^{\frac{1}{d}} & 1-(1-l_2)^{\frac{1}{d}} \\ 0 & 0 & 1 \end{bmatrix}, \tag{12}$$

where l_1 and l_2 are determined in (11). The no-migration matrix M_0 is simply the identity matrix I_3.

2.3 *Stochastic Simulations of the Short-Term Model*

For simulations of the short-term model, we use the migration matrices given in (10) and (12) with $(n_1, n_2, n_3) = (0.125, 0.2, 0.675)$, $l_3 = 0.25$, $q_1 = 0.3$, $q_2 = 0.7$, and $d = 90$ days. The values of l_2 and l_3 can be determined by (11). For the mixing matrix, the preferential parameters (ε_i) are chosen to be (0.95, 0.9, 0.95), which assumes that the peri-urban residents have a higher probability of having contacts with people from the other two patches. The per capita contact rates or activity levels for the three sub-populations are chosen to be (8, 5, 2) based on the assumption that the activity level for disease transmission is correlated with population density. The probability of infection per contact is assumed to be $\beta = 0.23$. The initial values for the short-term model are based on the immunity level of each patch estimated from long-term models, which are assumed to be 90 %, 87 %, 83 % of the total population, 1 million in the simulations.

One focus of the short-term vaccination policy is to vaccinate migrants from patches where density is lower (e.g., rural patch) who are entering patches with higher density (urban or peri-urban). We assume that it is possible to vaccinate these

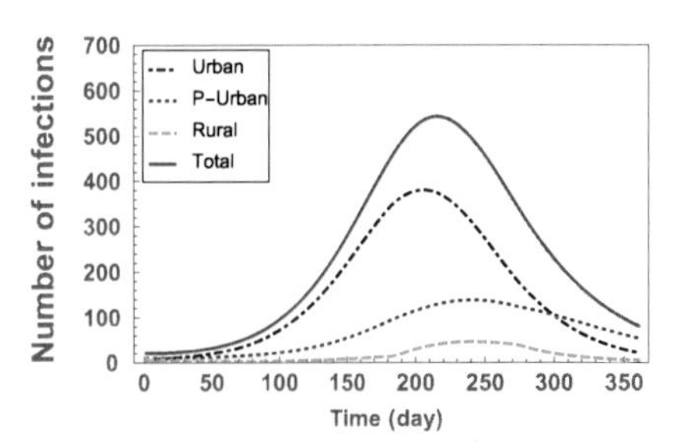

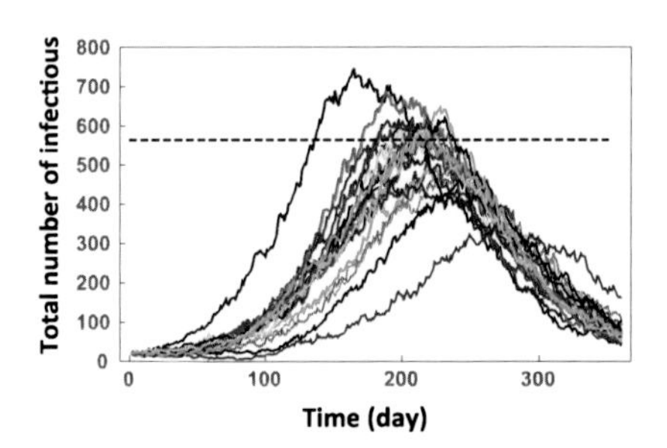

Fig. 4 Deterministic (*left*) and stochastic (*right*) simulations of the short-term model (5) over one year in the absence of supplementary vaccinations. The *left figure* shows the epidemic curves in the urban (*dot-dashed*), peri-urban (*dotted*), and rural patches (*dashed*), as well as the total number of infectious individuals in all three patches (*solid*). The *right figure* shows the epidemic curves from 20 stochastic realizations, each of which shows the total number of infectious individuals in all three patches. The *dashed line* indicates the mean of the total peak sizes (564)

immigrants (e.g., at bus stations) if needed. This policy (i.e., vaccinate migrants only) is compared to other policies including vaccinating (besides routine local vaccination) additional local populations. To identify a better vaccination strategy, we examine several measures including final epidemic and peak sizes. Because of the costs associated with vaccination programs, identification of the best policy will consider the total number of doses required to achieve a prescribed goal under the specific measures mentioned above.

We conducted simulations in both the deterministic and stochastic settings. Figure 4 shows the deterministic (left) and stochastic (right) outcomes of the short-term model in the absence of supplemental vaccinations. We examine how the outbreak can be affected by various vaccination policies. We compare outbreak sizes over a fixed period of time, one year in this case.

For ease of reference, we use the term "final size" to denote the number of infections over the entire period (one year in this case) in each patch, and use the term "total final size" to denote the final size over all three patches. Similarly, the total peak size denotes the peak size over the three patches. The measures used for comparison include the total final size, total peak size, and total number of vaccine doses used. For the deterministic outcome shown in Fig. 4 (left) the total final size is 12044, which is about 12 % of the total population, the total peak size is 540, and the total number of vaccine doses is zero (as this is the case of no supplemental vaccinations).

For stochastic simulations of the short-term model, events (e.g., migration, being vaccinated, etc.) occur based on their corresponding probabilities. In these simulations, for each fixed set of parameter values, the trajectories can be dramatically different, as illustrated in Fig. 4 for identical parameter values. This figure illustrates various levels of outbreaks in the three patches. It demonstrates the result of 20 realizations for the case of no supplementary vaccination. Each of the trajectories shows the total number of infectious individuals in all three patches at time t. We observe that these epidemic curves exhibit various outbreak as well as peak sizes. The mean of the total final sizes is 1.2 %, and the mean of the total peak sizes is 564.

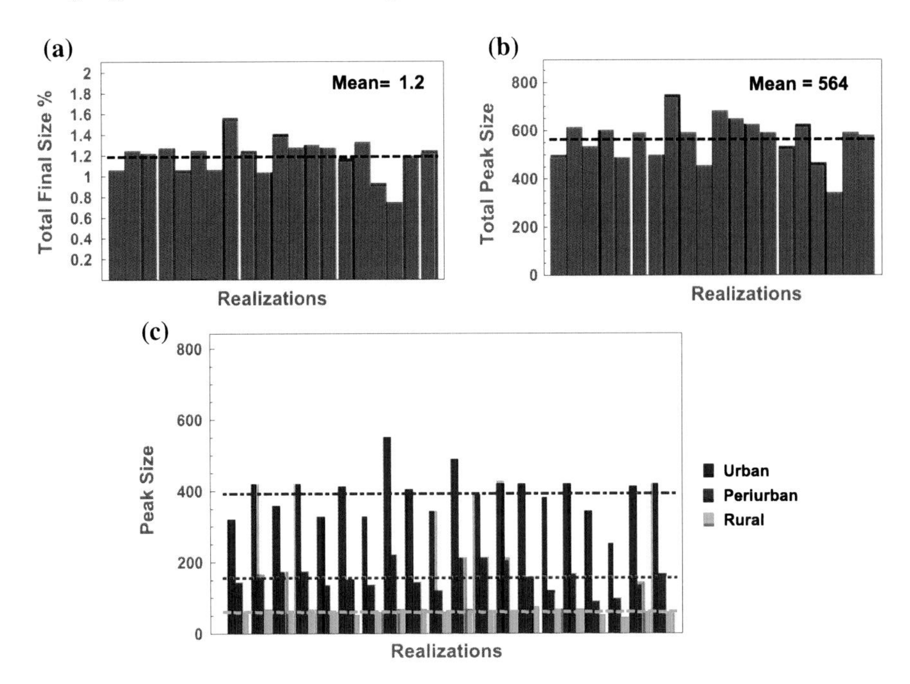

Fig. 5 Total final size (**a**) and peak size (**b**) from the 20 realizations of stochastic simulations shown in Fig. 4. Peak sizes in the three patches are shown in C. The dashed lines mark the mean values over the 20 realizations

The final and peak sizes of each of the 20 realizations are plotted in Fig. 5. as well as the mean values for the total final size and peak size among the 20 realizations (the dashed lines). Plots A and B illustrate the final size and peak size, respectively, and plot C shows the peak sizes in each patch. The dot-dashed, dotted and dashed lines mark the mean values of the peak sizes for urban, peri-urban and rural patches, respectively. In the peak sizes in each patch shown in plot C, we observe large variations, particularly in the urban patch, which vary between 150 and 515 with a mean value of about 400 (marked by the dot-dashed line). The mean peak sizes in the peri-urban and rural patches are 150 and 50, respectively.

3 Impact of Vaccination Policies on Short-Term Outbreaks

We can compare different ways of distributing supplemental vaccines to identify the best vaccination strategy. For local populations, we incorporate supplementary vaccination in the short-term model as initial conditions by moving the corresponding fraction of susceptible individuals (S_i) in patch i to the vaccinated class V_i^s. For migrants, supplementary vaccination is reflected in the daily vaccination probability η_{ji} of individuals migrating from patch j to patch i ($j \neq i$). Because we are focusing on migrations from rural to urban and peri-urban patches, we have $\eta_{ji} = 0$ for all i, j except η_{31} and η_{32}.

For ease of reference, let

$$\mathbf{h}_{\text{loc}} = (h_{\text{loc}1}, h_{\text{loc}2}, h_{\text{loc}3}), \quad \mathbf{h}_{\text{mig}} = (h_{\text{mig}1}, h_{\text{mig}2}),$$

where $h_{\text{loc}1}$, $h_{\text{loc}2}$ and $h_{\text{loc}3}$ denote the probabilities of local individuals in urban, peri-urban and rural, respectively, receiving supplementary vaccinations, and $h_{\text{mig}1}$ and $h_{\text{mig}2}$ denote the vaccination probabilities for migrants. We consider three types of supplementary vaccination:

Policy I. Vaccinate local populations only, i.e., $\mathbf{h}_{\text{loc}} > 0$ and $\mathbf{h}_{\text{mig}} = 0$;
Policy II. Vaccinate migrants only, i.e., $\mathbf{h}_{\text{loc}} = 0$, and $\mathbf{h}_{\text{mig}} > 0$;
Policy III. Vaccinate both local people and migrants, i.e., $\mathbf{h}_{\text{loc}} > 0$, $\mathbf{h}_{\text{mig}} > 0$.

Introduce the following vector notation

$$\mathbf{u} = (1, 1, 1), \quad \mathbf{v} = (a_1, a_2, a_3), \quad \mathbf{w} = (1, 1), \quad \mathbf{z} = (a_1, a_2), \tag{13}$$

where $a_i > 0$ are the activity levels in population i. For ease of reference, we define several terms based on the properties of $\mathbf{h}_{\text{loc}}$ and $\mathbf{h}_{\text{mig}}$ ($k_i > 0$ are constants):

(i) Homogeneous policy I (or Hom I) is a program with $\mathbf{h}_{\text{loc}} = k_1\mathbf{u}$, $\mathbf{h}_{\text{mig}} = 0$.
(ii) Heterogeneous policy I (or Het I) is a program with $\mathbf{h}_{\text{loc}} = k_2\mathbf{v}$, $\mathbf{h}_{\text{mig}} = 0$.
(iii) Homogeneous policy II (or Hom II) is a program with $\mathbf{h}_{\text{mig}} = k_3\mathbf{w}$, $\mathbf{h}_{\text{loc}} = 0$.
(iv) Heterogeneous policy II (or Het II) is a program with $\mathbf{h}_{\text{mig}} = k_4\mathbf{z}$, $\mathbf{h}_{\text{loc}} = 0$.
(v) Heterogeneous policy III (or Het III) is a program with $\mathbf{h}_{\text{loc}} > 0$, $\mathbf{h}_{\text{mig}} > 0$, and they are not multiples of $\mathbf{u}$ or $\mathbf{w}$.

We will compare both homogeneous and heterogeneous coverages. In addition to the cases mentioned above, we may also consider other heterogeneous programs for which $\mathbf{h}_{\text{mig}}$ is a non-zero multiple of neither $\mathbf{w}$ nor $\mathbf{z}$.

Figure 6 compares the outcomes of four vaccination programs under policies I and II. The activity levels are the same as in Figs. 4 and 5 (i.e., $a_1 = 8$, $a_2 = 5$, $a_3 = 2$). In this case, $\mathbf{v} = (8, 5, 2)$ and $\mathbf{z} = (8, 5)$. Rows 1 and 2 are for policy I with homogeneous coverage $\mathbf{h}_{\text{loc}} = 0.01\mathbf{u}$ (A1 and B1) and heterogeneous coverage $\mathbf{h}_{\text{loc}} = 0.0332\mathbf{v}$ (A2 and B2), and rows 3 and 4 are for policy II with homogeneous coverage $\mathbf{h}_{\text{mig}} = 0.547\mathbf{w}$ (A3 and B3) and heterogeneous coverage $\mathbf{h}_{\text{mig}} = 0.092\mathbf{z}$ (A4 and B4). For ease of comparison, the results are also summarized in Table 2 (see (a)–(d)). The h values are chosen such that all four programs described in rows (a)–(d) use a similar total number of vaccine doses: 15227, 15244, 15131 and 15091, respectively. However, the outcomes of these four programs are very different. The mean total final sizes are 0.47, 0.14, 0.14 and 0.07 % of the population, respectively, and the mean total peak sizes are 190, 57, 55 and 36, respectively. This suggests that heterogeneous policy II is most effective among the four programs in terms of reducing total final and peak sizes, while using fewer vaccine doses.

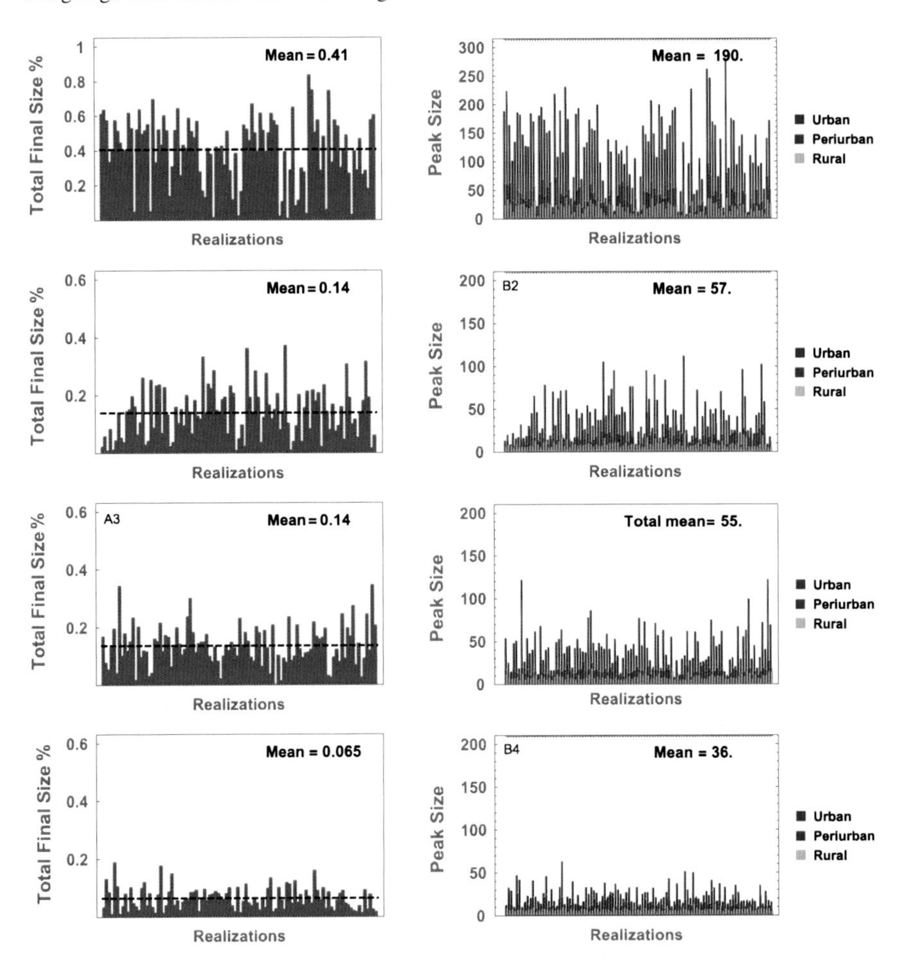

Fig. 6 Results of 100 stochastic realizations of the short-term model under homogeneous or heterogeneous policies I and II. See text for detailed descriptions

Table 2 Comparison of policies I and II under homogeneous and heterogeneous coverages

Policy type	Values	Mean final size (%)	Mean peak size	Mean total doses	Figure
None	$\mathbf{h}_{\text{loc}} = \mathbf{h}_{\text{mig}} = 0$	1.21	564	0	Fig. 5
(a) Hom I	$\mathbf{h}_{\text{loc}} = 0.1\mathbf{u}$	0.47	190	15227	Fig. 6 (A1, B1)
(b) Het I	$\mathbf{h}_{\text{loc}} = 0.0332\mathbf{v}$	0.14	57	15244	Fig. 6 (A2, B2)
(c) Hom II	$\mathbf{h}_{\text{mig}} = 0.547\mathbf{w}$	0.14	55	15131	Fig. 6 (A3, B3)
(d) Het II	$\mathbf{h}_{\text{mig}} = 0.092\mathbf{z}$	0.07	36	15091	Fig. 6 (A4, B4)
(e) Het I	$\mathbf{h}_{\text{loc}} = 0.01\mathbf{v}$	0.74	324	4591	Fig. 8 (A1, B1)
(f) Hom II	$\mathbf{h}_{\text{mig}} = 0.16\mathbf{w}$	0.75	316	4180	Fig. 8 (A2, B2)

Hom: Homogeneous policy. Het: Heterogeneous policy. Vectors **u**, **v**, **w**, **z** are defined in (13)

Although the mean values presented in Fig. 6 provide useful information, further insights can be obtained by examining the distribution of possible events shown in the stochastic results. Particularly important to policy decisions is the likelihood that the final size of an outbreak may exceed some prescribed level of severity under various vaccination programs. Figure 7 compares the four programs shown in Fig. 6 in terms of the frequencies of the 100 realizations (which is analogous to likelihood in a single outbreak) under each policy that corresponds to the final sizes being below some hypothetical prescribed thresholds. We observe that the homogeneous policy I with $\mathbf{h}_{\rm loc} = 0.1\mathbf{u}$ is less likely to reduce the final size to be below 0.2 % of the total population, while the heterogeneous policy II with $\mathbf{h}_{\rm mig} = 0.092\mathbf{z}$ is most likely (with a 80 % chance) to contain the final size to be below 0.1 %. The middle two programs (heterogeneous policy I with $\mathbf{h}_{\rm loc} = 0.0332\mathbf{v}$ and homogeneous policy II with $\mathbf{h}_{\rm mig} = 0.092\mathbf{z}$) have very similar likelihood for all threshold levels. Similarly, the heterogeneous policy II has a much higher likelihood than other three policies to contain the urban peak size to be below 25 or 50.

From Fig. 6, we also observe that, under the similar number of total vaccine doses, the heterogeneous policy II (A2 and B2) and homogeneous policy I (A3 and B3) have similar effects in reducing the final and peak sizes. Many of our simulations under other parameter values illustrate similar features. One such example is demonstrated in Fig. 8. The vaccination programs are represented by $\mathbf{h}_{\rm loc} = 0.01\mathbf{v}$ (Fig. 8 (A1 and B1)) and $\mathbf{h}_{\rm mig} = 0.15\mathbf{w}$ (A2 and B2). The average total numbers of vaccine doses over 20 realizations in these two cases are similar with 4591 in A1 and B1, and 4180 in A2 and B2. We observe that the mean final and peak sizes under these two programs are also similar: the mean total final sizes are 0.74 and 0.75 %, and the mean total peak sizes are 324 and 316. These comparison results are also listed in Table 2. From these and many other simulations, we observe that homogeneous policy I is least effective and heterogeneous policy II is most effective in terms of reducing the total final and peak sizes with a similar number of vaccine doses. However, it needs to be pointed out that the conclusion that heterogeneous policy II is more effective depends critically on the relative activity levels a_i $(i = 1, 2, 3)$.

We can also compare policies to identify the best strategy in the sense of using the fewest vaccine doses under a prescribed upper bound for the total final size. One such example is presented in Table 3. All parameter values are the same as in Table 2 except for the h_i values. The results presented in Table 3, however, are computed from the deterministic model. In rows (a)–(c), the three vaccination programs lead to the same total final size (0.43 %), but the number of vaccine doses required differ with program (c) being the most effective policy (6896 doses versus 9183 in (a) and 8905 in (b)). Similarly, the vaccination policies represented in (d)–(f) lead to the same final size (0.19 %) but the option (f) of heterogeneous policy II uses the least vaccine doses (10673 versus 13774 in (d) and 13915 in (e)).

To explore the effects of policy III, in which supplementary vaccination is given to both local populations and migrants, many factors can influence the allocation of supplementary vaccines among sub-groups, including the costs associated with vaccine distribution and administration. We present in Fig. 9 several scenarios based on two main objectives. One is to identify the policy that uses the least vaccine doses to

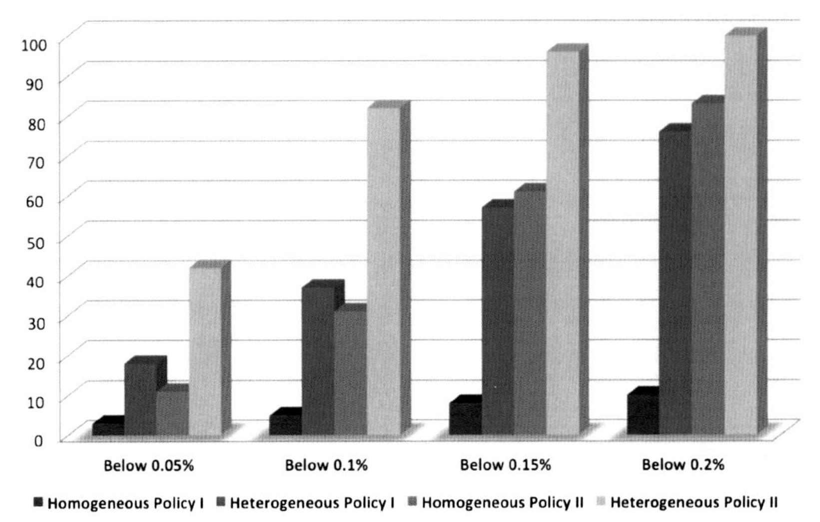

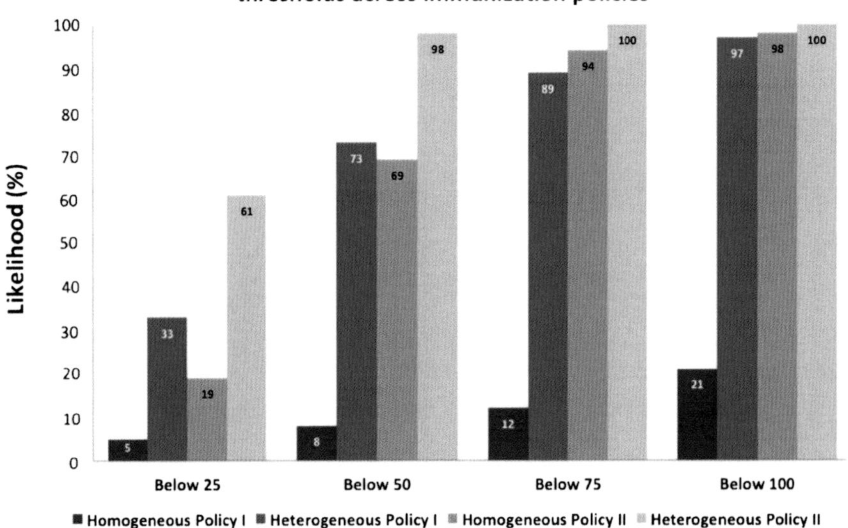

Fig. 7 Likelihood that the final size of an epidemic may exceed some prescribed level of severity (*top*) or the likelihood that the peak size in urban is below certain thresholds (*bottom*) under the four vaccination programs presented in Fig. 6 based on 100 stochastic realizations. The four policies correspond to the vaccination programs shown in A1–A4 in Fig. 6 or cases **a**–**d** in Table 2

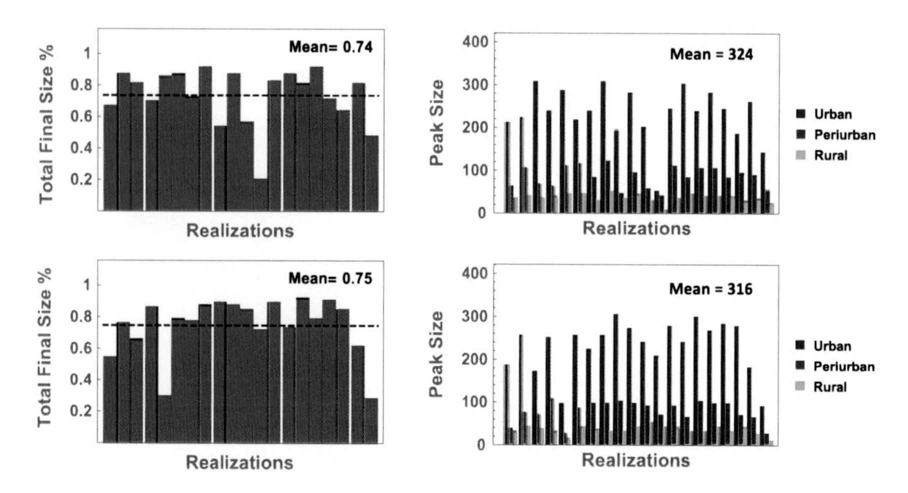

Fig. 8 Similar to Fig. 6 except the values of h_i. A1 and B1 are for the heterogeneous policy I with $\mathbf{h}_{\text{loc}} = 0.01\mathbf{v}$, and A2 and B2 are for the homogeneous policy II with $\mathbf{h}_{\text{mig}} = 0.15\mathbf{w}$. Similar numbers of vaccine doses, 4591 (*top*) and 4180 (*bottom*), were used

Table 3 Comparison of policy I and policy II (equal final size with fewer vaccine doses)

Policy type	Values	Mean final size (%)	Mean peak size	Mean total doses
(a) Het I	$\mathbf{h}_{\text{loc}} = 0.02\mathbf{v}$	0.43	147	9183
(b) Hom II	$\mathbf{h}_{\text{mig}} = 0.32\mathbf{w}$	0.43	144	8905
(c) Het II	$\mathbf{h}_{\text{mig}} = 0.042\mathbf{z}$	0.43	142	6896
(d) Het I	$\mathbf{h}_{\text{loc}} = 0.03\mathbf{v}$	0.19	55	13774
(e) Hom II	$\mathbf{h}_{\text{mig}} = 0.5\mathbf{w}$	0.19	54	13915
(f) Het II	$\mathbf{h}_{\text{mig}} = 0.065\mathbf{z}$	0.19	54	10673

Hom: Homogeneous policy. Het: Heterogeneous policy. Vectors $\mathbf{v}$, $\mathbf{w}$, $\mathbf{z}$ are defined in (13)

contain the final size at the same (or similar) level, and another is to identify a policy that reduces the final size the most with the same (or similar) vaccine doses. We compared various vaccination policies for local and migrant populations, including both homogeneous and heterogeneous coverages. Figure 9 (A1) is a baseline scenario, which corresponds to the combination of homogeneous local coverage with $\mathbf{h}_{\text{loc}} = 0.02\mathbf{u}$ and homogeneous migrant coverage with $\mathbf{h}_{\text{mig}} = 0.028\mathbf{z}$. It shows 20 realizations of the stochastic simulations. The top panel is for the case when local vaccinations are homogeneous with $\mathbf{h}_{\text{loc}} = 0.02\mathbf{u}$, and the bottom B panel is for the case of heterogeneous local coverage with $\mathbf{h}_{\text{loc}} = 0.07\mathbf{v}$. The six cases are for different coverages in migrants: homogeneous with $\mathbf{h}_{\text{mig}} = 0.2\mathbf{w}$ (A1); heterogeneous with $\mathbf{h}_{\text{mig}} = 0.28\mathbf{z}$ (A2); heterogeneous with $\mathbf{h}_{\text{mig}} = (0.54, 0.054)$ (A3); homogeneous with $\mathbf{h}_{\text{mig}} = 0.192\mathbf{w}$ (B1); heterogeneous with $\mathbf{h}_{\text{mig}} = 0.2\mathbf{z}$ (B2); and heterogeneous with $\mathbf{h}_{\text{mig}} = (0.52, 0.052)$ (B3). In each plot, the mean total final size and the mean total number of vaccine doses are listed. We observe again that, with the same or

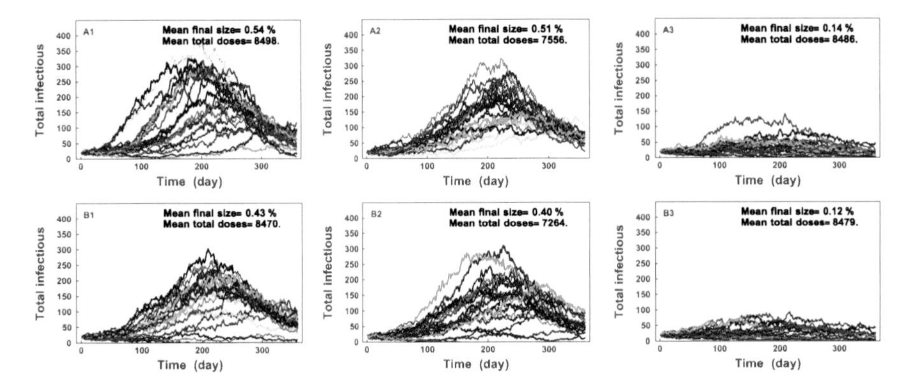

Fig. 9 Comparison of six scenarios under policy III. It shows the epidemic curves from 20 stochastic realizations in each scenario. The *top panel* is for the case when the local vaccinations are homogeneous with $\mathbf{h}_{\text{loc}} = 0.02\mathbf{u}$, whereas the *bottom panel* is for the heterogeneous local coverage with $\mathbf{h}_{\text{loc}} = 0.07\mathbf{v}$. The six cases are for different coverages in migrants. See the text for detailed information

similar vaccine doses (e.g., see A1, A3, B1 and B3)), heterogeneous coverage (A3 and B3) will likely lead to a lower final size than homogeneous coverage (A1). The greater effectiveness can be represented either by a lower final size with similar vaccine doses (A1 versus A3, or B1 versus B3) or by a lower number of vaccine doses when final sizes are similar (A1 versus A2, or B1 versus B2).

We need to point out that the assessments presented above are based only on the final and peak epidemic sizes or the number of vaccine doses needed to achieve a prescribed epidemic size. When other factors are considered, such as economic costs related to vaccinating local populations versus migrants, the conclusions might differ. In addition, parameter values may affect the relative effectiveness of these programs, including population density, migration patterns, infectious period, and others.

4 Discussion

The objective of this study is to evaluate vaccination policies for a vaccine-preventable disease using a meta-population model that explicitly incorporates migration between patches. This is an extension of the model considered in [3] (Chap. 8 in this volume), in which migrations are modeled implicitly. In model (5), seasonal spatial movements from one patch to another are included to capture the migration from rural to urban or peri-urban for employment opportunities and return home afterwards. The main findings of the study suggest that (because of the significant difference in population density, which directly influences the contact rate, affecting the rate of disease transmission), vaccinating migrants can be a very important means of preventing outbreaks. Particularly, heterogeneous coverages among migrants are likely the most effective vaccination strategies.

The model outcomes are generated by both deterministic and stochastic simulations. Various vaccination programs are compared in terms of three measures: number of vaccine doses used, final epidemic size, and peak epidemic size (either within individual patches or over all three patches). Deterministic simulations help identify suitable vaccination scenarios for comparison, and stochastic simulations with multiple realizations provide a range of possibilities in terms of epidemic sizes, for which the mean value of each measure also provides useful insights into possible outcomes of various vaccination policies.

Our comparisons focused on identifying the best vaccination strategy based on two objectives: Objective 1 is to apply fewer vaccine doses while bringing the epidemic size below a prescribed level, and Objective 2 is to reduce the outbreak size the most with a given number of vaccine doses. Three types of vaccination policies are considered in terms of the allocation of supplementary vaccines: policy I involves vaccinating only local populations; policy II involves vaccinating only migrants; and policy III involves combined vaccinations of both local and migrant populations. In all comparisons, we considered homogeneous and heterogeneous vaccination coverages in either local populations or migrants or both. One of the main results is that, in the case when the heterogeneity in population density is significant, the best vaccination strategy likely involves heterogeneous coverages among migrants. For example, Fig. 6(A1–A4) and the cases (a-d) in Table 2 present four policies that use similar vaccine doses. The homogeneous policy I (A1 and (a)) corresponds to a much higher final size than the other three policies, while the heterogeneous policy II (A4 and (d)) leads to the lowest final size. The results presented in Table 3 show two cases in which heterogeneous policy II is more effective then heterogeneous policy I in terms of using fewer doses while leading to similar final sizes.

In most cases, heterogeneous coverages are taken to be proportional to the activity levels $\mathbf{v} = (a_1, a_2, a_3)$, which are related to the population densities in urban, peri-urban and rural patches (i.e., $\mathbf{h}_{\text{loc}} = k\mathbf{v}$ or $\mathbf{h}_{\text{mig}} = k'\mathbf{z}$ for some positive constants k and k'). Results are shown for $\mathbf{v} = (a_1, a_2, a_3) = (8, 5, 2)$. For the set of parameter values used, simulation results show that the selection of vaccination policies should be guided by the objectives of outbreak prevention, and that for the evaluation of certain types of policy goals, stochastic models can provide more useful insights than deterministic ones. For example, based on 100 realizations from stochastic simulations of the short-term model (5) presented in Fig. 6 or the corresponding scenarios listed in (a)–(d) in Table 2, it is shown in Fig. 7 that the heterogeneous policy I is more likely than the homogeneous policy II to contain the outbreak within a small size (e.g., final size below 0.05 or 0.1 %, or urban peak size below 20 or 50), but that homogeneous policy II is more likely than the heterogeneous policy I to contain the outbreak within a medium to larger size (e.g., final size below 0.15 or 0.2 %, or urban peak size below 75 or 100). This illustrates that, while the deterministic model implies that these two vaccination policies are essentially identical, the stochastic model reveals meaningful differences.

It is important to emphasize that the conclusion that heterogeneous coverages among migrants are more effective is critically dependent on heterogeneity in contact and migration rates. If these heterogeneities are not very strong, vaccinating local populations could be more effective than vaccinating migrants. Which vaccination strategies are most effective may also depend on other characteristics of the population such as immunity (see [4]).

Acknowledgments We thank John Glasser for suggesting this study and for helpful comments and suggestions throughout the writing of this chapter.

Appendix

In this Appendix, we derive the reproduction numbers $\mathscr{R}_{vi}$ for model (1).

Denote the disease-free equilibrium by $U_i^0 = (M_i^0, V_i^0, S_i^0, E_i^0, I_i^0, R_i^0)$, $i = 1, 2, 3$. Then, $E_i^0 = I_i^0 = R_i^0 = 0$, and U^0 can be solved by the following equation:

$$\begin{aligned} M_i &= \theta_i \mu_i N_i + (1-\mu_i)(1-\sigma)M_i \\ V_i &= \alpha \nu_i^0 (1-\mu_i) S_i(n) + (1-\mu_i)(1-\chi)V_i \\ S_i &= (1-\theta_i)\mu_i N_i + (1-\mu_i)(1-\alpha\nu_i^0)S_i + \sigma(1-\mu_i)M_i(n) + \chi(1-\mu_i)V_i, \end{aligned}$$

with N_i being constants. Solving the above equations we obtain

$$\frac{M_i^0}{N_i} = \frac{\theta_i \mu_i}{1-(1-\mu_i)(1-\sigma)}, \quad \frac{S_i^0}{N_i} = \frac{\left[(1-\theta_i) + \theta_i \frac{\sigma(1-\mu_i)}{1-(1-\mu_i)(1-\sigma)}\right]\mu_i}{1-(1-\mu_i)(1-\alpha\nu_i^0) - \chi(1-\mu_i)\frac{\alpha\nu_i^0(1-\mu_i)}{1-(1-\mu_i)(1-\chi)}},$$

$$\frac{V_i^0}{N_i} = \frac{\alpha\nu_i^0(1-\mu_i)}{1-(1-\mu_i)(1-\chi)} \frac{\left[(1-\theta_i) + \theta_i \frac{\sigma(1-\mu_i)}{1-(1-\mu_i)(1-\sigma)}\right]\mu_i}{1-(1-\mu_i)(1-\alpha\nu_i^0) - \chi(1-\mu_i)\frac{\alpha\nu_i^0(1-\mu_i)}{1-(1-\mu_i)(1-\chi)}}.$$

Noticing that the Jacobian matrix at U_i^0 has the form $F + T$, where

$$F = \begin{bmatrix} 0 & (1-\mu_i)\beta_i^0 \frac{S_i^0}{N_i} \\ 0 & 0 \end{bmatrix}, \quad T = \begin{bmatrix} (1-\mu_i)(1-\gamma) & 0 \\ (1-\mu_i)\gamma & (1-\mu_i)(1-\rho) \end{bmatrix}.$$

Then

$$(1-T)^{-1} = \begin{bmatrix} \frac{1}{1-(1-\mu_i)(1-\gamma)} & 0 \\ \frac{(1-\mu_i)\gamma}{(1-(1-\mu_i)(1-\gamma))} \frac{1}{(1-(1-\mu_i)(1-\rho))} & \frac{1}{1-(1-\mu_i)(1-\rho)} \end{bmatrix},$$

and

$$F(1-T)^{-1} = \begin{bmatrix} \frac{(1-\mu_i)\gamma}{1-(1-\mu_i)(1-\gamma)} \frac{(1-\mu_i)\beta_i^0(S_i^0/N_i)}{1-(1-\mu_i)(1-\rho)} & \frac{(1-\mu_i)\beta_i^0(S_i^0/N_i)}{1-(1-\mu_i)(1-\rho)} \\ 0 & 0 \end{bmatrix}.$$

Therefore,

$$\mathscr{R}_{vi} = \varrho(F(1-T)^{-1}) = \frac{(1-\mu_i)\gamma}{1-(1-\mu_i)(1-\gamma)} \frac{(1-\mu_i)\beta_i^0(S_i^0/N_i)}{1-(1-\mu_i)(1-\rho)},$$

where $\frac{(1-\mu_i)\gamma}{1-(1-\mu_i)(1-\gamma)}$ is the probability that an infected individual survives the latent period, and $\frac{(1-\mu_i)\beta_i^0(S_i^0/N_i)}{1-(1-\mu_i)(1-\rho)}$ is the number of new infections that an infectious individual can generate during the entire infectious period in a population where the fraction of susceptibles is S_i^0/N_i.

References

1. Bogoch, I.I., Creatore, M.I., Cetron, M.S., Brownstein, J.S., Pesik, N., Miniota, J., Khan, K.: Assessment of the potential for international dissemination of Ebola virus via commercial air travel during the 2014 west African outbreak. The Lancet **385**(9962), 29–35 (2015)
2. Brauer, F., Feng, Z., Castillo-Chavez, C.: Discrete epidemic models. Math. Biosci. Eng. **7**(1), 1–16 (2010)
3. de Moraes, J. C., Camargo, M. C. C., de Mello, M. L. R., Hersh, B. S., and Glasser, J. W.: The 1997 Measles Outbreak in Metropolitan So Paulo, Brazil: Strategic Implications of Increasing Urbanization. Chapter 8, This volume
4. Feng, Z., Hill, A.N., Smith, P.J., Glasser, J.W.: An elaboration of theory about preventing outbreaks in homogeneous populations to include heterogeneity or preferential mixing. J. Theor. Biol. **386**, 177–187 (2015)
5. Gomes M.F.C., Pastore y Piontti A., Rossi L., Chao D., Longini I., Halloran M.E., Vespignani A.: Assessing the International Spreading Risk Associated with the 2014 West African Ebola Outbreak. PLoS Current Outbreaks, (2014). doi:10.1371/currents.outbreaks.cd818f63d40e24aef769dda7df9e0da5
6. Hernandez-Ceron, N., Feng, Z., Castillo-Chavez, C.: Discrete epidemic models with arbitrary stage distributions and applications to disease control. Bull. Math. Biol. **75**(10), 1716–1746 (2013a)
7. Hernandez-Ceron, N., Feng, Z., van den Driessche, P.: Reproduction numbers for discrete-time epidemic models with arbitrary stage distributions. J. Diff. Equ. Appl. **19**, 1671–1693 (2013b)
8. Lloyd-Smith, J.O., Galvani, A.P., Getz, W.M.: Curtailing transmission of severe acute respiratory syndrome within a community and its hospital. Proc. R. Soc. Lond. B **270**, 1979–1989 (2003)
9. Poletto, C., Gomes, M.F., y Piontti, A.P., Rossi, L., Bioglio, L., Chao, D.L., Vespignani, A.: Assessing the impact of travel restrictions on international spread of the 2014 West African Ebola epidemic. Eurosurveillance **19**(42) (2014)

Age of Infection Epidemic Models

Fred Brauer

Abstract The age of infection model, first introduced by Kermack and McKendrick in 1927, is a general structure for compartmental epidemic models, including models with heterogeneous mixing. It is possible to estimate the basic reproduction number if the initial exponential growth rate and the infectivity as a function of time since being infected are known, and this is also possible for models with heterogeneous mixing.

Keywords Epidemic models · Age of infection model · Heterogenous mixing · Basic reproduction number · Exponential growth rate · Infectivity

1 Introduction

Throughout recorded history diseases have emerged or re-emerged. Sometimes, as with SARS (Severe Acute Respiratory Syndrome) in 2002–2003, a disease has appeared once and not recurred. In other instances, as with the Black Death in the Middle Ages, seasonal influenza outbreaks, and Ebola since 1976, disease outbreaks have recurred. In most cases, the outbreaks have been of short duration, and it is appropriate to model them as epidemics without including demographic effects.

Many times throughout history it has been observed that an epidemic would invade a community but would eventually disappear without having infected the entire population. In 1927, W.O. Kermack and A.G. McKendrick formulated the first mathematical model for an epidemic that exhibited such behavior. In fact, such behavior was exhibited by a simple special case of their model, and for many years this special case was known as "the" Kermack–McKendrick epidemic model. However, the general model of Kermack and McKendrick included infectivity that could depend on the age of infection—the time since becoming infective.

F. Brauer (✉)
Department of Mathematics, University of British Columbia,
Vancouver, BC V6T 1Z2, Canada
e-mail: brauer@math.ubc.ca

G. Chowell and J.M. Hyman (eds.), *Mathematical and Statistical Modeling for Emerging and Re-emerging Infectious Diseases*,
DOI 10.1007/978-3-319-40413-4_13

The original formulation of the Kermack–McKendrick age of infection epidemic model given in [7] was

$$\begin{aligned} v(t) &= -x'(t) \\ x'(t) &= -x(t)\left[\int_0^t A(s)v(t-s)ds + A(t)y_0\right] \\ z'(t) &= \int_0^t C(s)v(t-s)ds + C(t)y_0 \\ y(t) &= \int_0^t B(s)v(t-s)ds + B(t)y_0. \end{aligned} \tag{1}$$

Here, $x(t)$ is the number of susceptibles, $y(t)$ is the number of infectious individuals, and $z(t)$ is the number of recovered individuals. Also $\varphi(s)$ is the recovery rate when the age of infection is s, $\psi(s)$ is the recovery rate at infection age s, and

$$B(s) = e^{-\int_0^t \psi(s)ds}, \quad A(s) = \varphi(s)B(s).$$

It is assumed that there are no disease deaths, so that the total population size remains constant. Kermack and McKendrick did not bring the basic reproduction number into their analysis, but were able to derive a final size relation in the form

$$\log \frac{1 - \frac{y_0}{N}}{1-p} = pN \int_0^\infty A(s)ds, \tag{2}$$

in which N is the total population size and p is the attack ratio

$$p = 1 - \frac{x_\infty}{N}.$$

If we define

$$S(t) = x(t), \quad A(s) = B(s) = e^{-\gamma s}, \quad I(t) = \frac{1}{\beta}y(t),$$

the model (1) can be reduced to the system

$$\begin{aligned} S' &= -\beta SI \\ I' &= \beta SI - \gamma I, \end{aligned} \tag{3}$$

which is the simple Kermack–McKendrick model.

In their later work on disease transmission models [8, 9], Kermack and McKendrick did not include age of infection, and age of infection models were neglected for many years. Age of infection reappeared in the study of HIV/AIDS, in which the infectivity of infected individuals is high for a brief period after becoming infected, then quite low for an extended period, possibly several years, before increasing rapidly with the onset of full-blown AIDS. Thus the age of infection described by Kermack and McKendrick for epidemics became very important in some endemic situations; see for example [11, 12].

Various disease outbreaks, including the *SARS* epidemic of 2002–2003, the concern about a possible $H5N1$ influenza epidemic in 2005, the $H1N1$ influenza pandemic of 2009, and the Ebola outbreak of 2014 have re-ignited interest in epidemic models, beginning with the reformulation of the Kermack–McKendrick model by Diekmann, Heesterbeek and Metz [6].

2 The Modern Infection Age Epidemic Model

In [6], Diekmann, Heesterbeek, and Metz rewrote the model (1) as

$$S'(t) = S(t) \int_0^\infty A(s)S'(t-s)ds, \tag{4}$$

with $S(t)$ denoting the density of susceptibles and $A(s)$ the expected infectivity of an individual that became infected s time units ago. In this general description, $A(s)$ includes factors describing the rate of secondary infections caused by a contact, the fraction of individuals still infected at infection age s and the infectivity of such individuals. This model is formulated under the same assumptions as for (1), namely

- a single infection triggers an autonomous process within the host,
- the disease results in either recovery with complete immunity or death,
- contacts are according to the law of mass action,
- all individuals are equally susceptible,
- the population is closed; at the time scale of disease transmission the influx of new susceptibles into the population and the outflow due to natural deaths are negligible,
- the population is large enough to warrant a deterministic description.

Here, we present a description and analysis of a model equivalent to (4), and an extension of this model to epidemics with heterogeneous mixing. The results in this section are not new but we believe that this approach will be useful for developing more general epidemic models.

We suppose that individuals in the population make an average of a contacts sufficient to transmit infection in unit time and that the total population size is a constant N (assuming no disease deaths). Then the rate of contacts made by a susceptible that produce a new infection is $a\varphi(t)/N$, where $\varphi(t)$ is the total infectivity of infected individuals, the number of infective individuals multiplied by their average relative infectivity. The number of new infections at time $(t-s)$ is $[-S'(t-s)]$ and on average the infectivity of these new infections at time t is $A(s)$. Thus the total infectivity at time t is

$$\varphi(t) = \int_0^\infty A(s)S'(t-s)ds.$$

Our formulation differs slightly from that of [6], by including in $A(s)$ only the fraction of individuals still infected at infection age s and the infectivity of such individuals, taking out the factor a/N describing the rate of contacts of such individuals.

Then

$$\begin{aligned} S'(t) &= -\frac{a}{N}S(t)\varphi(t) \\ \varphi(t) &= -\int_0^\infty A(s)S'(t-s)ds = \frac{a}{N}\int_0^\infty A(s)S(t-s)\varphi(t-s)ds. \end{aligned} \tag{5}$$

We may combine the two equations of (5) into a single equation

$$S'(t) = \frac{a}{N}S(t)\int_0^\infty A(s)S'(t-s)ds. \tag{6}$$

The model (6) or (5) is more general than the model (3) in two respects. It allows an arbitrary sequence of infective compartments and it allows an arbitrary distribution of stays in each compartment.

We assume that the disease outbreak begins at time $t = 0$, so that $S(u) = N$ for $u < 0$ and there may be a discontinuity in $S(u)$ at $u = 0$ corresponding to an initial infective distribution.

It is pointed out in [6] that the quantity

$$\mathcal{R}_0 = a\int_0^\infty A(s)ds \tag{7}$$

can be interpreted as the expected number of secondary disease cases produced by one typical primary case.

Further, there is an invasion criterion given in [6] and also in [14]. Initially, when $S(t)$ is close to N, we may replace $S(t)$ in (6) by its initial value N, giving a linear equation,

$$S'(t) = a\int_0^\infty A(s)S'(t-s)ds.$$

This equation is, in fact, the linearization of the system (5) at the equilibrium $S = N, \varphi = 0$. The condition that this linear equation has a solution $S(t) = S_0e^{rt}$ is

$$1 = a\int_0^\infty A(s)e^{-rs}ds. \tag{8}$$

Combination of (7) and (8) gives a relation between the initial exponential growth rate r and the basic reproduction number $\mathscr{R}_0$, namely

$$\mathscr{R}_0 = \frac{\int_0^\infty A(s)ds}{\int_0^\infty e^{-rs}A(s)ds}. \tag{9}$$

The relation (9) provides a means to estimate the basic reproduction number from measurements of the initial exponential growth rate provided the infectivity distribution is known. Also, it is clear from (9) that $r > 0$ if and only if $\mathscr{R}_0 > 1$. We may define an epidemic as a situation in which for the model (5) we have $r > 0$, so that initially the solution grows exponentially.

Division of the Eq. (6) by $S(t)$ and integration with respect to t from 0 to ∞ gives, with an interchange of order of integration

$$\log \frac{S_0}{S_\infty} = \frac{a}{N} \int_0^\infty [S(-s) - S_\infty]A(s)ds.$$

Since we are assuming that the epidemic does not begin until time $t = 0$, so that $S(-s) = N$ if $s < 0$, so that

$$\log \frac{S_0}{S_\infty} = a\frac{(N - S_\infty)}{N} \int_0^\infty A(s)ds,$$

and then, using (7) we obtain the final size relation

$$\log \frac{S_0}{S_\infty} = \mathscr{R}_0 \left[1 - \frac{S_\infty}{N}\right].$$

3 Example: The General *SEIR* Model

As an example of formulation of a model in age of infection form, we consider an *SEIR* model with general distributions of stay in both the exposed and infectious period. Here, we consider the exposed period to be the time period from the acquisition of infection to the time when an individual can transmit infection, and the infective period to be the time period during which an individual can transmit infection.

Suppose the fraction of exposed individuals who are still in the exposed class s time units after being exposed is $P_E(s)$ and the fraction of individuals who are still in the infectious class s time units after entering the infectious class is $P_I(s)$, with $P_E(s), P_I(s)$ non-negative, non-increasing functions such that

$$P_E(0) = 1, \quad \int_0^\infty P_E(s)ds < \infty,$$

$$P_I(0) = 1, \quad \int_0^\infty P_I(s)ds < \infty.$$

Then P_E and P_I represent survival probabilities in the classes E and I respectively.

We assume that E_0 newly exposed members enter the exposed class at time $t = 0$. Then

$$S' = -a\frac{S}{N}I$$
$$E(t) = E_0 P_E(t) + \int_0^t [-S'(s)]P_E(t-s)ds.$$

If we assume that $S(u) = N$ for $u < 0$ and that $S(u)$ has a jump of $-E_0$ at $u = 0$, then we may write the equation for $E(t)$ as

$$E(t) = \int_0^\infty [-S'(s)]P_E(t-s)ds.$$

Differentiation of the equation for $E(t)$ shows that the output from E to I at time t is

$$-E_0 P_E'(t) - \int_0^t [-S'(s)]P_E'(t-s)ds = -\int_0^\infty [-S'(s)]P_E'(t-s)ds.$$

Then

$$I(t) = -\int_0^\infty \int_0^\infty [-S'(s)]P_E'(t-s-u)P_I(u)duds, \tag{10}$$

and

$$I(t) = \int_0^\infty [-S'(s)]A_I(t-s)ds,$$

with

$$A_I(z) = -\int_0^\infty P_E'(z-v)P_I(v)dv,$$

The model is

$$\begin{aligned} S' &= -a\frac{S}{N}I \\ E(t) &= \int_0^\infty [-S'(s)]P_E(t-s)ds \\ I(t) &= \int_0^\infty [-S'(s)]A_I(t-s)ds, \end{aligned} \tag{11}$$

which is in age of infection form with $\varphi = I$ and $A(z) = A_I(z)$. Then

$$\begin{aligned}\mathscr{R}_0 &= a\int_0^\infty A(z)dz\\ &= -a\int_0^\infty\int_0^z P_E'(z-u)P_I(u)dudz\\ &= a\int_0^\infty P_I(u)du,\end{aligned}$$

using $-\int_0^\infty P_E'(v)dv = P_E(0) - P_E(\infty) = 1$.

The initial exponential growth rate of the general *SEIR* model (11) satisfies

$$a\int_0^\infty e^{-rs}\int_0^s [-P_E'(s-u)]P_I(u)duds = 1,$$

which reduces to

$$\begin{aligned}1 &= a\int_0^\infty [-P_E(v)e^{-rv}dv\int_0^\infty e^{-ru}P_I(u)du\\ &= a\left[1 - r\int_0^\infty e^{-rv}P_E(v)dv\right]\int_0^\infty e^{-ru}P_I(u)du,\end{aligned} \quad (12)$$

with the aid of integration by parts.

4 A Heterogeneous Mixing Age of Infection Model

The basic age of infection model (6) extends the simple *SIR* epidemic model by allowing an arbitrary number of stages in the model and arbitrary distributions of stay in each stage. However, it does not include the possibility of subgroups with different activity levels and heterogeneous mixing between subgroups. This possibility can be included in a heterogeneous mixing age of infection model as in [3, 4]. As in homogeneous mixing models, the age of infection approach is more general than simpler models in several respects. For an epidemic model, in which we assume the time scale is short enough that members do not age over the course of the epidemic, the grouping could be by age. However, for a longer term disease transmission model with age-dependent transmission it would be necessary to use an age-structured model that includes the passage of members between age classes.

We consider two subpopulations of sizes N_1, N_2 respectively, each divided into susceptibles and infected members with subscripts to identify the subpopulation. Suppose that $A_i(s)$ is the mean infectivity of individuals in the subgroup i who have been infected s time units previously, and that a_1, a_2 are the contact rates of the two subpopulations. By contact, we mean contact sufficient to transmit infection, but we may include infectivity factors in the infectivity distributions $A_i(s)$. If the two groups also have different susceptibilities this may be indicated by including susceptibility factors σ_i in the model.

A two-group model may describe a population with groups differing by activity levels and possibly by vulnerability to infection, but not by infectivity, so that $a_1 \neq a_2$ but $A_1(s) = A_2(s)$. It may also describe a population with one group which has been vaccinated against infection, so that the two groups have the same activity level but different disease model parameters. In this case, $a_1 = a_2$ but $A_1(s) \neq A_2(s)$, $\sigma_1 \neq \sigma_2$.

It is necessary to describe also the mixing between the two groups. Suppose that the fraction of contacts made by a member of group i that is with a member of group j is p_{ij}, $i, j = 1, 2$. Then

$$p_{11} + p_{12} = p_{21} + p_{22} = 1.$$

For the properties of the mixing matrix, see [10]

An age of infection model with two subgroups is

$$\begin{aligned} S_1' &= -a_1\sigma_1 S_1 \left[\frac{p_{11}}{N_1}\varphi_1 + \frac{p_{12}}{N_2}\varphi_2\right] \\ \varphi_1(t) &= \int_0^\infty [-S_1'(t-\tau)A_1(\tau)]d\tau \\ S_2' &= -a_2\sigma_2 S_2 \left[\frac{p_{21}}{N_1}\varphi_1 + \frac{p_{22}}{N_2}\varphi_2\right] \\ \varphi_1(t) &= \int_0^\infty [-S_2'(t-\tau)A_2(\tau)]d\tau. \end{aligned} \tag{13}$$

Here, $\varphi_i(t)$ is the total infectivity of infected members of group i and σ_i is the relative susceptibility to infection of group i.

Just as for the homogeneous mixing model, we may write this model using only the equations for S_1, S_2,

$$\begin{aligned} S_1'(t) &= -a_1\sigma_1 S_1(t) \left[\frac{p_{11}}{N_1}\int_0^\infty A_1(s)S_1'(t-s)ds + \frac{p_{12}}{N_2}\int_0^\infty A_2(s)S_2'(t-s)ds\right] \\ S_2'(t) &= -a_2\sigma_2 S_2(t) \left[\frac{p_{21}}{N_1}\int_0^\infty A_1(s)S_1'(t-s)ds + \frac{p_{22}}{N_2}\int_0^\infty A_2(s)S_2'(t-s)ds\right] \end{aligned} \tag{14}$$

The next generation matrix [13] is

$$P = \begin{bmatrix} a_1\sigma_1 p_{11}\int_0^\infty A_1(s)ds & a_1\sigma_1 p_{12}\frac{N_1}{N_2}\int_0^\infty A_2(s)ds \\ a_2\sigma_2 p_{21}\frac{N_2}{N_1}\int_0^\infty A_1(s)ds & a_2\sigma_2 p_{22}\int_0^\infty A_2(s)ds \end{bmatrix}.$$

The matrix P is similar to the matrix $Q = R^{-1}PR$, with

$$R = \begin{bmatrix} N_1 & 0 \\ 0 & N_2 \end{bmatrix}$$

and

$$Q = \begin{bmatrix} a_1\sigma_1 p_{11} \int_0^\infty A_1(\tau)ds & a_1\sigma_1 p_{12} \int_0^\infty A_2(s)ds \\ a_2\sigma_2 p_{21} \int_0^\infty A_1(s)ds & a_2\sigma_2 p_{22} \int_0^\infty A_2(s)ds \end{bmatrix}.$$

Thus $\mathscr{R}_0$ is the largest root of

$$\det \begin{bmatrix} a_1\sigma_1 p_{11} \int_0^\infty A_1(s)ds - \lambda & a_1\sigma_1 p_{12} \int_0^\infty A_2(s)ds \\ a_2\sigma_2 p_{21} \int_0^\infty A_1(s)ds & a_2\sigma_2 p_{22} \int_0^\infty A_2(s)ds - \lambda \end{bmatrix} = 0, \qquad (15)$$

and

$$\mathscr{R}_0 = \frac{p_{11}a_1\sigma_1\hat{A}_1 + p_{22}a_2\sigma_2\hat{A}_2 + \sqrt{\left(p_{11}a_1\sigma_1\hat{A}_1 - p_{22}a_2\sigma_2\hat{A}_2\right)^2 + 4p_{12}p_{21}a_1\sigma_1a_2\sigma_2\hat{A}_1\hat{A}_2}}{2}$$

Here, we have written $\hat{A}_i$ for $\int_0^\infty A_i(s)ds$.

In order to obtain a more useful expression for $\mathscr{R}_0$, it is necessary to make some assumptions about the nature of the mixing between the two groups. The mixing is determined by the two quantities p_{12}, p_{21} since $p_{11} = 1 - p_{12}$ and $p_2 = 1 - p_{21}$. However, these quantities are not completely arbitrary. The total number of contacts made in unit time by members of group 1 with members of group 2 is $a_1 p_{12} N_1$ and because this must equal the total number of contacts by members of group 2 with members of group 1, we have a balance relation

$$\frac{p_{12}a_1}{N_2} = \frac{p_{21}a_2}{N_1}.$$

There has been much study of mixing patterns, see for example [1, 2, 5]. One possibility is proportionate mixing, that is, that the number of contacts between groups is proportional to the relative activity levels. In other words, mixing is random but constrained by the activity levels [10]. Under the assumption of proportionate mixing,

$$p_{ij} = \frac{a_j N_j}{a_1 N_1 + a_2 N_2},$$

and we may write

$$p_{11} = p_{21} = p_1, \quad p_{12} = p_{22} = p_2,$$

with $p_1 + p_2 = 1$. In particular,

$$p_{11}p_{22} - p_{12}p_{21} = 0,$$

and thus

$$\mathscr{R}_0 = p_1 a_1 \sigma_1 \hat{A}_1 + p_2 a_2 \sigma_2 \hat{A}_2.$$

Another possibility is preferred mixing [10], in which a fraction π_i of each group mixes randomly with its own group and the remaining members mix proportionately. Thus, preferred mixing is given by

$$\begin{aligned} p_{11} &= \pi_1 + (1-\pi_1)p_1, \quad p_{12} = (1-\pi_1)p_2 \\ p_{21} &= (1-\pi_2)p_1, \quad p_{22} = \pi_2 + (1-\pi_2)p_2, \end{aligned} \tag{16}$$

with

$$p_i = \frac{(1-\pi_i)a_i N_i}{(1-\pi_1)a_1 N_1 + (1-\pi_2)a_2 N_2}.$$

Proportionate mixing is the special case of preferred mixing with $\pi_1 = \pi_2 = 0$.

It is also possible to have like-with-like mixing, in which members of each group mixes only with members of the same group. This is the special case of preferred mixing with $\pi_1 = \pi_2 = 1$. For like-with-like mixing,

$$p_{11} = p_{22} = 1, \quad p_{12} = p_{21} = 0.$$

Then the roots of (15) are $a_1\sigma_1\hat{A}_1$ and $a_2\sigma_2\hat{A}_2$, and the reproduction number is

$$\mathscr{R}_0 = \max\left[a_1\sigma_1\hat{A}_1, a_2\sigma_2\hat{A}_2\right].$$

By calculating the partial derivatives of $p_{11}, p_{12}, p_{21}, p_{22}$ with respect to π_1, π_2, we may show that p_{11} and p_{22} increase when either π_1 or π_2 is increased, while p_{12} and p_{21} decrease when either π_1 or π_2 is increased. From this, we may see from the general expression for $\mathscr{R}_0$ that increasing either of the preferences π_1, π_2 increases the basic reproduction number.

5 The Invasion Criterion

In order to obtain an invasion criterion, initially when $S_1(t)$ is close to $S_1(0) = N_1$ and $S_2(t)$ is close to $S_2(0) = N_2$, we replace $S_1(t)$ and $S_2(t)$ by N_1, N_2 respectively to give a linear system, and the condition that this linear system have a solution $S_1(t) = N_1 e^{rt}, S_2(t) = N_2 e^{rt}$ is

$$\begin{aligned} 1 &= a_1\sigma_1 p_{11}\int_0^\infty e^{-rs}A_1(s)ds + a_1\sigma_1 p_{12}\int_0^\infty e^{-rs}A_2(s)ds \\ 1 &= a_2\sigma_2 p_{21}\int_0^\infty e^{-rs}A_1(s)ds + a_2\sigma_2 p_{22}\int_0^\infty e^{-rs}A_2(s)ds. \end{aligned} \tag{17}$$

The initial exponential growth rate is the solution r of the equation

$$\det \begin{bmatrix} a_1\sigma_1 p_{11}\int_0^\infty e^{-rs}A_1(s)ds - 1 & a_1\sigma_1 p_{12}\int_0^\infty e^{-rs}A_2(s)ds \\ a_2\sigma_2 p_{21}\int_0^\infty e^{-rs}A_1(s)ds & a_2\sigma_2 p_{22}\int_0^\infty e^{-rs}A_2(s)ds - 1 \end{bmatrix} = 0. \qquad (18)$$

In the special case in which the two groups have the same infectivity distribution but may have different activity levels and possibly vulnerability to infection, so that $A_1(s) = A_2(s) = A(s)$, $\mathscr{R}_0$ is the largest root of

$$\det \begin{bmatrix} a_1\sigma_1 p_{11}\int_0^\infty A(s)ds - \lambda & a_1\sigma_1 p_{12}\int_0^\infty A(s)ds \\ a_2\sigma_2 p_{21}\int_0^\infty A(s)ds & a_2\sigma_2 p_{22}\int_0^\infty A(s)ds - \lambda \end{bmatrix} \qquad (19)$$

and the initial exponential growth rate is the solution r of the equation

$$\det \begin{bmatrix} a_1\sigma_1 p_{11}\int_0^\infty e^{-rs}A(s)ds - 1 & a_1\sigma_1 p_{12}\int_0^\infty e^{-rs}A(s)ds \\ a_2\sigma_2 p_{21}\int_0^\infty e^{-rs}A(s)ds & a_2\sigma_2 p_{22}\int_0^\infty e^{-rs}A(s)ds - 1 \end{bmatrix} = 0. \qquad (20)$$

Comparing the Eqs. (19) and (20), we see that each of $\mathscr{R}_0/\int_0^\infty A(s)ds$ and $1/\int_0^\infty e^{-rs}A(s)ds$ is the largest root of the equation

$$x^2 - (a_1p_{11}\sigma_1 + a_2p_{22}\sigma_2)x + a_1a_2\sigma_1\sigma_2(p_{11}p_{22} - p_{12}p_{21}) = 0.$$

Thus

$$\frac{\mathscr{R}_0}{\int_0^\infty A(s)ds} = \frac{1}{\int_0^\infty e^{-rs}A(s)ds},$$

which implies the same relation as for the homogeneous mixing model. Thus, if we assume heterogeneous mixing, we obtain the same estimate of the reproduction number from observation of the initial exponential growth rate. The estimate of the basic reproduction number from the initial exponential growth rate does not depend on heterogeneity of the model. This result does not generalize to the case $A_1(s) \neq A_2(s)$, but it does remain valid for an arbitrary number of groups with different contact rates.

In the special case of proportionate mixing, in which $p_{11} = p_{21}$, $p_{12} = p_{22}$, so that $p_{12}p_{21} = p_{11}p_{22}$, the basic reproduction number is given by

$$\mathscr{R}_0 = a_1\sigma_1 p_{11}\int_0^\infty A_1(s)ds + a_2\sigma_2 p_{22}\int_0^\infty A_2(s)ds,$$

and the Eq. (18) reduces to

$$a_1\sigma_1 p_{11}\int_0^\infty e^{-rs}A_1(s)ds + a_2\sigma_2 p_{22}\int_0^\infty e^{-rs}A_i(s)ds = 1. \tag{21}$$

There is an epidemic if and only if $\mathscr{R}_0 > 1$.

6 The Final Size of a Heterogeneous Mixing Epidemic

With homogeneous mixing, knowledge of the basic reproduction number translates into knowledge of the final size of the epidemic. However, with heterogeneous mixing the size of the epidemic is not determined uniquely by the basic reproduction number.

For the heterogeneous mixing model (14) there is a pair of final size relations. We divide the first equation of the model by $S_1(t)$ and integrate with respect to t from 0 to ∞. Much as in the derivation of the final size relation for the homogeneous mixing model we obtain

$$\begin{aligned}\log\frac{S_1(0)}{S_1(\infty)} &= a_1\sigma_1\frac{p_{11}}{N_1}[N_1 - S_1(\infty)]\int_0^\infty A_1(s)ds\\ &+a_1\sigma_1\frac{p_{12}}{N_2}[N_2 - S_2(\infty)]\int_0^\infty A_2(s)ds.\end{aligned}$$

The same process applied to the second equation gives

$$\begin{aligned}\log\frac{S_2(0)}{S_2(\infty)} &= a_2\sigma_2\frac{p_{21}}{N_1}[N_1 - S_1(\infty)]\int_0^\infty A_1(s)ds\\ &+a_2\sigma_2\frac{p_{22}}{N_2}[N_2 - S_2(\infty)]\int_0^\infty A_2(s)ds.\end{aligned}$$

Thus we have a pair of final size relations which may be solved for $S_1(\infty)$, $S_2(\infty)$.

$$\begin{aligned}\log\frac{S_1(0)}{S_1(\infty)} &= a_1\sigma_1\frac{p_{11}}{N_1}[N_1 - S_1(\infty)]\int_0^\infty A_1(s)ds\\ &+ a_1\sigma_1\frac{p_{12}}{N_2}[N_2 - S_2(\infty)]\int_0^\infty A_2(s)ds\\ \log\frac{S_2(0)}{S_2(\infty)} &= a_2\sigma_2\frac{p_{21}}{N_1}[N_1 - S_1(\infty)]\int_0^\infty A_1(s)ds\\ &+ a_2\sigma_2\frac{p_{22}}{N_2}[N_2 - S_2(\infty)]int_0^\infty A_2(s)ds.\end{aligned} \tag{22}$$

The system of equations (22) has a unique solution $(S_1(\infty), S_2(\infty))$.

In order to prove the existence of a unique solution of (22), we define

$$g_1(x_1, x_2) = \log \frac{S_1(0)}{x_1} - a_1\sigma_1 \sum_{j=1}^{2} p_{1j} \left[1 - \frac{x_j}{N_j}\right] \int_0^\infty A_j(s)$$

$$g_2(x_1, x_2) = \log \frac{S_1(0)}{x_2} - a_2\sigma_2 \sum_{j=1}^{2} p_{1j} \left[1 - \frac{x_j}{N_j}\right] \int_0^\infty A_j(s)ds.$$

A solution of (22) is a solution (x_1, x_2) of the system

$$g_1(x_1, x_2) = 0, \quad g_2(x_1, x_2) = 0.$$

For each x_2, $g_1(0+, x_2) > 0$, $g_1(S_1(0), x_2) < 0$. Also, as a function of x_1, $g_1(x_1, x_2)$ either decreases or decrease initially and then increases to a negative value when $x_1 = S_1(0)$. Thus for each $x_2 < S_2(0)$, there is a unique $x_1(x_2)$ such that $g_1(x_1(x_2), x_2) = 0$. Also, since $g_1(x_1, x_2)$ is an increasing function of x_2, the function $x_1(x_2)$ is increasing. Now, since $g_2(x_1, 0+) > 0$, $g_2(x_1, S_2(0)) < 0$, there exists x_2 such that $g_2(x_1(x_2), x_2) = 0$. Also, $g_2(x_1(x_2), x_2)$ either decreases monotonically or decreases initially and then increases to a negative value when $x_2 = S_2(0)$. Therefore this solution is also unique. This implies that

$$(x_1(x_2), x_2)$$

is the unique solution of the final size relations.

7 Conclusions

The age of infection model is a general framework for epidemic models. It allows arbitrary compartmental structure as well as arbitrary distributions of stay in a compartment. In addition, it can be extended to situations with heterogeneous mixing. For a given disease outbreak, if we understand the compartmental structure and the distribution of stay in each compartment, it is possible to estimate the basic reproduction number.

If the mixing structure between groups is also known, the final size of the epidemic can be estimated. The reproduction number of an epidemic model is not sufficient to determine the size of the epidemic if there is heterogeneity in the model. Numerical simulations indicate that models with heterogeneous mixing may give very different epidemic sizes than models with the same basic reproduction number and homogeneous mixing. We conjecture that for a given value of the basic reproduction number the maximum epidemic size for any mixing is obtained with homogeneous mixing. This would suggest that the assumption of homogeneous mixing would be appropriate for estimating the worst case scenario in an epidemic. Since the public health approach is to hope for the best but prepare for the worst, use of a homogeneous mixing age of infection model with measurement of the initial exponential growth rate to estimate the basic reproduction number and the epidemic final size would be a good first step in planning control strategies. When more data are obtained we suggest that the number of groups to be considered for different treatment rates should determine the number of groups to be used in the model. On the other hand, the number of groups to be considered should also depend on the amount and reliability of data, and these two criteria may be contradictory. A model with fewer groups and parameters chosen as weighted averages of the parameters for a model with more groups may give predictions that are quite similar to those of the more detailed models. We suggest also that use of the final size relations for a model with total population size assumed constant is a good time-saving procedure for making predictions if the disease death rate is small.

Acknowledgments This work was supported by the Natural Sciences and Engineering Research Council of Canada.

References

1. Blythe, S.P., Busenberg, S., Castillo-Chavez, C.: Affinity and paired-event probability. Math. Biosci. **128**, 265–284 (1991)
2. Blythe, S.P., Castillo-Chavez, C., Palmer, J., Cheng, M.: Towards a unified theory of mixing and pair formation. Math. Biosci. **107**, 379–405 (1991)
3. Brauer, F.: Epidemic models with heterogeneous mixing and treatment. Bull. Math. Biol. **70**, 1869–1885 (2008)
4. Brauer, F., Watmough, J.: Age of infection epidemic models with heterogeneous mixing. J. Biol. Dyn. **3**, 324–330 (2009)
5. Busenberg, S., Castillo-Chavez, C.: Interaction, pair formation and force of infection terms in sexually transmitted diseases. In: Castillo-Chavez, C. (ed.) Mathematical and Statistical Approaches to AIDS Epidemiology. Lecture Notes in Biomathematics, vol. 83, pp. 289–300. Springer, Berlin (1989)
6. Diekmann, O., Heesterbeek, J.A.P., Metz, J.A.J.: The legacy of Kermack and McKendrick. In: Mollison, D. (ed.) Epidemic Models: Their Structure and Relation to Data, pp. 95–115. Cambridge University Press, Cambridge (1995)
7. Kermack, W.O., McKendrick, A.G.: A contribution to the mathematical theory of epidemics. Proc. R. Soc. Lond. **115**, 700–721 (1927)
8. Kermack, W.O., McKendrick, A.G.: Contributions to the mathematical theory of epidemics, part. II. Proc. R. Soc. Lond. **138**, 55–83 (1932)
9. Kermack, W.O., McKendrick, A.G.: Contributions to the mathematical theory of epidemics, part. III. Proc. R. Soc. Lond. **141**, 94–112 (1933)
10. Nold, A.: Heterogeneity in disease transmission modeling. Math. Biosci. **52**, 227–240 (1980)
11. Thieme, H.R., Castillo-Chavez, C.: On the role of variable infectivity in the dynamics of the human immunodeficiency virus. In: Castillo-Chavez, C. (ed.) Mathematical and Statistical Approaches to AIDS Epidemiology. Lecture Notes in Biomathematics, pp. 200–217. Springer, Berlin (1989)
12. Thieme, H.R., Castillo-Chavez, C.: How may infection-age dependent infectivity affect the dynamics of HIV/AIDS? SIAM J. Appl. Math. **53**, 1447–1479 (1993)
13. van den Driessche, P., Watmough, J.: Reproduction numbers and sub-threshold endemic equilibria for compartmental models of disease transmission. Math. Biosci. **180**, 29–48 (2002)
14. Wallinga, J., Lipsitch, M.: How generation intervals shape the relationship between growth rates and reproductive numbers. Proc. R. Soc. B **274**, 599–604 (2007)

Optimal Control of Vaccination in an Age-Structured Cholera Model

K. Renee Fister, Holly Gaff, Suzanne Lenhart, Eric Numfor, Elsa Schaefer and Jin Wang

Abstract A cholera model with continuous age structure is given as a system of hyperbolic (first-order) partial differential equations (PDEs) in combination with ordinary differential equations. Asymptomatic infected and susceptibles with partial immunity are included in this epidemiology model with vaccination rate as a control; minimizing the symptomatic infecteds while minimizing the cost of the vaccinations represents the goal. With the method of characteristics and a fixed point argument, the existence of a solution to our nonlinear state system is achieved. The representation and existence of a unique optimal control are derived. The steps to justify the optimal control results for such a system with first order PDEs are given. Numerical results illustrate the effect of age structure on optimal vaccination rates.

Keywords Cholera · Optimal control · Mathematical model · Partial differential equation · Waning immunity

K.R. Fister
Department of Mathematics and Statistics,
Murray State University, Murray, KY 42071, USA
e-mail: renee.fister@murraystate.edu

H. Gaff
Department of Biological Sciences, Old Dominion University, Norfolk, VA 23929, USA
e-mail: hgaff@odu.edu

S. Lenhart (✉)
Department of Mathematics, University of Tennessee, Knoxville, TN 37996, USA
e-mail: lenhart@math.utk.edu

E. Numfor
Department of Mathematics, Augusta University, Augusta, GA 30912, USA
e-mail: enumfor@augusta.edu

E. Schaefer
Department of Mathematics, Marymount University, Arlington, VA 22207, USA
e-mail: elsa.schaefer@marymount.edu

J. Wang
Department of Mathematics, University of Tennessee at Chattanooga,
Chattanooga, TN 37403, USA
e-mail: jin-wang02@utc.edu

G. Chowell and J.M. Hyman (eds.), *Mathematical and Statistical Modeling for Emerging and Re-emerging Infectious Diseases*,
DOI 10.1007/978-3-319-40413-4_14

1 Introduction

Cholera is a diarrhoeal disease that affects millions of residents annually in regions with poor sanitation across the world. The bacterium responsible for the outbreaks, *Vibrio cholerae*, is environmentally endemic throughout Asia and Africa, and hence without proper control strategies, we can well expect cholera to continue to plague human populations indefinitely.

Populations with clean water and adequate sanitation are not vulnerable to a cholera epidemic, even if an individual manages to contract the disease through environmental interaction. However, when sanitation is lacking, there is a fecal-environmental amplification of the bacteria in the human environment, and an outbreak ensues [36]. Once an outbreak is present, oral rehydration therapy is extremely effective in preventing death, but the cost of the associated morbidity is quite large [38]. Unfortunately, administration, especially prophylactically, of antibiotics may lead to bacterial resistance quickly [24]. While antibiotic resistance is indeed an issue, there remain effective antibiotics for treating cholera (like azithromycin in Haiti), and their usage is frequently advocated as part of the effort to combat cholera [48]. Other key tools for decreasing morbidity by safely slowing the spread of cholera are sanitation (clean water, waste treatment, food safety), vaccination, or perhaps quarantine. Recent studies have sought to consider which of these control measures, or which combination of measures, might be most cost-effective in reducing the financial and societal cost of cholera outbreaks in affected regions [20, 38]. Because cholera results in symptomatic infections more often for the very young or old, one concern is whether age-based vaccination protocols that target priority populations can effectively slow the spread of disease while limiting the costs of intervention.

There have been many developments in cholera modeling over the past fifteen years. In 2001, Codeço formulated an ODE cholera model which considered the interplay between infected humans and the concentration of cholera bacteria in the surrounding environment and the resulting disease dynamics [6]. The next year Merrell and Butler reported that freshly shed cholera bacteria from human intestines are as much as 700 times more infectious than bacteria shed only hours previously [31]. Thus, to model this pathway of infection, Hartley et al. [18] proposed a model with hyperinfective vibrios introduced into the water reserves by the infected people in the population; that new model explained the frequent explosive nature of the disease due to the human-environmental amplification [36].

King et al. [22] proposed a two-patch cholera ODE model including classes for 'inapparent' infections and the feature of varying periods of waning immunity. The work by Miller Neilan et al. [32] incorporated several ideas from the paper by King et al. [22] into a model influenced by Hartley et al., [18], investigating the optimal control balancing of three strategies to slow the spread of the disease in an ODE model with hyperinfectious vibrios, both symptomatic and asymptomatic infected populations, and waning immunity.

Other recent work includes a four compartment modeling approach that tracks pathogen in the water; this system of four ODEs has been used to simulate cholera in the 19th century in London [44, 45]. The ODE system was further extended to a multi-patch model to study the recent cholera outbreak in Haiti [46]. Mukandavire et al. proposed another model that incorporated both direct and indirect transmission pathways and applied it to the 2008–2009 Zimbabwean cholera outbreak [33]. A more general modeling framework for cholera was proposed in [43, 47], and later extended to a periodic environment for the investigation of seasonal impact [39]. Some discussion of the influence of human behavior on cholera dynamics was conducted in a recent study [49]. In addition, more sophisticated multi-group and multi-patch cholera models incorporating general incidence functions appeared in [9, 42].

Cholera dynamics such as the risk for contracting the disease and then for becoming symptomatic [36] may depend on the age of the humans and amount of previous exposure to this disease. The immunity from vaccination may also depend on age [34] and previous exposure. To investigate optimal control of vaccination for cholera, we use an age-structured model, a system with first order partial differential equations (PDEs) and ordinary differential equations (ODEs).

We want to illustrate how optimal control can be applied to an age-structured PDE and ODE coupled model for this specific disease application. Optimal control of a first order PDE system is quite different from optimal control applied on second order PDE systems, due to the difference in regularity of the state solutions. Specifically elliptic and parabolic systems with nonlinearities in the lower order terms have H^1 regularity in the spatial variable, while solutions of first order systems usually do not have such regularity. The H^1 regularity gives some additional compactness, which usually gives a more straightforward path to obtain the existence of an optimal control. One can see the background of optimal control of second order PDE in [28, 29] and see some specific applications in [25, 27, 35]. To obtain the existence of an optimal control in the first order PDE case, the foundation was laid by Barbu [4, 5] with the use of Ekeland Principle's [10] to obtain the existence of an optimal control. See related applications of this technique in [2, 3, 5, 11, 12, 37]. We will point out the steps in our analysis that are needed to use Ekeland's Principle and this technique.

Our age-structured model includes seven human classes. There is one group of humans who experience disease (susceptible $S \rightarrow$ infected $I \rightarrow$ recovered R) with no prior immunity, while the remainder of the population has some partial immunity as it moves through the $S \rightarrow I \rightarrow R$ process. We assume that both classes of susceptible humans are equally likely to become infected after contact with cholera bacteria, but that partially immune individuals will experience asymptomatic infections, while fully susceptible individuals can either have symptomatic or asymptomatic infections. The length of illness is much shorter for asymptomatic infections than for symptomatic infections, and additionally immunity from asymptomatic infections wanes more quickly than for symptomatic infections [22, 36]. Vaccinated humans are placed in a vaccinated class, which is assumed to wane more slowly than either recovered class due to the multi-strain nature of cholera vaccines. The bacteria are modeled following Hartley et al. and Miller-Neilan et al. with hyper- and low-infectious bacterial classes, [18, 32].

This paper provides a discussion of an age-structured cholera model in Sect. 2, as well as, the incorporation of intervention as a control. In Sect. 3, we prove the existence of a solution in L^1 and L^∞ to our PDE system using a fixed point argument on a representation derived from the method of characteristics. In Sect. 4, the conditions for optimal control representation are determined and the characterization of the control is developed. Section 5 provides the analysis of the characterization and the uniqueness of the optimal control. In Sects. 5 and 6 respectively, we discuss parameter choices and then illustrate some numerical results. Some conclusions are given at the end.

2 The Model and Optimal Control Formulation

In our cholera model, the susceptible human population is compartmentalized into those who are fully susceptible S and those with partial immunity $\hat{S}$. We assume that some age-varying proportion $p(a)$ of the fully susceptible humans who become infected will have symptomatic infections I_S, while the remainder of those and the partially immune humans, who become infected, will be asymptomatic I_A. Humans who recover from symptomatic infections enter one recovered class R_S, while those who recover from asymptomatic infections enter a separate class R_A. Humans who are in either susceptible class may become vaccinated V. All human classes are modeled as functions of time, measured in weeks, and age, measured in years.

Infection occurs as a result of human contact with the cholera bacteria. As we mentioned in the introduction, contact with freshly shed vibrios may be 700 times more likely to result in infection than for contact with bacteria that have been shed five or more hours in the past. Thus, we model the density of both low-infectious and high-infectious bacteria in the environment using classes B_L and B_H, respectively, depending only on time.

Figure 1 suggests the key interactions and corresponding rates assumed for this cholera model, with parameter definitions given in Table 1.

In this work, we analyze the behaviors that result from an outbreak in a population with separate fully susceptible and partially immune dynamics. We then propose an intervention $u(a,t)$ that represents a time- and age-based movement of humans from susceptible classes to the vaccinated class. Formally, we consider the age-time domain, $Q = (0,A) \times (0,T)$, with vaccination rates u in

$$\Gamma = \{\, u \in L^\infty(Q) \mid 0 \le u(a,t) \le N_1, \quad \text{a.e. in } Q\}, \tag{1}$$

where $N_1 \le 1$ denotes the maximum rate of vaccination. Given a control $u \in \Gamma$, the corresponding state variables,

$$(S, I_S, R_S, \hat{S}, I_A, R_A, V, B_H, B_L) = (S, I_S, R_S, \hat{S}, I_A, R_A, V, B_H, B_L)(u)$$

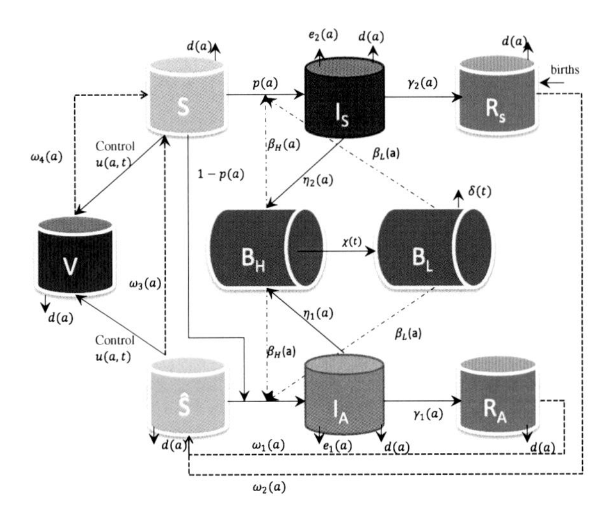

Fig. 1 Diagram of cholera dynamics. The *solid arrows* show movement through the *S–I–R* stages of disease within and between the two human tracks, as well as the intervention moving humans from susceptible classes to the vaccinated class. The *dot-dashed lines* in the figure refer to the coefficient describing the infection resulting from contact between infected vibrios and humans. The four *dashed lines* show the four routes in which immunity is lost

satisfy the state system as follows:

$$\frac{\partial S}{\partial t} + \alpha \frac{\partial S}{\partial a} = -\left[\beta_L(a)\frac{B_L(t)}{\kappa_L(a) + B_L(t)} + \beta_H(a)\frac{B_H(t)}{\kappa_H(a) + B_H(t)}\right] S(a,t)$$

$$- d(a)S(a,t) + \omega_3(a)\hat{S}(a,t) + \omega_4(a)V(a,t) - u(a,t)S(a,t), \tag{2}$$

$$\frac{\partial I_S}{\partial t} + \alpha \frac{\partial I_S}{\partial a} = p(a)\left[\beta_L(a)\frac{B_L(t)}{\kappa_L(a) + B_L(t)} + \beta_H(a)\frac{B_H(t)}{\kappa_H(a) + B_H(t)}\right] S(a,t)$$

$$- [d(a) + \gamma_2(a) + e_2(a)]\, I_S(a,t) \tag{3}$$

$$\frac{\partial R_S}{\partial t} + \alpha \frac{\partial R_S}{\partial a} = -[d(a) + \omega_2(a)]\, R_S(a,t) + \gamma_2(a) I_S(a,t), \tag{4}$$

$$\frac{\partial \hat{S}}{\partial t} + \alpha \frac{\partial \hat{S}}{\partial a} = -\left[\beta_L(a)\frac{B_L(t)}{\kappa_L(a) + B_L(t)} + \beta_H(a)\frac{B_H(t)}{\kappa_H(a) + B_H(t)}\right] \hat{S}(a,t) \tag{5}$$

$$- [d(a) + \omega_3(a) + u(a,t)]\, \hat{S}(a,t) + \omega_1(a) R_A(a,t)$$

$$+ \omega_2(a) R_S(a,t), \tag{6}$$

$$\frac{\partial I_A}{\partial t} + \alpha \frac{\partial I_A}{\partial a} = \left[\beta_L(a)\frac{B_L(t)}{\kappa_L(a) + B_L(t)} + \beta_H(a)\frac{B_H(t)}{\kappa_H(a) + B_H(t)}\right] \hat{S}(a,t)$$

$$- [d(a) + \gamma_1(a) + e_1(a)]\, I_A(a,t)$$

$$+ (1 - p(a))\left[\frac{B_L(t)}{\kappa_L(a) + B_L(t)} + \beta_H(a)\frac{B_H(t)}{\kappa_H(a) + B_H(t)}\right] S(a,t), \tag{7}$$

$$\frac{\partial R_A}{\partial t} + \alpha \frac{\partial R_A}{\partial a} = -[d(a) + \omega_1(a)]\, R_A(a,t) + \gamma_1(a) I_A(a,t), \tag{8}$$

Table 1 Summary of notation for parameters

Parameter	Description
u	Rate of vaccination for S and $\hat{S}$
A_1	Weight for human morbidity in OC
A_2, A_3	Weights for cost in OC
p	Prob. of indiv. in S to be symp. when infected
β_L	Ingestion rate of non-HI vibrio from environment
β_H	Ingestion rate of HI vibrio from environment
κ_L	Half saturation constant of non-HI vibrios
κ_H	Half saturation constant of HI vibrios
e_1	Cholera-related death rate for asymp. infecteds
e_2	Cholera-related death rate for symp. infecteds
γ_1	Cholera recovery rate for asymptomatic infecteds
γ_2	Cholera recovery rate for symptomatic infecteds
ω_1	Rate of waning cholera immunity from R_A to $\hat{S}$
ω_2	Rate of waning cholera immunity from R_S to $\hat{S}$
ω_3	Rate of waning cholera immunity from $\hat{S}$ to S
ω_4	Rate of waning cholera immunity from V to S
η_1	Rate of contribution to HI vibrios in environment by asymptomatic infecteds
η_2	Rate of contribution to HI vibrios in environment by symptomatic infecteds
χ	Transition rate of vibrios from HI to non-HI state
δ	Death rate of vibrios from HI to non-HI state
f	fecundity rate of humans
d	Natural death rate of humans

$$\frac{\partial V}{\partial t} + \alpha \frac{\partial V}{\partial a} = u(a,t)\left[S(a,t) + \hat{S}(a,t)\right] - [\omega_4(a) + d(a)]\, V(a,t), \tag{9}$$

$$\frac{dB_H}{dt} = \int_0^A \eta_1(a) I_A(a,t)da + \int_0^A \eta_2(a) I_S(a,t)da - \chi(t) B_H(t), \tag{10}$$

$$\frac{dB_L}{dt} = \chi(t) B_H(t) - \delta(t) B_L(t). \tag{11}$$

In the above equations, $\alpha = \frac{1}{52} \frac{\text{weeks}}{\text{years}}$ is a coefficient introduced to balance the units of age a in years and time t in weeks. Also, A which appears in the equation for B_H is an upper bound on the age of people in the model (here $A = 72$ years). The human compartments have units of number of individuals, while the two bacteria compartments have units of number of vibrios/ml.

The boundary and initial conditions are given below. Since there are low disease rates in infants, due perhaps to breastfeeding or cross-protection from *Escherichia coli* infections that are caused by a similar toxin, [14, 40], we choose to place newborns in the symptomatic recovered class.

$$S(0,t) = 0, \tag{12}$$
$$I_S(0,t) = 0, \tag{13}$$
$$R_S(0,t) = \int_0^A (S(a,t) + \hat{S}(a,t) + I_S(a,t) + I_A(a,t) + R_S(a,t) + R_A(a,t) + V(a,t))f(a)da, \tag{14}$$
$$\hat{S}(0,t) = 0, \tag{15}$$
$$I_A(0,t) = 0, \tag{16}$$
$$R_A(0,t) = 0, \tag{17}$$
$$V(0,t) = 0, \tag{18}$$
$$B_H(0) = B_{H0},\ B_L(0) = B_{L0}, \tag{19}$$

where the fecundity function f is modeled as

$$f(a) = \begin{cases} \frac{1}{5}\sin^2\left[\left(\frac{a-15}{30}\right)\pi\right], & 15 < a < 45, \\ 0, & \text{otherwise.} \end{cases} \tag{20}$$

$$S(a,0) = S_0(a),\quad I_S(a,0) = I_{S0}(a),\quad R_S(a,0) = R_{S0}(a)$$

$$\hat{S}(a,0) = \hat{S}_0(a),\quad I_A(a,0) = I_{A0}(a),$$

$$R_A(a,0) = R_{A0}(a),\quad V(a,0) = V_0(a),\quad B_H(0) = B_{H0} = 0,\quad B_L(0) = B_{L0}. \tag{21}$$

We wish to suggest an age- and time-based vaccination strategy that is effective in decreasing the morbidity due to a cholera outbreak while being mindful of cost. Thus, we seek to minimize the functional,

$$\mathcal{J}(u) = \int_0^T \int_0^A A_1 I_S(a,t) + A_2\, u(a,t)(S(a,t) + \hat{S}(a,t) + I_A(a,t) + R_A(a,t))\, da\, dt + \frac{1}{2}\int_0^T \int_0^A A_3\, u^2(a,t)\, da\, dt, \tag{22}$$

over $u \in \Gamma$, where A_1, A_2 and A_3 are weight factors. The weight A_1 is a balancing term suggesting our emphasis on mitigating morbidity within the population. The weight A_2 balances the cost of the intervention on the two susceptible populations and the two asymptomatic populations. Thus there is a cost associated with vaccinating humans who may be unaware of recent asymptomatic infections though the model does not assume movement to the vaccinated class V from the asymptomatic classes I_A and R_A. If the vaccination of those persons in the two asymptomatic classes affects their immune status, one could move them into the vaccinated class V, but we did not include this feature in our model. To clarify in our minimization problem, an optimal control u^* in Γ will satisfy

$$\mathcal{J}(u^*) = \inf_{u \in \Gamma} \mathcal{J}(u).$$

3 Existence of the Solution to the State System

Given a control, the existence of the corresponding state solution can be obtained by using a fixed point theorem and the representation of solution by the method of characteristics, [4, 50]. Then we prove the existence of a using a contraction mapping principle.

We let M be chosen such that

$$0 \leq S_0(a),\ I_{S0}(a),\ R_{S0}(a),\ \hat{S}_0(a),\ I_{A0}(a),\ R_{A0}(a),\ V_0(a) \text{ a.e.,} \tag{23}$$

$$\int_0^A S_0(a)da \leq M, \int_0^A I_{S0}(a)da \leq M, \int_0^A R_{S0}(a)da \leq M, \tag{24}$$

$$\int_0^A \hat{S}_0(a)da \leq M, \int_0^A I_{A0}(a)da \leq M, \int_0^A R_{A0}(a)da \leq M, \tag{25}$$

$$\int_0^A V_0(a)da \leq M, 0 \leq B_{H0}, B_{L0} \leq M. \tag{26}$$

We define our state solution space as

$$\begin{aligned} X = \Bigg\{ &(S, I_S, R_S, \hat{S}, I_A, R_A, V, B_H, B_L) \in (L^\infty(0,T; L^1(0,A)))^7 \times (L^\infty(0,T))^2 | \\ &\sup_t \int_0^A |S(a,t)|da \leq 2M, \sup_t \int_0^A |I_S(a,t)|da \leq 2M, \sup_t \int_0^A |R_S(a,t)|da \leq 2M, \\ &\sup_t \int_0^A |\hat{S}(a,t)|da \leq 2M, \sup_t \int_0^A |I_A(a,t)|da \leq 2M, \sup_t \int_0^A |R_A(a,t)|da \leq 2M, \\ &\sup_t \int_0^A |V(a,t)|da \leq 2M, |B_H(t)| \leq 2M, |B_L(t)| \leq 2M \text{ a.e. } t \Bigg\}. \end{aligned}$$

To illustrate the structure of the representation of the solution from the method of characteristics (including the birth terms), see the two terms below.

$$R_S(a,t) = \begin{cases} e^{-\int_0^t d(\alpha\tau-\alpha t+a)d\tau} R_{S0}(a-\alpha t) \\ +\int_0^t e^{-\int_s^t d(\alpha\tau-\alpha t+a)d\tau} \times & \text{if } a > \alpha t \\ (\omega_2(\alpha s+a-\alpha t)R_S(\alpha s+a-\alpha t, s)+ \\ \gamma_2(\alpha s+a-\alpha t)I_S(\alpha s+a-\alpha t, s))\, ds \\ \\ (\frac{1}{\alpha})\int_0^a e^{-\int_s^a \frac{d(\tau)}{\alpha}d\tau} \times \\ \int_0^A \left[S+\hat{S}+V+I_S+I_A+R_S+R_A\right](s, \frac{\alpha t-a}{\alpha})f(s)\, ds \\ +(\frac{1}{\alpha})\int_0^a e^{-\int_s^a \frac{d(\tau)}{\alpha}d\tau} \times & \text{if } a < \alpha t, \\ \omega_2(s)R_S(s, \frac{s+\alpha t-a}{\alpha}) + \gamma_2(s)I_S(s, \frac{s+\alpha t-a}{\alpha})\, ds \end{cases} \quad (27)$$

and

$$B_H(t) = B_{H0}e^{-\chi t} + \int_0^t \int_0^A e^{-\chi(t-s)} \left[\eta_1(a)I_A(a,t) + \eta_2(a)I_s(a,t)\right] da\, ds. \quad (28)$$

To prove the following existence theorem, one would have a representation of each state variable similar to the representation above for R_S. To use a fixed point theorem, define a map as

$$L : X \to X \text{ such that}$$

where for $N = (S, I_S, R_S, \hat{S}, I_A, R_A, V, B_H, B_L) \in X$, we define

$$L(N) = (L_1(N), L_2(N), L_3(N), L_4(N), L_5(N), L_6(N), L_7(N), L_8(N), L_9(N)).$$

Then the right side of (27) is $L_3(N)$. In a fixed point argument for the operator L, the third component would be $R_S = L_3(N)$. A fixed point argument (similar to [11]) would give the existence of a solution as stated in this theorem. From results in Chap. 2 in Webb [50] with the specific structure of the right hand sides of the state equations, we can obtain the non-negativity of the solutions.

Theorem 1 (Existence of solutions) *For $u \in \Gamma$ as defined in (1) and T sufficiently small, there exists a solution $(S, I_S, R_S, \hat{S}, I_A, R_A, V, B_H, B_L)$ to the state system (2)–(11) with boundary and initial conditions (12)–(19) and (21).*

In order to prove the optimality conditions and to prove the existence of an optimal control, we require estimates involving Lipschitz conditions of the solutions in terms of the control.

Theorem 2 *For T sufficiently small, the map:*

$$u \in \Gamma \to N = N(u) \in X.$$

is Lipschitz in the following ways where the dependence on age and time is suppressed:

$$\int_Q (|S_1 - S_2| + |I_{S1} - I_{S2}| + |R_{S1} - R_{S2}| + |\hat{S}_1 - \hat{S}_2|$$
$$+|I_{A1} - I_{A2}| + |R_{A1} - R_{A2}| + |V_1 - V_2|)\,da\,dt$$
$$+ \int_0^T (|B_{H1} - B_{H2}| + |B_{L1} - B_{L2}|)\,dt \le C_1 T \left(\int_Q |u_1 - u_2|(a,t)\,da\,dt \right)$$

and

$$\|S_1 - S_2\|_{L^\infty(Q)} + \|I_{S1} - I_{S2}\|_{L^\infty(Q)} + \|R_{S1} - R_{S2}\|_{L^\infty(Q)} + \|\hat{S}_1 - \hat{S}_2\|_{L^\infty(Q)}$$
$$+\|I_{A1} - I_{A2}\|_{L^\infty(Q)} + \|R_{A1} - R_{A2}\|_{L^\infty(Q)} + \|B_{H1} - B_{H2}\|_{L^\infty(0,T)}$$
$$+\|B_{L1} - B_{L2}\|_{L^\infty(0,T)} \le C_2 T \left(\|u_1 - u_2\|_{L^\infty(Q)} \right),$$

where $(S_i, I_{Si}, R_{Si}, \hat{S}_i, I_{Ai}, R_{Ai}, V_i, B_{Hi}, B_{Li}) = (S_i, I_{Si}, R_{Si}, \hat{S}_i, I_{Ai}, R_{Ai}, V_i, B_{Hi}, B_{Li})(u_i)$ *for* $i = 1, 2$ *and for* u_1 *and* u_2 *in* Γ.

The proof of these estimates follow similarly as in the corresponding result found in Fister and Lenhart, [11, 12]. The proof utilizes the representations of the state solution system coming from the method of characteristics. The representations for the state vectors corresponding to two controls, u_1 and u_2, are subtracted and then the differences are estimated. Additionally, one must use care in the order in which these estimates are determined, especially for the case when age is larger than time. From the representations found through the method of characteristics, we first find the L^1 estimate. Then we estimate L^1 integral of the difference of the state variables depending on age and time in the age variable to obtain the L^∞ estimate.

4 Conditions for Optimality

We derive the sensitivity functions which provide the differentiability of the solution map of $u \to N = N(u)$ where $N = (S, I_S, R_S, \hat{S}, I_A, R_A, V, B_H, B_L)$. These functions provide the information necessary to differentiate the objective functional with respect to the control. The sensitivity functions are then used to determine the adjoint equations.

Theorem 3 *The map*

$$u \in \Gamma \to N = N(u) \in X$$

is differentiable in the following sense:

$$\frac{N(u + \varepsilon l) - N(u)}{\varepsilon} \to (\phi, \psi_S, r_S, \hat{\phi}, \psi_A, r_A, v, \theta_H, \theta_L)$$

in $(L^\infty(Q))^7 \times (L^\infty(0,T))^2$, *for* $(u+\varepsilon l)$, $u \in \Gamma$ *and* $\varepsilon \to 0$, *with* $l \in L^\infty(Q)$. *Furthermore, the sensitivities* $(\phi, \psi_S, r_S, \hat{\phi}, \psi_A, r_A, v, \theta_H, \theta_L)$ *satisfy*

$$
\begin{aligned}
\frac{\partial \phi}{\partial t} + \alpha \frac{\partial \phi}{\partial a} &= -\beta_L(a)\left[\frac{B_L(t)}{\kappa_L(a)+B_L(t)}\phi(a,t) + \frac{S(a,t)\kappa_L(a)\theta_L(t)}{(\kappa_L(a)+B_L(t))^2}\right] \\
&\quad - \beta_H(a)\left[\frac{B_H(t)}{\kappa_H(a)+B_H(t)}\phi(a,t) + \frac{S(a,t)\kappa_H(a)\theta_H(t)}{(\kappa_H(a)+B_H(t))^2}\right] \\
&\quad - d(a)\phi(a,t) + \omega_3\hat{\phi}(a,t) + \omega_4 v(a,t) \\
&\quad - u(a,t)\phi(a,t) - l(a,t)S(a,t) \qquad (29) \\
\frac{\partial \psi_S}{\partial t} + \alpha \frac{\partial \psi_S}{\partial a} &= p(a)\beta_L(a)\left[\frac{B_L(t)}{\kappa_L(a)+B_L(t)}\phi(a,t) + \frac{S(a,t)\kappa_L(a)\theta_L(t)}{(\kappa_L(a)+B_L(t))^2}\right] \\
&\quad + p(a)\beta_H(a)\left[\frac{B_H(t)}{\kappa_H(a)+B_H(t)}\phi(a,t) + \frac{S(a,t)\kappa_H(a)\theta_H(t)}{(\kappa_H(a)+B_H(t))^2}\right] \\
&\quad - [d(a)+\gamma_2(a)+e_2(a)]\,\psi_S(a,t) \qquad (30) \\
\frac{\partial r_S}{\partial t} + \alpha \frac{\partial r_S}{\partial a} &= -[d(a)+\omega_2(a)]\,r_S(a,t) + \gamma_2(a)\psi_S(a,t) \qquad (31) \\
\frac{\partial \hat{\phi}}{\partial t} + \alpha \frac{\partial \hat{\phi}}{\partial a} &= -\beta_L(a)\left[\frac{B_L(t)}{\kappa_L(a)+B_L(t)}\hat{\phi}(a,t) + \frac{\hat{S}(a,t)\kappa_L(a)\theta_L(t)}{(\kappa_L(a)+B_L(t))^2}\right] \\
&\quad - \beta_H(a)\left[\frac{B_H(t)}{\kappa_H(a)+B_H(t)}\hat{\phi}(a,t) + \frac{\hat{S}(a,t)\kappa_H(a)\theta_H(t)}{(\kappa_H(a)+B_H(t))^2}\right] \\
&\quad - [d(a)+\omega_3(a)+u(a,t)]\,\hat{\phi}(a,t) - l(a,t)\hat{S}(a,t) \\
&\quad + \omega_1(a)r_A(a,t) + \omega_2(a)r_S(a,t), \qquad (32) \\
\frac{\partial \psi_A}{\partial t} + \alpha \frac{\partial \psi_A}{\partial a} &= \beta_L(a)\left[\frac{B_L(t)}{\kappa_L(a)+B_L(t)}\hat{\phi}(a,t) + \frac{\hat{S}(a,t)\kappa_L(a)\theta_L(t)}{(\kappa_L(a)+B_L(t))^2}\right] \\
&\quad + \beta_H(a)\left[\frac{B_H(t)}{\kappa_H(a)+B_H(t)}\hat{\phi}(a,t) + \frac{\hat{S}(a,t)\kappa_H(a)\theta_H(t)}{(\kappa_H(a)+B_H(t))^2}\right] \\
&\quad - [d(a)+\gamma_1(a)+e_1(a)]\,\psi_A(a,t) \\
&\quad + (1-p(a))\beta_L(a)\left[\frac{B_L(t)}{\kappa_L(a)+B_L(t)}\phi(a,t) + \frac{S(a,t)\kappa_L(a)\theta_L(t)}{(\kappa_L(a)+B_L(t))^2}\right] \\
&\quad + (1-p(a))\beta_H(a)\left[\frac{B_H(t)}{\kappa_H(a)+B_H(t)}\phi(a,t) + \frac{S(a,t)\kappa_H(a)\theta_H(t)}{(\kappa_H(a)+B_H(t))^2}\right] \qquad (33)
\end{aligned}
$$

$$
\begin{aligned}
\frac{\partial r_A}{\partial t} + \alpha \frac{\partial r_A}{\partial a} &= -[d(a)+\omega_1(a)]\,r_A(a,t) + \gamma_1(a)\psi_A(a,t), \qquad (34) \\
\frac{\partial v}{\partial t} + \alpha \frac{\partial v}{\partial a} &= u(a,t)\left[\phi(a,t)+\hat{\phi}(a,t)\right] + l(a,t)\left[S(a,t)+\hat{S}(a,t)\right] \\
&\quad - [\omega_4(a)+d(a)]\,v(a,t), \qquad (35) \\
\frac{d\theta_H}{dt} &= \int_0^A \eta_1(a)\psi_A(a,t)da + \int_0^A \eta_2(a)\psi_S(a,t)da - \chi(t)\theta_H(t), \qquad (36) \\
\frac{d\theta_L}{dt} &= \chi(t)\theta_H(t) - \delta(t)\theta_L(t), \qquad (37)
\end{aligned}
$$

with initial and boundary conditions

$$
\begin{aligned}
&\textit{For } a \in (0, A),\\
&\quad \phi(a,0) = 0,\ \psi_S(a,0) = 0,\ r_S(a,0) = 0,\ \hat{\phi}(a,0) = 0,\ \psi_A(a,0) = 0,\\
&\quad r_A(a,0) = 0, v(a,0) = 0;\\
&\textit{for } t \in (0, T),\\
&\quad \phi(0,t) = 0,\ \psi_S(0,t) = 0,\ \hat{\phi}(0,t) = 0,\ \psi_A(0,t) = 0,\\
&\quad r_A(0,t) = 0,\ v(0,t) = 0,\\
&\quad r_S(0,t) = \int_0^A f(a)\left[\phi + \hat{\phi} + \psi_S + \psi_A + r_S + r_A\right](a,t)\,da;\\
&\quad \theta_H(0) = 0, \theta_L(0) = 0.
\end{aligned} \tag{38}
$$

Proof We see that the map of the control to the solution, $u \to N$ is Lipschitz in L^∞ by Theorem 2, Thus, the Gateaux derivative for each of the sensitivity variables exists. [4]. We pass to the limit in the equations satisfied by the quotients (like $\frac{(S^\epsilon - S)(a,t)}{\epsilon}$) We find that $(\phi, \psi_S, r_S, \hat{\phi}, \psi_A, r_A, v, \theta_H, \theta_L)$ satisfies our system (29–37) with boundary conditions (38). □

To derive the optimal control representation, we incorporate adjoint variables and an adjoint operator coming from the sensitivity functions. Using the following notation:

$$
\begin{aligned}
\zeta(a,t) &= \beta_L(a)\frac{B_L(t)}{\kappa_L(a) + B_L(t)} + \beta_H(a)\frac{B_H(t)}{\kappa_H(a) + B_H(t)},\\
H(a,t) &= \frac{\beta_H(a)\kappa_H(a)}{(\kappa_H(a) + B_H(t))^2}, \text{ and } K(a,t) = \frac{\beta_L(a)\kappa_L(a)}{(\kappa_L(a) + B_L(t))^2},
\end{aligned} \tag{39}
$$

the adjoint system associated with control $u(a,t)$ and state variables

$$(S, I_S, R_S, \hat{S}, I_A, R_A, V, B_H, B_L)$$

is

$$
\begin{aligned}
-\left(\frac{\partial \lambda_1}{\partial t} + \alpha\frac{\partial \lambda_1}{\partial a}\right) &= -\zeta(a,t)\lambda_1(a,t) - (d(a) + u(a,t))\lambda_1(a,t)\\
&\quad + p(a)\zeta(a,t)\lambda_2(a,t)\\
&\quad + (1 - p(a))\zeta(a,t)\lambda_5(a,t) + u(a,t)\lambda_7(a,t)\\
&\quad + A_2u(a,t) + \lambda_3(0,t)f(a)
\end{aligned} \tag{40}
$$

$$
\begin{aligned}
-\left(\frac{\partial \lambda_2}{\partial t} + \alpha\frac{\partial \lambda_2}{\partial a}\right) &= -(d(a) + \gamma_2(a) + e_2(a))\lambda_2(a,t) + \gamma_2(a)\lambda_3(a,t)\\
&\quad + \eta_2(a)\lambda_8(t) + \lambda_3(0,t)f(a) + A_1
\end{aligned} \tag{41}
$$

$$
\begin{aligned}
-\left(\frac{\partial \lambda_3}{\partial t} + \alpha\frac{\partial \lambda_3}{\partial a}\right) &= -\left[d(a) + \omega_2(a)\right]\lambda_3(a,t) + \omega_2(a)\lambda_4(a,t)\\
&\quad + \lambda_3(0,t)f(a),
\end{aligned} \tag{42}
$$

$$-\left(\frac{\partial \lambda_4}{\partial t}+\alpha\frac{\partial \lambda_4}{\partial a}\right) = -\zeta(a,t)\lambda_4(a,t) - (d(a)+\omega_3(a))\lambda_4(a,t) - u(a,t)\lambda_4(a,t) + \omega_3(a)\lambda_1(a,t) + \zeta(a,t)\lambda_5(a,t) + u(a,t)\lambda_7(a,t) + A_2u(a,t) + \lambda_3(0,t)f(a) \quad (43)$$

$$-\left(\frac{\partial \lambda_5}{\partial t}+\alpha\frac{\partial \lambda_5}{\partial a}\right) = -(d(a)+e_1(a)+\gamma_1(a))\lambda_5(a,t) + \gamma_1(a)\lambda_6(a,t) + \eta_1(a)\lambda_8(t) + \lambda_3(0,t)f(a) + A_2u(a,t), \quad (44)$$

$$-\left(\frac{\partial \lambda_6}{\partial t}+\alpha\frac{\partial \lambda_6}{\partial a}\right) = -\left[d(a)+\omega_1(a)\right]\lambda_6(a,t) + \omega_1(a)\lambda_4(a,t) + \lambda_3(0,t)f(a) + A_2u(a,t), \quad (45)$$

$$-\left(\frac{\partial \lambda_7}{\partial t}+\alpha\frac{\partial \lambda_7}{\partial a}\right) = -(d(a)+\omega_4(a))\lambda_7(a,t) + \omega_4(a)\lambda_1(a,t) + \lambda_3(0,t)f(a) \quad (46)$$

$$-\frac{d\lambda_8}{dt} = \chi(t)(\lambda_9(t)-\lambda_8(t)) + \int_0^A H(a,t)\left[-\lambda_1(a,t)+p(a)\lambda_2(a,t)+(1-p(a))\lambda_5(a,t)\right]S(a,t)\,da + \int_0^A H(a,t)(\lambda_5(a,t)-\lambda_4(a,t))\hat{S}(a,t)\,da \quad (47)$$

$$-\frac{d\lambda_9}{dt} = \int_0^A K(a,t)\left[-\lambda_1(a,t)+p(a)\lambda_2(a,t)+(1-p(a))\lambda_5(a,t)\right]S(a,t)\,da + \int_0^A K(a,t)(\lambda_5(a,t)-\lambda_4(a,t))\hat{S}(a,t)\,da - \delta(t)\lambda_9(t), \quad (48)$$

with the initial and boundary conditions as

$$\lambda_i(a,T)=0 \quad \text{for } a\in[0,A] \text{ and } i=1,\dots,7$$
$$\lambda_i(A,t)=0 \quad \text{for } t\in[0,T] \text{ and } i=1,\dots,7$$
$$\lambda_8(T)=\lambda_9(T)=0 \quad (49)$$

We note that the existence of the adjoint solutions can be proven through a fixed point argument mapping principle [4]. The solution to the adjoint system satisfies a Lipschitz condition, which needed in the proof of the existence and uniqueness of our optimal control.

Theorem 4 *For $u \in \Gamma$, the adjoint system (40)–(49) has a weak solution*

$$(\lambda_1, \lambda_2, \lambda_3, \lambda_4, \lambda_5, \lambda_6, \lambda_7, \lambda_8, \lambda_9)$$

in $(L^\infty(Q))^7 \times (L^\infty(0,T))^2$ *such that*

$$\begin{aligned}
&\|\lambda_1 - \hat{\lambda}_1\|_{L^\infty(Q)} + \|\lambda_2 - \hat{\lambda}_2\|_{L^\infty(Q)} + \|\lambda_3 - \hat{\lambda}_3\|_{L^\infty(Q)} + \|\lambda_4 - \hat{\lambda}_4\|_{L^\infty(Q)} \\
&\quad + \|\lambda_5 - \hat{\lambda}_5\|_{L^\infty(Q)} + \|\lambda_6 - \hat{\lambda}_6\|_{L^\infty(Q)} + \|\lambda_7 - \hat{\lambda}_7\|_{L^\infty(Q)} \\
&\quad + \|\lambda_8 - \hat{\lambda}_8\|_{L^\infty(0,T)} + \|\lambda_9 - \hat{\lambda}_9\|_{L^\infty(0,T)} \\
&\le C_5 T \left(\|u_1 - u_2\|_{L^\infty(Q)}\right),
\end{aligned} \tag{50}$$

with adjoint solutions $(\lambda_1, \lambda_2, \lambda_3, \lambda_4, \lambda_5, \lambda_6, \lambda_7, \lambda_8, \lambda_9)$ *and* $(\hat{\lambda}_1, \hat{\lambda}_2, \hat{\lambda}_3, \hat{\lambda}_4, \hat{\lambda}_5, \hat{\lambda}_6, \hat{\lambda}_7, \hat{\lambda}, \hat{\lambda}_9)$ *corresponding to control* $u_1(a,t)$ *and* $u_2(a,t)$, *respectively.*

We next determine the characterization of our optimal control.

Theorem 5 *If* u^* *in* Γ *is an optimal control that minimizes* $\mathcal{J}(u)$ *and*

$$(S, I_S, R_S, \hat{S}, I_A, R_A, V, B_H, B_L; \lambda_1, \lambda_2, \lambda_3, \lambda_4, \lambda_5, \lambda_6, \lambda_7, \lambda_8, \lambda_9)$$

are the corresponding state and adjoint variables, then

$$u^*(a,t) = \min\left[N_1, \max\left[0, \left(\tfrac{\lambda_1 S + \lambda_4 \hat{S} - \lambda_7 (S + \hat{S}) - A_2(S + \hat{S} + I_A + R_A)}{A_3}\right)\right]\right] \tag{51}$$

a.e. in $L^\infty(Q)$.

Proof Since u^* is an optimal control, then we have

$$\begin{aligned}
0 &\le \lim_{\varepsilon \to 0^+} \frac{\mathcal{J}(u^* + \epsilon l) - \mathcal{J}(u^*)}{\epsilon} \qquad (52) \\
&= \int_0^T \int_0^A \left(A_1 \psi_S + A_2 u^* \phi + A_2 u^* \hat{\phi} + A_2 u^* \psi_A + A_2 u^* r_A\right) da\, dt \\
&\quad + \int_0^T \int_0^A \left[A_2 l(a,t)\left(S + \hat{S} + I_A + R_A\right) + A_3 u^* l(a,t)\right] da\, dt \\
&= \int_0^T \int_0^A \left(\lambda_1(-l(a,t)S) + \lambda_4(-l(a,t)\hat{S}) + \lambda_7 l(a,t)(S + \hat{S})\right) da\, dt \\
&\quad + \int_0^T \int_0^A \left[A_2 l(a,t)\left(S + \hat{S} + I_A + R_A\right) + A_3 u^* l(a,t)\right] da\, dt \\
&= \int_0^T \int_0^A l(a,t)\left[A_2\left(S + \hat{S} + I_A + R_A\right) + A_3 u^* - \lambda_1 S - \lambda_4 \hat{S} + \lambda_7 (S + \hat{S})\right], \qquad (53)
\end{aligned}$$

where we simplify terms through the adjoint and the sensitivity functions and using integration by parts. The optimal control characterization result follows from standard optimality arguments with choosing the variation l. □

5 Existence of the Optimal Control

We next prove the result of this manuscript that shows the key difference in obtaining existence of optimal controls in first order PDEs versus parabolic PDEs. The difficulty is to find a sequence of controls and corresponding states that converges to the optimal control and states. There is a lack of compactness in this setting and one can use Ekeland's Principle [4, 10] to use the convergence of minimizing sequences of approximate functionals. We note that $\mathscr{J}(u)$ is lower semi-continuous with respect to strong $L^1(Q)$ convergence. However, it is not so with respect to weak $L^1(Q)$ convergence. To use Ekeland's Principle for our functional $\mathscr{J}$, we need that $\mathscr{J}$ is bounded below and lower semicontinuous in $L^1(Q)$. Note that 0 is a lower bound on $\mathscr{J}$ here. The lower semicontinuity follows from the Lipschitz properties.

For $\epsilon > 0$, there exists (u_ϵ) in $L^1(Q)$ such that

$$(i) \quad \mathscr{J}(u_\epsilon) < \inf_{u \in \Gamma} \mathscr{J}(u) + \epsilon \tag{54}$$

$$(ii) \quad \mathscr{J}(u_\epsilon) = \min \left\{ \mathscr{J}(u) + \sqrt{\epsilon} \|u_\epsilon - u\|_{L^1(Q)} \right\}. \tag{55}$$

Note that u_ϵ is a minimizer for $\mathscr{J}_\varepsilon$ defined by

$$\mathscr{J}_\epsilon(u) = \mathscr{J}(u) + \sqrt{\epsilon} \left(\|u_\epsilon - u\|_{L^1(Q)} \right). \tag{56}$$

For completeness, we provide the representation of the approximate optimal control through the theorem below. This proof can be obtained similar to the proof of Theorem 5 by differentiating $\mathscr{J}_\epsilon(u)$.

Theorem 6 *If u_ϵ is an optimal control minimizing the functional $\mathscr{J}_\epsilon(u)$, then*

$$u_\epsilon = \min \left[N_1, \max \left[0, \left(\frac{\lambda_1^\epsilon S^\epsilon + \lambda_4^\epsilon \hat{S}^\epsilon - \lambda_7^\epsilon (S^\epsilon + \hat{S}^\epsilon) - A_2 (S^\epsilon + \hat{S}^\epsilon + I_A^\epsilon + R_A^\epsilon) - \sqrt{\epsilon}\theta^\epsilon}{A_3} \right) \right] \right]$$

where the function θ^ϵ belongs to $L^\infty(Q)$ such that $|\theta^\epsilon(a,t)| \le 1$ for all $(a,t) \in Q$.

The existence of a unique optimal control is proven below using the L^∞ Lipschitz estimates for the states and the adjoints in terms of the control and the approximate minimizing sequence through the use of Ekeland's principle.

Theorem 7 *If $\dfrac{T}{A_3}$ is sufficiently small, there exists a unique optimal control u^* minimizing $\mathscr{J}(u)$.*

Proof First we define a function $F(u)$ as

$$F : \Gamma \to \Gamma \quad \text{by}$$

$$F(u) = \max \left[N_1, \min \left[0, \left(\frac{\lambda_1 S + \lambda_4 \hat{S} - \lambda_7 (S + \hat{S}) - A_2 (S + \hat{S} + I_A + R_A)}{A_3} \right) \right] \right]$$

with the corresponding state and adjoint variables associated with control $u(a,t)$. Consider two controls, $u_1(a,t)$ and $u_2(a,t)$, and corresponding states, with the terms corresponding to u_2 having subscripts 2 on the states and hats on the adjoints. All of the norms are in $L^\infty(Q)$ in the work below unless otherwise noted. With use of Lipschitz properties, we have

$$\begin{aligned}
\|F(u_1) - F(u_2)\| \le \Bigg\| &\left(\frac{\lambda_1 S + \lambda_4 \hat{S} - \lambda_7(S+\hat{S}) - A_2(S+\hat{S}+I_A+R_A)}{A_3}\right) \\
&- \left(\frac{\hat{\lambda}_1 S_2 + \hat{\lambda}_4 \hat{S}_2 - \hat{\lambda}_7(S_2+\hat{S}_2) - A_2(S_2+\hat{S}_2+I_{A2}+R_{A2})}{A_3}\right)\Bigg\| \\
&\le \|\lambda_1\|\,\|S - S_2\| + \|S_2\|\,\left\|\lambda_1 - \hat{\lambda}_1\right\| + \|\lambda_4\|\,\left\|\hat{S} - \hat{S}_2\right\| + \left\|\hat{S}_2\right\|\,\left\|\lambda_4 - \hat{\lambda}_4\right\| \\
&\quad + \left\|\hat{S} + S\right\|\,\left\|\lambda_7 - \hat{\lambda}_7\right\| + \left\|\hat{\lambda}_7\right\|\left(\left\|\hat{S} - \hat{S}_2\right\| + \|S - S_2\|\right) \\
&\quad + \|A_2\|_{L^\infty(0,A)}\left(\left\|\hat{S} - \hat{S}_2\right\| + \|S - S_2\| + \|I_A - I_{A2}\|\,\|R_A - R_{A2}\|\right) \\
&\le \frac{C_6 T}{A_3}\|u_1 - u_2\|_{L^\infty(Q)}
\end{aligned} \tag{57}$$

where the constant C_6 depends on the L^∞ bounds on the state and adjoint solutions and the Lipschitz constants. If $\frac{C_6 T}{A_3} < 1$, then $F(u)$ has a unique fixed point, called u^*.

To prove this fixed point is an optimal control, we use the approximate sequence u_ϵ generated through Ekeland's principle with its associated state and adjoint variables having superscripts of ϵ and obtain

$$\begin{aligned}
&\left\| F(u_\epsilon) - \min\left[N_1, \max\left[0, \left(\frac{\lambda_1^\epsilon S^\epsilon + \lambda_4^\epsilon \hat{S}^\epsilon - \lambda_7^\epsilon(S^\epsilon+\hat{S}^\epsilon) - A_2(S^\epsilon+\hat{S}^\epsilon+I_A^\epsilon+R_A^\epsilon) - \sqrt{\epsilon}\theta^\epsilon}{A_3}\right)\right]\right]\right\| \\
&= \Bigg\|\left(\frac{\lambda_1^\epsilon S^\epsilon + \lambda_4^\epsilon \hat{S}^\epsilon - \lambda_7^\epsilon(S^\epsilon+\hat{S}^\epsilon) - A_2(S^\epsilon+\hat{S}^\epsilon+I_A^\epsilon+R_A^\epsilon)}{A_3}\right) \\
&\quad - \left(\frac{\lambda_1^\epsilon S^\epsilon + \lambda_4^\epsilon \hat{S}^\epsilon - \lambda_7^\epsilon(S^\epsilon+\hat{S}^\epsilon) - A_2(S^\epsilon+\hat{S}^\epsilon+I_A^\epsilon+R_A^\epsilon) - \sqrt{\epsilon}\theta^\epsilon}{A_3}\right)\Bigg\| \\
&\le \frac{\sqrt{\epsilon}\theta^\epsilon}{A_3} \le \frac{\sqrt{\epsilon}}{A_3}.
\end{aligned} \tag{58}$$

We use the fixed point estimate (57) and the estimate with the approximate minimizer (58) to show the convergence of the approximate minimizer to our fixed point $u^*(a,t)$ in $L^\infty(Q)$. We have

$$\begin{aligned}
&\|u^* - u_\epsilon\| \\
&= \left\|F(u^*) - \min\left[N_1, \max\left[0, \left(\frac{\lambda_1^\epsilon S^\epsilon + \lambda_4^\epsilon \hat{S}^\epsilon - \lambda_7^\epsilon(S^\epsilon+\hat{S}^\epsilon) - A_2(S^\epsilon+\hat{S}^\epsilon+I_A^\epsilon+R_A^\epsilon) - \sqrt{\epsilon}\theta^\epsilon}{A_3}\right)\right]\right]\right\| \\
&\le \|F(u^*) - F(u_\epsilon)\| \\
&\quad + \left\|F(u_\epsilon) - \min\left[N_1, \max\left[0, \left(\frac{\lambda_1^\epsilon S^\epsilon + \lambda_4^\epsilon \hat{S}^\epsilon - \lambda_7^\epsilon(S^\epsilon+\hat{S}^\epsilon) - A_2(S^\epsilon+\hat{S}^\epsilon+I_A^\epsilon+R_A^\epsilon) - \sqrt{\epsilon}\theta^\epsilon}{A_3}\right)\right]\right]\right\|
\end{aligned}$$

$$\leq \frac{C_6 T}{A_3} \|u^* - u_\epsilon\|_{L^\infty(Q)} + \frac{\sqrt{\epsilon}}{A_3}. \tag{59}$$

For $\dfrac{T}{A_3}$ small, we have

$$\left\|u^* - u_\epsilon\right\| \leq \frac{\sqrt{\epsilon}}{A_3} \times \frac{1}{1 - C_6 T \left(\frac{1}{A_3}\right)}$$

for which the convergence follows.

Since our approximate minimizer converges to our fixed point, we need to show that our fixed point minimizes the objective functional. Using Ekeland's principle, we pass to the limit in $\mathscr{J}(u_\epsilon) < \inf_{u \in \Gamma} \mathscr{J}(u) + \epsilon$ as $\epsilon \to 0$ and we see that $\mathscr{J}(u_*) \leq \inf_{u \in \Gamma} \mathscr{J}(u)$. □

With our representation of our now unique optimal control, we have a solution of our optimality system which is our state system (2–11) coupled with our adjoint system (40–47) with the corresponding initial and boundary conditions found in (21) and (49).

6 Parameter Choices

One of the difficulties in trying to create meaningful models is that we have many unknown parameters and a limited amount of observational data. There are a number of parameter assumptions that deserve discussion. While this initial work shows the potential for optimal control to shed light on age-based vaccination strategies for a cholera epidemic, we believe future work should be informed by the uncertainty within our parameter choices. Given a specific dataset, one could alternatively fit many of the model parameters using data.

Our choices for the initial state of the populations are in Table 2. If a cholera epidemic affects a long-affected region, we expect $\hat{S}$ to be large, but in epidemiologically naive populations we expect $\hat{S}$ to be zero; here we choose an initial $\hat{S}$ population in the middle of those two cases. The assumptions are summarized in Table 2.

6.1 Proportion of Symptomatic Infections *p*

An interesting aspect of the spread of cholera is that only some humans will have symptomatic infections. The number of severe infections depends on the bacterial biotype [21], genetic factors [36], as well as perhaps nutrition (see [36] versus [15]). Prior exposure to the disease is known to lead to complete or partial immunity,

Table 2 Initial conditions and age distributions

State variable	Age distribution
$S(a,0)$	$450a,\ 0 \leq a \leq 2,\ -0.4289a^2 + 18.1373a + 867.402,\ 2 < a \leq 72$
$\hat{S}(a,0)$	$-0.381a^2 + 14.2381a + 900,\ 0 \leq a \leq 72$
$I_A(a,0)$	$0.02\hat{S}(a,0)$
$I_S(a,0)$	$0.02S(a,0)$
$R_A(a,0)$	0
$R_S(a,0)$	0
$V(a,0)$	0
$B_L(0)$	$\frac{K_L}{100}$
$B_H(0)$	0

[30, 36], so that minimally recovery from symptomatic cholera should provide short-term protection from a severe case of cholera [13]. Data prove that in areas for which the disease occurs frequently, there are fewer symptomatic illnesses [36].

Prior studies leave the role of asymptomatic individuals in the spread of cholera a somewhat open question with a variety of values of the proportion of asymptomatic infections [13, 22, 36, 41]. Our choice for values of $p(a)$, the proportions of individuals of age a in the fully susceptible class S who will experience symptomatic cholera infections, is complicated and seeks to explain some proportion of asymptomatic illness through the mechanism of gaining partial immunity through recovery from symptomatic disease.

A Bangladeshi study found that children under the age of five infected with *Vibrio cholerae* O1 El Tor were two to three times more likely to become symptomatic than older-age individuals [36]. In our simulations, we hypothesized that a large majority of fully susceptible youth and elderly would be likely to experience symptoms, while a smaller portion of the remaining population would experience symptoms. We assume for the purposes of this illustration that

$$p(a) = 0.75 - 0.021a + 0.00029a^2,$$

with a given in years.

6.2 Transmission Rates β_L and β_H

Compounding the misunderstanding of the numbers of asymptomatic infections is a lack of understanding of the environmental contribution of humans who are unknowingly shedding infectious bacteria, albeit in smaller quantities than for their infectious counterparts. Some researchers suggest the inapparent infections may drive the spread of disease [22, 41], while others claim the impact from this class of individuals is minimal [36]. As with many models, the contact rates β_L and β_H of humans with low-infectious and hyper-infectious bacteria, are practically impossible to identify. While previously many models, perhaps following [6], where the contact rate is 1.5, have based the values of β_L and β_H (or only one of these depending on the model) on the amount of water that an average human would drink in a day, the reality is that the contact with the bacteria additionally comes from contamination of food and household items [36]. In various cholera models, we observe ranges of beta from 0.023 to 2.1 [33] versus 0.00108–0.00285 [8].

In areas of endemicity, cases of cholera are concentrated in children aged 2–9 with a secondary peak in women in their childbearing years (15–35) [21]. For our simulations, we hypothesize that infants are protected through breast-feeding, and elderly are protected through less environmental contact. We suppose that youth and those caring for youth would be subject to the highest bacterial contact. We define $M = 1.5$ milliliters per day, and we assume a piecewise linear function allowing no contact for infants, heading to a contact rate of M at age 7, decreasing to the rate of $\frac{M}{10}$ contact at age of 15, increasing once more to $\frac{M}{2}$ at age 25, and finally decreasing to $\frac{M}{2}$ at our terminal age of 72:

$$\beta_L(a) = \begin{cases} 0, & \text{if } a < 2 \\ \frac{M}{5}(a-2), & \text{if } 2 \le a \le 7 \\ \frac{M}{80}(143 - 9a), & \text{if } 7 < a \le 15 \\ \frac{M}{50}(2a - 25), & \text{if } 15 < a \le 25 \\ \frac{M}{470}(335 - 4a) & \text{otherwise} \end{cases}, \tag{60}$$

$$\beta_H = 1.5\beta_L. \tag{61}$$

6.3 *Waning Immunity*

Given the disagreement in the literature regarding the proportions of the population who experience symptomatic infections, it is not surprising that choices for the length of immunity for humans in each class (denoted by ω_1 and ω_2 in our model) are in doubt.

Although statistical pairing of data from Bangladesh with a mathematical model for cholera suggested that the immunity from an asymptomatic infection most likely lasts a significantly shorter period of time than does the immunity from symptomatic infection [22], it is difficult to validate this idea from a microbiological viewpoint. Multiple sources suggest that length of immunity from symptomatic cholera is likely at least 3 years [21, 41]. We will assume that symptomatic and asymptomic infections result in equivalent waning immunity.

Additionally, we have not found an estimate for the rate of waning of partial immunity outside of that deduced from a mathematical model (10 years [23]). We assume that partial immunity wanes over a period of 5 years. Due to our boundary conditions and our intention to remove infants from the susceptible class for only a short time period, we assume age-based waning is only slow after age 3.

Finally, we have to approximate immunity due to vaccination using the fact that the World Health Organization estimates 50 % efficacy over 3–5 years and 67 % after 2 years. A study by the International Vaccine Institute suggests 85 % protective efficacy in the first 6 months, and 60 % after 18 months.

As a mechanistic tool to allow protection for infants, we assume that infants are born with immunity, but that the immunity quickly wanes. In addition, there is evidence that young children do not retain immunity from vaccination as long as older children and adults [34].

Our assumptions governing immunity are summarized in the equations below: Waning immunity to the partially immune class following asymptomatic or symptomatic infection:

$$\omega_1(a) = \omega_2(a) = \begin{cases} \frac{2}{365}, & \text{if } 0 \le a \le 1 \\ \frac{11-5a}{3\cdot 365}, & \text{if } 1 < a \le 2 \\ \frac{1}{3\cdot 365}, & \text{otherwise} \end{cases} \tag{62}$$

Waning immunity from partially immune to fully susceptible:

$$\omega_3(a) = \begin{cases} \frac{2}{365} & \text{if } 0 \le a \le 2 \\ \frac{28-9a}{5\cdot 365}, & \text{if } 2 < a \le 3 \\ \frac{1}{5\cdot 365}, & \text{otherwise} \end{cases} \tag{63}$$

Waning immunity from vaccinated to fully susceptible:

$$\omega_4(a) = \begin{cases} \frac{a}{365}, & \text{if } 0 \le a \le 2 \\ \frac{2}{365}, & \text{if } 2 < a \le 5 \\ \frac{33-5a}{4\cdot 365}, & \text{if } 5 < a \le 6 \\ \frac{3}{4\cdot 365}, & \text{otherwise} \end{cases} \tag{64}$$

6.4 Death Rates

We chose to have our simulations reflect the expectation of a higher cholera-related death rate for symptomatic young and elderly humans:

$$e_2(a) = \frac{4\hat{e}_2}{A^2}a^2 - \frac{4\hat{e}_2}{A}a + 2\hat{e}_2, \tag{65}$$

where $\hat{e}_2 = 0.004$. We would expect no deaths from asymptomatic class, and thus $e_1 = 0$. For this illustration, the natural death rate is $d(a) = \frac{0.16}{(10)365}$ for $a \leq 2$ and $d(a) = (\frac{1}{10} - \frac{19(a-2)}{700})\frac{0.16}{365}$ for $a > 2$, which starts out flat and then linearly goes down.

6.5 *Michaelis Constants κ_L and κ_H*

It is a frequent assumption that the Michaelis constant for our density-based infection should be chosen as 10^6 (see [18, 32], for example), although there are circumstances when other choices may be preferred (see [36], for example). For the purposes of illustration in this age-based model, we hypothesize that younger individuals would require a lower concentration of cholera vibrios to become ill, although we do not base this hypothesis on a microbiological study. Accordingly, we define the Michaelis constant as

$$\kappa_L(a) = \begin{cases} \frac{a}{15} \times 10^6, & \text{if } 0 \leq a < 15 \\ 10^6, & \text{if } a \geq 15 \end{cases}. \tag{66}$$

Following [18, 32], and based on a microbiological study by [31], we assume that freshly-shed vibrios are hyperinfectious and thus 700 times more infectious than they will be in about 5 h:

$$\kappa_H(a) = \frac{1}{700}\kappa_L(a). \tag{67}$$

6.6 *Shedding Rates η_1 and η_2*

In Sect. 6.2 we explored the difficulty in quantifying transmission rates in general, and in particular to choose contact/transmission rates for contact with hyperinfectious versus low-infectious bacteria. It is similarly difficult to quantify the so-called "shedding rate," the rate of fecal-oral environmental contamination resulting from symptomatic and asymptomatic infected individuals (i.e., the parameter values for η_1 and η_2). First, although certainly we can quantify the daily numbers of bacteria that are shed from the infected humans [21], we cannot quantify the number that might be leaked into the environment due to inadequate sanitation, nor can we view the reservoir as having fixed and known value so that the amount of shed bacteria can be converted to describe an increment to the density of infectious bacteria in the water. Considering the *relative* values of the two shedding parameters, we note that although we can quantify the difference in shedding rates between the symptomatic and asymptomatic humans [36], we suspect that symptomatic individuals could be more likely to be careful about protecting the environment from their waste, while unknowing carriers may unwittingly spread their disease in a larger environment.

In the literature we observe a wide variety of choices for the shedding rate, measured in cells per milliliter per day. For example, we observe a shedding rate of 10

[7], or 0.5 for asymptomatic versus 50 to symptomatic [32]. For these simulations, we chose to set the shedding rates at $\eta_1 = 5$ and $\eta_2 = 50$ per milliliter per day.

6.7 Vibrio Rates

Varying the parameter values in current models can cause a very big change in model predictions [16, 41]. However, for this current study, we use an often-cited assumption that the vibrios are not viable after about 30 days in the environment [1, 18] with $\delta = \frac{7}{30}, week^{-1}$.

From [31], we took the transition rate from hyperinfectious to low-infectious bacteria to be $\chi = 7 * 5, week^{-1}$.

6.8 Maximum Daily Vaccination Rate

Note that the vaccination rates are based on factors such as the level of development of the infrastructure. In areas without infrastructure we might see 1–2 % as a vaccination rate but in areas with infrastructure, such as a refuge camp, we expect up to a 4 % daily vaccination rate with $N_1 = 0.04$. For some data on vaccination rates in Haiti, see the paper by Iver et al. [19].

7 Numerical Results

Our numerical scheme for the age-structured model (2)–(11) is based on a semi-implicit finite-difference scheme for partial differential equations based on finding solutions along characteristic lines [37]. The corresponding backwards scheme is used for the adjoint system. Starting with initial age distributions defined in Table 2 for susceptible, infectious, recovered and vaccinated humans; using finite difference schemes, and the forward-backward sweep numerical method [17, 26], we obtain simulations for our optimality system.

We chose a large value of the weight A_1, the importance of reducing symptomatic infections, to see the possible impact of wide-spread vaccination. Thus the weights in the objective functional are $A_1 = 2000$ and $A_2 = A_3 = 1$. In the code, units on the rates are calculated using the units of age a and of time t as years and weeks, respectively.

Figure 2 portrays the dynamics of all susceptible individuals (including both fully and partially-immune) in the population in the absence/presence of vaccination. In the presence of vaccination, we see only a modest decrease in the number of susceptible in the population.

Figure 3 shows the dynamics of asymptomatic and symptomatic infected individuals in the absence/presence of vaccination in the population. Because the infections in the epidemic occur early in time and our ability to vaccinate quickly is limited, we again see only modest improvements in both cases with our control.

Figure 4 indicates the number of humans with vaccinated immunity given by $u(a,t)(S(a,t) + \hat{S}(a,t) + I_A(a,t) + R_A(a,t))$. The figure shows the clear dependence on age in the number who are vaccinated, reflecting the age structure of the

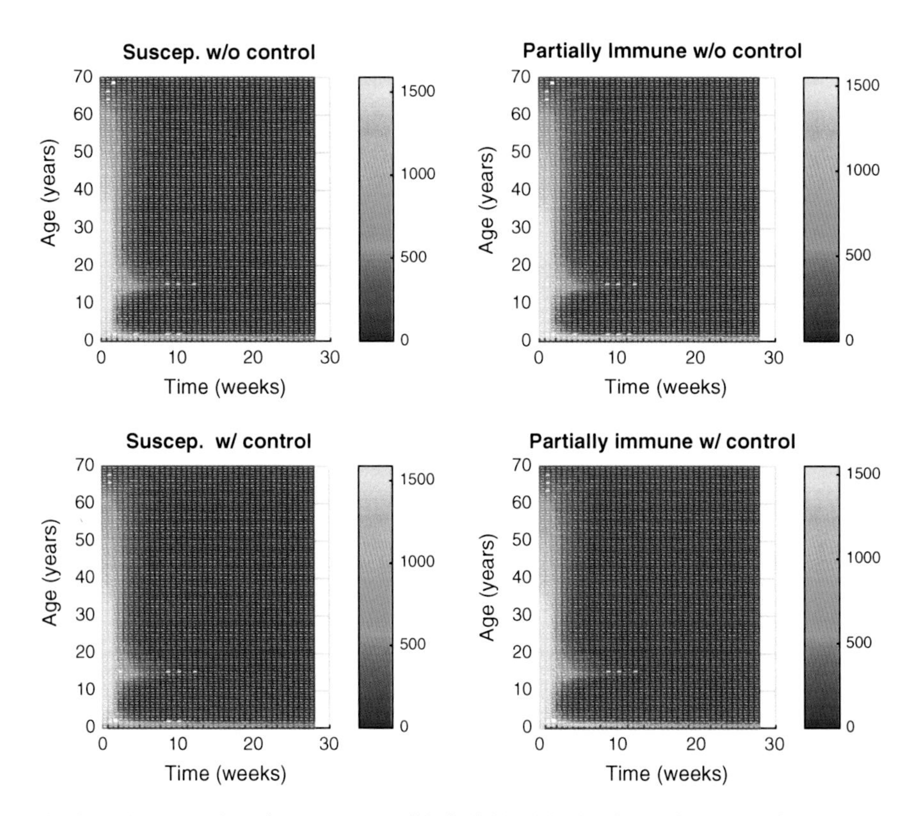

Fig. 2 Fully and partially-immune susceptible individuals in the absence/presence of control

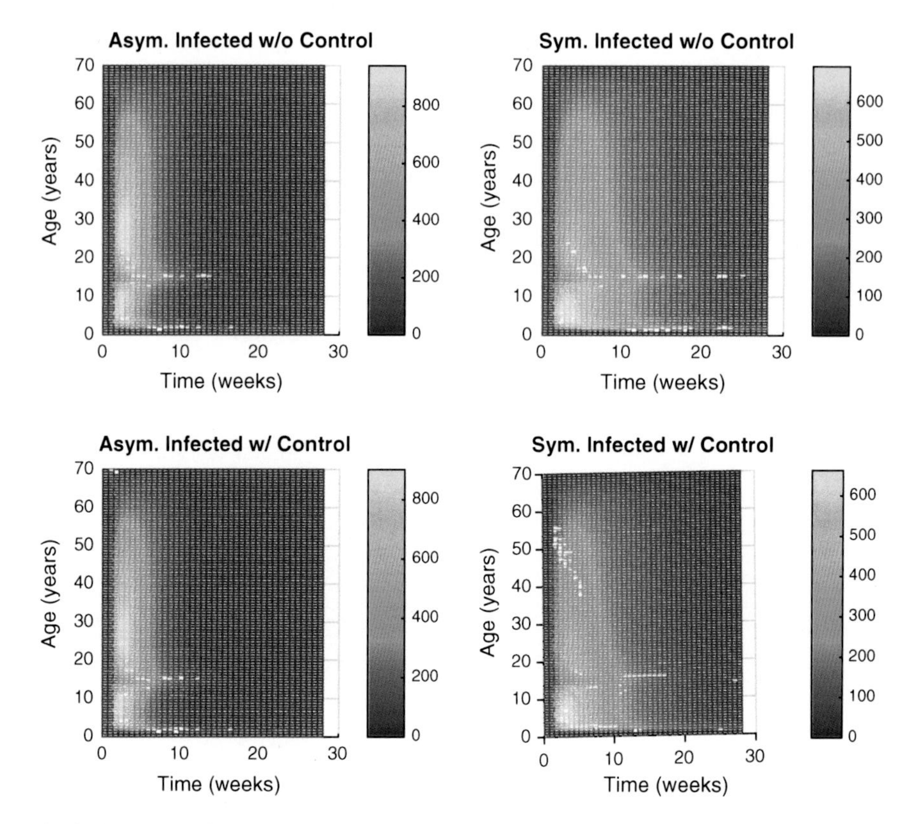

Fig. 3 Asymptomatic and symptomatic infected individuals in the absence/presence of control

population. The rate of control is essentially at the maximum wherever control is applied; thus, the effect of age structure on the control is evident with the times at which vaccination is recommended for each age group, with less vaccination recommended for ages near 10 and 30.

The optimal vaccination is shown in Fig. 5. In this figure, our simulations suggest vaccinating all age groups within the first few weeks followed by less vaccination for individuals of ages in the neighborhood of 10 and 30 as indicated in Fig. 4. The rate of control is mostly at the maximum wherever control is applied; thus, the effect of age structure on the control is evident with the times at which vaccination is recommended for each age group. The contact rate decreasing about ages 7–15 may cause the decrease in the control at later times for those ages.

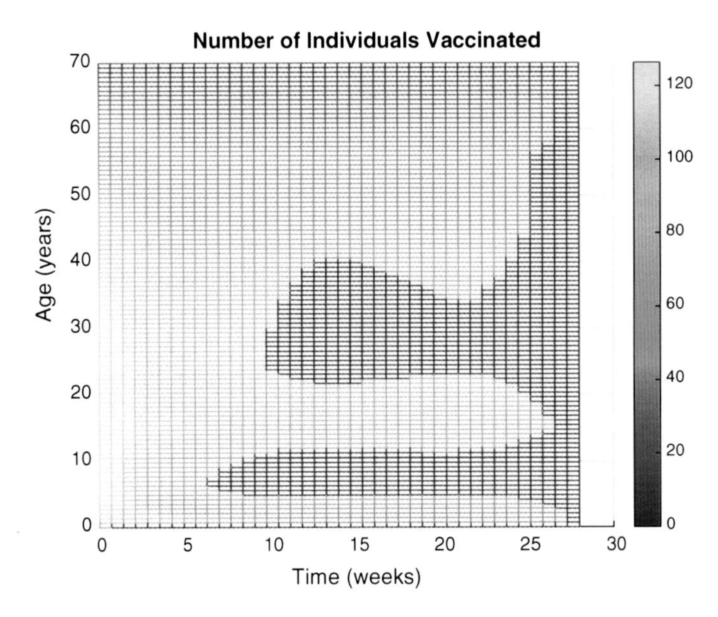

Fig. 4 Humans with vaccinated immunity: This figure shows the number of individuals who are moved to the vaccinated class as determined by $u(a,t)(S(a,t) + \hat{S}(a,t) + I_A(a,t) + R_A(a,t))$. This graph shows the number of vaccinations given to each age at each time

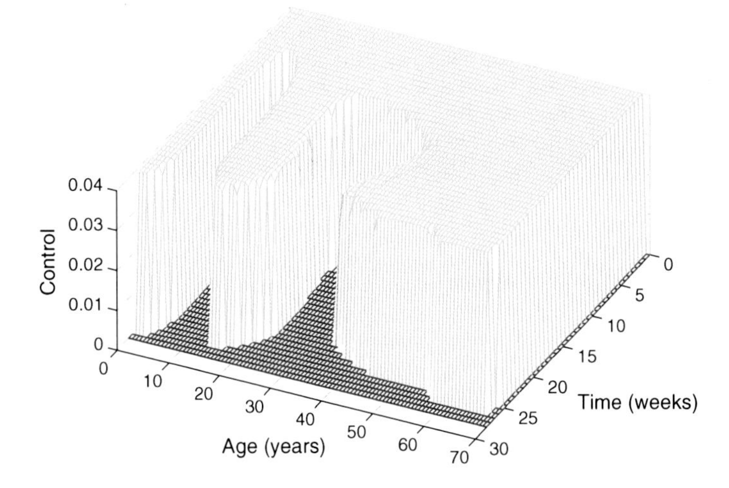

Fig. 5 Optimal vaccination control

8 Conclusions

We formulated an age-structured model with human population compartmentalized into fully susceptible and individuals with partial immunity. An optimal vaccination problem with the goal of minimizing symptomatic infected humans is formulated and analyzed. We established a Lipschitz property for the state solutions in terms of the vaccination function, and sensitivity and adjoint equations are derived. We obtained an optimal control characterization and established the existence of optimal control using Ekeland's Principle. Using a minimizing sequence obtained via Ekeland's Principle, we established uniqueness results.

The steps for this optimal control analysis were shown for this model. Illustrating the steps in the technique of optimal control of such age-structured models can serve to facilitate more applications of these techniques.

Numerical results indicate a clear dependence on age in the number of individuals vaccinated, and suggest less vaccination for individuals in the young and middle-aged adults, which is expected from the choices of our rates depending on age. In a situation with better known rates in terms of age and more well-informed assumptions, this work could provide a useful tool for suggesting vaccination strategies.

Due to uncertainty in some of the parameters, an interesting future direction would be to perform a sensitivity analysis of the objective functional value and the structure of the optimal control as the parameters are varied. Other types of control actions could also be incorporated.

Acknowledgments This work was funded by the National Science Foundation DMS-0813563. Lenhart's support also included funding from the National Institute for Mathematical and Biological Synthesis NSF EF 0832858. Wang's work was partially supported by National Science Foundation DMS-1412826. We thanks Boloye Gomero for her initial work with the graphic for the description of the model.

References

1. Andrews, J.R., Basu, S.: Transmission dynamics and control of cholera in haiti: an epidemic model. Lancet **377**, 1248–1255 (2011)
2. Anita, S.: Optimal harvesting for a nonlinear age-dependent population dynamics. J. Math. Anal. Appl. **226**, 6–22 (1998)
3. Anita, S.: Analysis and Control of Age-Dependent Population Dynamics. Kluwer Academic Publishers, Dordretcht (2000)
4. Barbu, V.: Mathematical Methods in Optimization of Differential Systems. Kluwer Academic Publishers, Dordrecht (1994)
5. Barbu, V., Iannelli, M.: Optimal control of population dynamics. J Optim. Theory Appl. **102**, 1–14 (1999)
6. Codeco, C.T.: Endemic and epidemic dynamics of cholera: the role of the aquatic reservoir. BMC Infect. Dis. **1**, 1 (2001)
7. Codeco, C.T., Coelho, F.C.: Trends in cholera epidemiology. PLoS Med **3**, e42 (2006)

8. Eisenberg, M.C., Kujbida, G., Tuite, A.R., Fisman, D.N., Tien, J.H.: Examining rainfall and cholera dynamics in Haiti using statistical and dynamic modeling approaches. Epidemics **5**, 197–207 (2013)
9. Eisenberg, M.C., Shuai, Z., Tien, J.H., van den Driessche, P.: A cholera model in a patchy environment with water and human movement. Math. Biosci. **246**, 105–112 (2013)
10. Ekeland, I.: On the variational principle. J. Math. Anal. Appl. **47**, 324–353 (1974)
11. Fister, K.R., Lenhart, S.: Optimal control of a competitive system with age-structure. J. Math. Anal. **291**, 526–537 (2004)
12. Fister, K.R., Lenhart, S.: Optimal harvesting in an age-structured predator-prey model. Appl. Math. Optim. **54**, 1–15 (2006)
13. Glass, R.I., Becker, S., Huq, M.I., Stoll, B.J., Khan, M.U., Merson, M.H., Lee, J.V., Black, R.E.: Endemic cholera in rural Bangladesh, 1966–1980. Am. J. Epidemiol. **116**, 959–970 (1982)
14. Glass, R.I., Svennerholm, A.M., Stoll, B.J., Khan, M.R., Hossain, K.M., Huq, M.I., Holmgren, J.: Protection against cholera in breast-fed children by antibodies in breast milk. New Engl. J. Med. **308**, 1389–1392 (1983)
15. Glass, R.I., Svennerholm, A.M., Stoll, B.J., Khan, M.R., Huda, S., Huq, M.I., Holmgren, J.: Effects of undernutrition on infection with vibrio cholerae o1 and on response to oral cholera vaccine. Pediatr. Infect. Dis. J. **8**, 105–109 (1989)
16. Grad, Y.H., Miller, J.C., Lipsitch, M.: Cholera modeling: challenges to quantitative analysis and predicting the impact of interventions. Epidemiology (Cambridge, Mass) **23**, 523 (2012)
17. Hackbush, W.K.: A numerical method for solving parabolic equations with opposite orientation. Computing, pp. 229–240 (1978)
18. Hartley, D.M., Morris Jr., J.G., Smith, D.L.: Hyperinfectivity: A critical element in the ability of v. cholerae to cause epidemics? PLoS Med **3**, e7 (2005)
19. Ivers, L.C., Teng, J.E., Lascher, J., Raymond, M., Weigel, J., Victor, N., Jerome, J.D., Hilaire, I.J., Amazor, C.P., Ternier, R., Cadet, J., Francois, J., Guillaume, F.D., Farmer, P.E.: Use of oral cholera vaccine in Haiti: a rural demonstration project. Am. J. Trop. Med. Hyg. **89**, 617–624 (2013)
20. Jeuland, M., Cook, J., Poulos, C., Clemens, J., Whittington, D.: Cost effectiveness of new generation oral cholera vaccines: a multisite analysis. Value Health **12**, 899–907 (2009)
21. Kaper, J.B., Morris Jr., J.G., Levine, M.M.: Cholera. Clin. Microbio. Rev. **8**, 48–86 (1995)
22. King, A.A., Ionides, E.L., Pascual, M., Bouma, M.J.: Inapparent infections and cholera dynamics. Nature **454**, 877–880 (2008)
23. Koelle, K., Rodo, X., Nad Md Yunus, M.P., Mostafa, G.: Refractory periods and climate forcing in cholera dynamics. Nature **436**, 696–700 (2005)
24. Laxminarayan, R.: Bacterial resistance and the optimal use of antibiotics. Technical Report 1–23 (2001)
25. Lenhart, S., Liang, M., Protopopescu, V.: Optimal control of boundary habitat hostility of interacting species. Math. Methods Appl. Sci. **22**, 1061–1077 (1999)
26. Lenhart, S., Workman, J.T.: Optimal Control Applied to Biological Models. Chapman Hall/CRC, Boca Raton (2007)
27. Leung, A.W.: Optimal harvesting coefficient control of a steady-state prey-predator diffusive Lotka-Volterra system. Appl. Math. Optim. **31**, 219–241 (1995)
28. Lions, J.L.: Optimal Control of Systems Governed by Partial Differential Equations. Springer, New York (1971)
29. Lions, X., Yong, J.: Optimal Control Theory for Infinite Dimensional Systems. Birkhauser, Boston (1995)
30. Longini, I.M., Yunus, M., Zaman, K., Siddique, A., Sack, R.B., Nizam, A.: Epidemic and endemic cholera trends over a 33-year period in bangladesh. J. Infect. Dis. **186**, 246–251 (2002)
31. Merrell, D., Butler, S., Qadri, F., Dolganov, N., Alam, A., Cohen, M., Calderwood, S., Schoolnik, G., Camilli, A.: Host-induced epidemic spread of the cholera bacterium. Nature **417**, 642–5 (2002)

32. Miller Neilan, R.L., Schaefer, E., Gaff, H., Fister, K.R., Lenhart, S.: Modeling optimal intervention strategies for cholera. Bull. Math. Biol. **72**, 2004–2018 (2010)
33. Mukandavire, Z., Liao, S., Wang, J., Gaff, H., Smith, D.L., Morris, J.G.: Estimating the reproductive numbers for the 20082009 cholera outbreaks in Zimbabwe. Proc. Nat. Acad. Sci. **108**, 8767–8772 (2011)
34. Naficy, A., Rao, M.R., Paquet, C., Antona, D., Sorkin, A., Clemens, J.D.: Treatment and vaccination strategies to control cholera in sub-saharan refugee settings. JAMA J. Am. Med. Assoc. **279**, 521–525 (1998)
35. Neilan, R.M., Lenhart, S.: Optimal vaccine distribution in a spatiotemporal epidemic model with an application to rabies and raccoons. J. Math. Anal. Appl. **378**, 603–619 (2011)
36. Nelson, E.J., Harris, J.B., Morris, J.G., Calderwood, S.B., Camilli, A.: Cholera transmission: the host, pathogen and bacteriophage dynamic. Nat. Rev. Microbiol. **7**, 693–702 (2009)
37. Numfor, E., Bhattacharya, S., Lenhart, S., Martcheva, M.: Optimal control applied in coupled within-host and between-host models. Math. Modell. Nat. Phenom. **9**, 171–203 (2014)
38. Organization, W.H.: Cholera vaccines: who position paper. Wkly. Epidemiol. Rec. **85**, 117–128 (2010)
39. Posny, D., Wang, J.: Modelling cholera in periodic environments. J. Biol. Dyn. **8**, 1–19 (2014)
40. Qureshi, K., Molbak, K., Sandstrom, A., Kofoed, P.E., Rodrigues, A., Dias, F., Aaby, P., Svennerholm, A.M.: Breast milk reduces the risk of illness in children of mothers with cholera: observations from an epidemic of cholera in guinea-bissau. Pediatr. Infect. Dis. J. **25**, 1163–1166 (2006)
41. Rinaldo, A., Bertuzzo, E., Mari, L., Righetto, L., Blokesch, M., Gatto, M., Casagrandi, R., Murray, M., Vesenbeckh, S.M., Rodriguez-Iturbe, I.: Reassessment of the 2010–2011 Haiti cholera outbreak and rainfall-driven multiseason projections. Proc. Natl. Acad. Sci. **109**, 6602–6607 (2012)
42. Shuai, Z., van den Driessche, P.: Global stability of infectious disease models using lyapunov functions. SIAM J. Appl. Math. **73**, 1513–1532 (2013)
43. Tian, J.P., Wang, J.: Global stability for cholera epidemic models. Math. Biosci. **232**, 31–41 (2011)
44. Tien, J., Earn, D.: Multiple transmission pathways and disease dynamics in a waterborne pathogen model. Bull. Math. Biol. **72**, 1506–1533 (2010)
45. Tien, J.H., Poinar, H.N., Fisman, D.N., Earn, D.J.D.: Herald waves of cholera in nineteenth century London. J. R. Soc. Interface **8**, 756–760 (2011)
46. Tuite, A.R., Tien, J., Eisenberg, M., Earn, D.J., Ma, J., Fisman, D.N.: Cholera epidemic in Haiti, 2010: using a transmission model to explain spatial spread of disease and identify optimal control interventions. Ann. Intern. Med. **154**, 593–601 (2011)
47. Wang, J., Liao, S.: A generalized cholera model and epidemic-endemic analysis. J. Biol. Dyn. **6**, 568–589 (2012)
48. Walton, D., Suri, A., Farmer, P.: Cholera in Haiti: fully integrating prevention and care. Ann. Intern. Med. **154**, 635–637 (2011)
49. Wang, X., Gao, D., Wang, J.: Influence of human behavior on cholera dynamics. Math. Biosci. **267**, 41–52 (2015)
50. Webb, G.: Theory of Nonlinear Age-dependent Population Dynamics. Marcel Dekker, New York (1985)

A Multi-risk Model for Understanding the Spread of Chlamydia

Asma Azizi, Ling Xue and James M. Hyman

Abstract Chlamydia trachomatis, CT, infection is the most frequently reported sexually transmitted infection in the United States. To better understand the recent increase in disease prevalence, and help guide in mitigation efforts, we created and analyzed a multi-risk model for the spread of chlamydia in the heterosexual community. The model incorporates the heterogeneous mixing between men and women with different number of partners and the parameters are defined to approximate the disease transmission in the 15–25 year-old New Orleans African American community. We use sensitivity analysis to assess the relative impact of different levels of screening interventions and behavior changes on the basic reproduction number. Our results quantify, and validate, the impact that reducing the probability of transmission per sexual contact, such as using prophylactic condoms, can have on CT prevalence.

Keywords Mathematical modeling · Sexually transmitted infection · STI · Chlamydia · Epidemic model · Basic reproduction number · Sensitivity analysis

1 Introduction

Over 1.8 million cases of chlamydia trachomatis, CT, are reported each year [35] in the United States. This sexually transmitted infection (STI) is a major cause of infertility, pelvic inflammatory disease, and ectopic pregnancy among women [7, 8, 14, 15, 17, 28, 32, 40, 41], and has been associated with increased HIV acquisition and transmission [7, 13, 14, 17, 28, 31, 32, 39–41]. Untreated, an estimated 16 % of, women with CT will develop PID [33], and 6 % will have tubal infertility [38]. We

A. Azizi · L. Xue · J.M. Hyman (✉)
Department of Mathematics, Tulane University, New Orleans, LA 70118, USA
e-mail: mhyman@tulane.edu

A. Azizi
e-mail: aazizibo@tulane.edu

L. Xue
e-mail: lxue2@tulane.edu

G. Chowell and J.M. Hyman (eds.), *Mathematical and Statistical Modeling for Emerging and Re-emerging Infectious Diseases*,
DOI 10.1007/978-3-319-40413-4_15

developed and analyzed a multicompartmental risk-based heterosexual transmission model that can be used to help understand the spread of the disease and quantify the relative effectiveness of different mitigation efforts.

Mathematical models create frameworks for understanding underling epidemiology of diseases and how they are correlated to the social structure of the infected population [9, 11, 12, 18–25]. Transmission-based models can help the medical/scientific community to understand and to anticipate the spread of diseases in different populations, and help them to evaluate the potential effectiveness of different approaches for bringing the epidemic under control. The primary goal of our modeling effort is to create a model that can be used to understand the spread of CT and to predict the impact of screening, sexual contact tracing, and treatment programs on mitigating the CT epidemic.

In modeling the spread of CT, the population is divided into the susceptible sexually active population (S), the exposed infected, but not infectious, population (E), and the infectious population (I). Once a person has recovered from CT infection, they are again susceptible to infection. Therefore, the models all have a S→E→I→S (SEIS) structure, or an SIS structure if the exposed state is combined with the infectious state. The SEIRS CT transmission model developed by Althaus et al. [1] captured the most essential transitions through an infection with CT to assess the impact of CT infection screening programs. Using sensitivity analysis, they identified the time to recover from infection and duration of the asymptomatic period as the two most important model parameters governing the disease prevalence. Longer recovery times diminishes the effect of screening, however longer duration of the asymptomatic period results in a more pronounced impact of program. They also used their model to improve the estimates for the duration of the asymptomatic period by reanalyzing previously published data on persistence of CT in asymptomatically infected women. This model did not divide the population into separate risk groups and assumed that all men and women had the same number of partners.

Our model is also closely related to the deterministic population-based model developed by Clarke et al. [6] to explore the short-term impacts of increasing screening and contact tracing. They investigated how control plans can affect observable quantities and demonstrated that partner positivity (the probability that the partner of an infected person is infected) is insensitive to changes in screening coverage or contact tracing efficiency. They also evaluated the cost-effectiveness of increasing contact tracing versus screening and concluded that partner notification along with screening is the most cost effective mitigation approach.

The number of partners a person has (his/her risk), and the number of partners that their partners have (his/her partner's risk) both affect the spread of CT. That is, different assumptions about the distribution of risk behavior for the population will result in different disease forecasts. We use the selective sexual mixing STI model developed by Hyman et al. [19] to capture the heterogenous mixing among people with different number of partners. This model is well-described by Del Valle et al. [10] to investigate the impact of different mixing assumptions on spread of infectious diseases and how sensitivity analysis can be used to prioritize different possible mitigation efforts.

Kretzschmar et al. and Turner et al. [26, 27] evaluated different screening and partner referral methodologies in controlling CT. They compared their RIVM model to evaluate the effectiveness of opportunistic CT screening program in the Netherlands [27]; the ClaSS model to evaluate proactive, register-based CT screening using home sampling in the UK [29]; and the HPA model to evaluate opportunistic national CT screening program in England [36]. We relied on these studies in formulating our differential equation compartmental model.

Our model is closely related to the STI models for the spread of the HIV/AIDS virus in a heterosexual network [23, 24]. These models account for the distribution of risk in a population based on realistic sexual contact networks [9, 11, 12, 21–24]. Although age, ethnicity, economic statues, and the spatial location of the individuals all influence the assortative mixing of sexual contacts, the risk of contracting CT is primarily a function of the number of partners a person has, number of contacts per partner, the probability that a partner is infected, and the use of prophylactics (e.g. condoms).

In our ordinary differential equation model (ODE), we considered defining the risk categories based on either the number of partners a person has, or their total number of sexual contacts. The relative importance of the number of partners and the number of contacts per partner on the spread of an STI depends on the disease infectiousness. CT is a very infectious and the probability of transmission, per contact, from an infected person to uninfected one is high; one contact with an infected person is enough to catch the infection. Therefore, the number of people a person infects, and a person's risk, depends mostly upon the number of partners he/she has.

Parameters in the model were estimated within a reasonable level of accuracy in order for results to give qualitative and quantitative understanding of how the disease is spreading [19]. We use local sensitivity analysis to identify the relative importance of the model parameters and numerical examples to illustrate how we can prioritize mitigation strategies based on their predicted effectiveness.

After formulating the mathematical model, we derived the basic reproduction number, $\mathbb{R}_0$ for two main risk groups (high-risk and low-risk) for men and women. We then use sensitivity analysis of $\mathbb{R}_0$ and the equilibrium points with respect to the model parameters to study how the heterogeneous mixing affects the spread of CT. Our numerical simulations illustrate the behavior of the model system and the effectiveness of screening to reduce the spread of CT.

2 Mathematical Model

Because the exposed (infected, but not infectious) time period is short compared to time in the infectious stage, we do not include an exposed stage in our model. Recovered individuals are immediately susceptible to reinfection; We divide men and women into n risk groups based on the number of partners an individual has in a year. This SIS model can be written as the system of $2n$ ordinary differential equations:

$$\frac{dS_k}{dt} = \mu(N_k^o - N_k) - \lambda_k S_k + \rho_k I_k, \tag{1}$$

$$\frac{dI_k}{dt} = \lambda_k S_k - \rho_k I_k - \mu I_k, \tag{2}$$

where $k = 1, \ldots, n$ denotes men with risk from 1 to n, and $k = n + 1, \ldots, 2n$ denotes women with risk from 1 to n. The migration rate, μ, determines the rate at which people enter and leave the population, $N_k = S_k + I_k$ is the total population of group k, N_k^o is total population of group k in the absence of infection, λ_k is the rate at which a susceptible person in risk group k is being infected, and ρ_k is the rate that a person recovers either through treatment, screening, or natural recovery.

2.1 Migration Rate

We model a population of 15–25 year-old individuals and assume that the primary mechanism for migration is by aging into, and out of, the population, where migration rate $\mu = 0.1 = [(25 - 15) \text{ years}]^{-1}$, with the assumption that death is negligible compared to the rate that people enter and leave the modeled population. We assume that, in the absence of infection, equilibrium population N_k^o for each risk group of men and women is given, and that everyone aging into the model population enters as a susceptible person.

2.2 Disease Recovery Rate

The rate the infected population is treated, ρ_k, depends upon the sex of the person and their risk level. The treatment can be initiated when infection is identified through screening, contact tracing, or a medical check-up. Most infected people are asymptomatic and, when a significant fraction of a population is infected, then screening has been found to be a cost-effective approach to identify, and treat, infected people.

We separate the recovery rate into two parts, $\rho_k = \rho_k^n + \rho_k^s$, where the natural recovery rate ρ_k^n depends only on the sex of the infected person, and the screening rate ρ_k^s depends upon both the sex and risk level of an individual. Natural recovery rate, ρ_k^n, is determined by assuming an exponential distribution for the average time to recovery $1/\rho_k^n$. We define the probablity that an individual is screened each day, ρ_k^s, in terms of the fraction of the population that will be screened at least once within a year as f_k^s. That is,

$$\rho_k^s = 1 - (1 - f_k^s)^{1/365}. \tag{3}$$

2.3 Disease Transmission Rate

We will derive the disease transmission rate for the heterosexual case where a susceptible person in group k can be infected by someone of the opposite sex in any of the infected groups j. This force of infection, λ_k, is the rate that people in risk group k are infected through sexual contacts. Here a contact is any sexual act that can transmit the disease between individuals. We define λ_i as the sum of the rate of disease transmission from each infected group, I_j, to the susceptible group, S_k:

$$\lambda_k = \sum_{j=1}^{n} \lambda_{kj}. \tag{4}$$

The rate of disease transmission from the infected people I_j in group j to the susceptible individuals S_k in group k, λ_{kj}, is defined as the product of three factors:

$$\begin{aligned}\lambda_{kj} &= \begin{pmatrix}\text{Number of partners}\\ \text{a susceptible in group } k\\ \text{has with someone in}\\ \text{group } j \text{ per unit time}\end{pmatrix} \begin{pmatrix}\text{Probability of}\\ \text{disease transmission}\\ \text{per partner}\end{pmatrix} \begin{pmatrix}\text{Probability that}\\ \text{partner in group } j\\ \text{that is infected}\end{pmatrix}\\ &= p_{kj}\ \beta_{kj}\ \left(\frac{I_j}{N_j}\right).\end{aligned}$$

These terms are defined as:

- the number of sexual partners per unit time that each individual in group k has with someone in group j, (p_{kj}), and
- the probability of disease transmission per partner, β_{kj}, for a susceptible person in group k with their partner in group j, and
- the probability of that the person in group j is infectious.

For this last factor, we assume that the partners in group j are all equally likely to be infected. That is, the probability of that the person in group j is infected is the same as the fraction of the people in group j that are infected, (I_j/N_j).

2.3.1 Partnership Formation

The extent that CT spreads through a population is sensitive to the heterogenous mixing (partnership selection) among the different risk groups. The models approximates the mixing through the mixing probabilities, p_{kj}, that define how many partners a typical person in group k has with someone in group j. These mixing functions must dynamically change to account for variations in the size of the groups [4, 10, 18].

The force of infection, λ_k, depends on how many partners people in group k have, the number of contacts they have per partner, and the probability that their partners are infected. The mixing is biased since people who only have a few sexual partners (low-risk) typically have partners who are also at low-risk.

We define the model parameters so that someone in group k has, on average, p_{kj} partners who are in group j per day. Therefore, the total number of partnerships per day between people in group k and group j is then $p_{kj}N_k = p_{jk}N_j$. Since each partnership may have more than one contact, we define c_k as the average number of contacts per partner for people in group k. We define $\bar{\beta}$ as the average probability of transmitting the infection per contact. Both c_k and $\bar{\beta}$ will then be used to define the average transmission rate β_k per partnership. Finally, the product, $p_{kj}\beta_k$, is the rate that the susceptible people in group k are infected by an infected person in group j.

To determine p_{kj}, we use a heterogenous mixing algorithm developed in [18]. This approach starts by defining $\bar{p}_k$ as the *desired* number of partnerships someone in group k wishes to have per unit time. Because there may not be sufficient available partners for everyone to have their desired number of partners, the actual number of partners could be different.

We define the *proportional* partnership (mixing) as the desired fraction d_{kj} of these partnerships that a person in group k wants to have with someone in group j. That is, a person in group k wants to have an average of $d_{kj}\bar{p}_k$ partnerships per unit time with someone in group j. Unfortunately, there is no guarantee that the total number of desired partnership people in group k want to have with people in group j will be the same as the total number of desired partnerships that people in group j want to have with people in group k. That is, in general $d_{kj}\bar{p}_kN_k \neq d_{jk}\bar{p}_jN_j$, and this must be reconciled.

Since not everyone can have their desired number of partners distributed exactly as they wish, the different heterogenous mixing algorithms represent different compromises to resolve these conflicts. All of the heterogenous mixing algorithms maintain the detailed balance for mixing where the total number of partnerships for people in group k with people in group j is the same as the total number of partnerships that people in group j have with people in group k. In our model, we use the heterogenous mixing algorithm based on the algorithm described in [10, 18] to determine p_{kj}.

The population in group k desires $d_{kj}\bar{p}_kN_k$ partners from group j, and the population in group j desires $d_{jk}\bar{p}_jN_j$ partners from group k. As a compromise, we set the total number of partners the people in group k have with people in group j, and visa versa, to be the harmonic mean

$$p_{kj}N_k = p_{jk}N_j = \frac{2(d_{kj}\bar{p}_kN_k)(d_{jk}\bar{p}_jN_j)}{(d_{kj}\bar{p}_kN_k) + (d_{jk}\bar{p}_jN_j)}. \quad (5)$$

Other possibilities include the geometric mean or minimum of $(d_{kj}\bar{p}_kN_k)$ and $(d_{jk}\bar{p}_jN_j)$. All of these averages satisfy the balance condition to have the property that if $d_{jk} = 0$ then $p_{kj} = p_{jk} = 0$, where if one group refuses to have a partnership with another group, then this partnership does not happen. In our model, we use the harmonic mean and define

$$p_{kj} = \frac{1}{N_k} \frac{2(d_{kj}\bar{p}_k N_k)(d_{jk}\bar{p}_j N_j)}{(d_{kj}\bar{p}_k N_k) + (d_{jk}\bar{p}_j N_j)}. \tag{6}$$

Hence, $p_k = \sum_j p_{kj}$ is the actual average number of partners someone in group k has per day.

Note that this approach is only appropriate if the desired number of partners between any two groups is in close agreement, that is, $d_{kj}\bar{p}_k N_k \approx d_{jk}\bar{p}_j N_j$. This is because, the approach assumes that if the partners are not available from the desired group, then the individuals will not change their preferences to seek partners in other risk groups. The model can be extended to handle these situations where the people adjust their desires to be in closer alignment with the availability of partners through a simple iterative algorithm. However, we avoid this complication in our simulations and initialize the populations so the groups desires are close to the availability of partnerships.

2.3.2 Disease Transmission per Partnership

The probability of a susceptible person catches infection from their infected partners depends upon the number of contacts between the people. We allow the number of contacts per partner for a person in group k, c_k, to depend upon the number of his (her) actual partners,(p_k), and his (her) total number of contacts per unit time, (C_k), i.e. $C_k = c_k p_k$.

However, the number of contacts for a person in group k, should be the same as the number of contacts per partner for their partner in group j, c_j. To make it compatible, we define harmonic average c_{kj} (Fig. 1):

$$c_{kj} = \frac{2c_k c_j}{c_k + c_j},$$

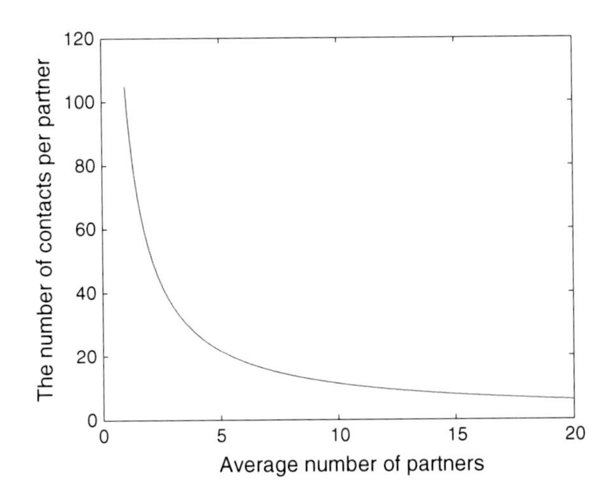

Fig. 1 The number of contacts per partnership per year, c_k, is a decreasing function of $\bar{p}_{kj}$, that is people with more partners have fewer contacts per partner than people with fewer partners. If C_k is total number of contacts for a person in group k, c_k is defined as $c_k = \frac{C_k}{p_k} = \frac{C_k}{\sum_j p_{kj}}$

Table 1 The values of variables and parameters in the simulations

Parameters or variables	Description	Value
N_1	Population for group 1 (high-risk men)	695
N_2	Population for group 2 (low-risk men)	6257
N_3	Population for group 3 (high-risk women)	652
N_4	Population for group 4 (low-risk women)	1239
$\bar{\beta}$	Probability of transmission per contact	0.1100
C_1	Total number of contacts per day for group 1	0.1400
C_2	Total number of contacts per day for group 2	0.0740
C_3	Total number of contacts per day for group 3	0.0750
C_4	Total number of contacts per day for group 4	0.0410
$\bar{P}_1$	Desired number of partners for group 1	0.1400
$\bar{P}_2$	Desired number of partners for group 2	0.0312
$\bar{P}_3$	Desired number of partners for group 3	0.0570
$\bar{P}_4$	Desired number of partners for group 4	0.0180
d_{13}	Desired fraction of partners by group 1 with group 3	0.7500
d_{31}	Desired fraction of partners by group 3 with group 1	0.7500
d_{24}	Desired fraction of partners by group 2 with group 4	0.8000
d_{42}	Desired fraction of partners by group 4 with group 2	0.8000
ρ_i	Natural recovery rate for group i	0.0056
μ	Migration rate	0.0003

as number of contacts between a person in group k and their partner in group j. The probability of transmission per contact, $\bar{\beta}$, can be used to define the probability that a susceptible person will not be infected by a single contact with an infected person, $1-\bar{\beta}$. Therefore, the probability of someone in group k not being infected after c_{kj} contacts with an infected partner in group j is $(1-\bar{\beta})^{c_{kj}}$. Hence, the probability of being infected per partner is [22]

$$\beta_{kj} = 1 - (1-\bar{\beta})^{c_{kj}}. \tag{7}$$

With this definition, we have $\beta_{kj} = \beta_{jk}$.

Tables 1 and 2 contain a complete list of the model parameters and their baseline values.

3 Basic Reproduction Number

The basic reproduction number is the number of new infected introduced if a newly infectous person is introduced into a disease free population at the $(S_k = N_k,\ I_k =$

Table 2 Variables and parameters in the model and their dimensions

Variables	Description	Unit
S_j	Number of susceptible humans in risk group j	Number
I_j	Number of infectious humans in risk group j	Number
N_j	Total human population in risk group j	Number
μ	Migration rate	Time^{-1}
ρ_j	Per capita recovery rate for humans from the infectious state to the susceptible state	Time^{-1}
$\bar{\beta}$	Probability of transmission of infection from an infectious human to a susceptible one per contact per time	Time^{-1}
C_j	Total number of contacts for a person in risk group j per time	Time^{-1}
$\bar{p}_j$	Desired number of contacts for a person in group j	Dimensionless
$\bar{d}_{jk}$	Desired fraction of contacts for a person in group j wants to have with group k	Dimensionless

Numerical values for these parameters are provided in Table 1

0). After using a branching process approach to describe how the infections move through the population, we will use the next generation matrix approach [16, 37] to derive $\mathbb{R}_0$.

3.1 Branching Process Analysis

The equation for the nondimensionalized infected population can be written as

$$\frac{\mathrm{d}I_k}{\mathrm{d}t} = \sum_j \alpha_{kj} I_j - \tau_k^{-1} I_k. \tag{8}$$

Here $\tau_k = 1/(\rho_k + \mu)$ is the average time that an infected person stays in the kth infection compartment. The force from infection, $\alpha_{kj} = \beta_{kj} q_{kj} S_j$, is the rate (per day) that a typical infected person in group j infects a susceptible in group k. Here the factor q_{kj} is defined as $q_{kj} = (p_{kj}/N_j)$ and because we had $p_{kj} N_k = p_{jk} N_j$, therefore, $(p_{kj}/N_j) = (p_{jk}/N_k)$, and that means $q_{kj} = q_{jk}$ is the fraction of people in group j someone in group k has as a partner.

We define the group j-to-group k reproduction number, $\mathbb{R}_0^{j \to k} = \alpha_{jk} \tau_j$, as the average number of people that a new infected person in group j will infect someone in group k at the DFE. Note that in our model, if group j and group k are of the same sex, then $\mathbb{R}_0^{j \to k} = 0$.

Consider the situation where the first infection is in group j, then the number of secondary infections over all possible groups is $\mathbb{R}_0^{j \to *} = \sum_k \mathbb{R}_0^{j \to k}$. Each of these secondary infections in group k then infect $\mathbb{R}_0^{k \to *}$ others. That is, the total number of new infections is a branching process and grows geometrically.

The reproduction numbers measure the average number of new infected cases over a *single* infection cycle and is defined as the square-root of the number of new infections over two cycles. We can define the basic reproduction number for group j as

$$\mathbb{R}_0^j = \sqrt{\sum_k \left(\mathbb{R}_0^{j\to k}\mathbb{R}_0^{k\to *}\right)} = \sqrt{\sum_k \left(\mathbb{R}_0^{j\to k}\sum_i \mathbb{R}_0^{k\to i}\right)}\,.$$

3.2 Next Generation Derivation of Basic Reproduction Number

We will derive the basic reproduction number, $\mathbb{R}_0$, using the next generation approach for situations with two risk levels for men and women labeled: $1 =$ (high-risk men), $2 =$ (low-risk men), $3 =$ (high-risk women) and $4 =$ (low-risk women). The differential equations (8) for the infected populations, $x = (I_1, I_2, I_3, I_4)^T$, can be written as a matrix equation for the rate of production of new infections, F, minus the removal rate of individuals from that population class, V,

$$\frac{dx}{dt} = \mathbf{F}x - \mathbf{V}x, \tag{9}$$

where the klth element of the matrix $\mathbf{F}_{kl} = \alpha_{kl}$ and V is diagonal matrix $V_{kk} = \tau_k^{-1}$, for $k, l = 1, 4$.

At the DFE, $\alpha_{kj} = \beta_{kj} q_{kj} N_k$ and the Jacobian matrices, $\mathbf{J}_F$ and $\mathbf{J}_V^{-1}$, of Fx and Vx are

$$J_F = \begin{pmatrix} 0 & 0 & \alpha_{13} & \alpha_{14} \\ 0 & 0 & \alpha_{23} & \alpha_{23} \\ \alpha_{31} & \alpha_{32} & 0 & 0 \\ \alpha_{41} & \alpha_{42} & 0 & 0 \end{pmatrix}, \quad J_V = \begin{pmatrix} \tau_1 & 0 & 0 & 0 \\ 0 & \tau_2 & 0 & 0 \\ 0 & 0 & \tau_3 & 0 \\ 0 & 0 & 0 & \tau_4 \end{pmatrix},$$

We define $\mathbb{R}_0$ as spectral radius of $J_F J_V^{-1}$ or (equivalently) $J_V^{-1} J_F$,

$$J_F J_V^{-1} = \begin{bmatrix} 0 & 0 & \alpha_{13}\tau_3 & \alpha_{14}\tau_4 \\ 0 & 0 & \alpha_{23}\tau_3 & \alpha_{24}\tau_4 \\ \alpha_{31}\tau_1 & \alpha_{32}\tau_2 & 0 & 0 \\ \alpha_{41}\tau_1 & \alpha_{42}\tau_2 & 0 & 0 \end{bmatrix}, \quad J_V^{-1} J_F = \begin{bmatrix} 0 & 0 & \alpha_{13}\tau_1 & \alpha_{14}\tau_1 \\ 0 & 0 & \alpha_{23}\tau_2 & \alpha_{24}\tau_2 \\ \alpha_{31}\tau_3 & \alpha_{32}\tau_3 & 0 & 0 \\ \alpha_{41}\tau_4 & \alpha_{42}\tau_4 & 0 & 0 \end{bmatrix}. \tag{10}$$

Note that jkth element of $J_F J_V^{-1}$ is $\mathbb{R}_0^{j\to k} = \alpha_{jk}\tau_k$.

Based on a result of Sylvester's inertia theorem [34],[1] if a matrix K can be factored into the product of a diagonal positive definite matrix A and a symmetric matrix B, then eigenvalues of K are the same as eigenvalues of $A^{\frac{1}{2}}BA^{\frac{1}{2}}$. To apply this result, we rewrite $J_V^{-1}J_F = AB$ where A is a diagonal positive definite matrix and B is symmetric,

$$A = \begin{bmatrix} N_1\tau_1 & 0 & 0 & 0 \\ 0 & N_2\tau_2 & 0 & 0 \\ 0 & 0 & N_3\tau_3 & 0 \\ 0 & 0 & 0 & N_4\tau_4 \end{bmatrix}, \quad B = \begin{bmatrix} 0 & 0 & \beta_{13}q_{13} & \beta_{14}q_{14} \\ 0 & 0 & \beta_{23}q_{23} & \beta_{24}q_{24} \\ \beta_{31}q_{31} & \beta_{32}q_{32} & 0 & 0 \\ \beta_{41}q_{41} & \beta_{42}q_{42} & 0 & 0 \end{bmatrix}. \quad (11)$$

Therefore, eigenvalues of $J_V^{-1}J_F$ are the same as eigenvalues of symmetric block anti-diagonal generation matrix

$$A^{\frac{1}{2}}BA^{\frac{1}{2}} = \begin{bmatrix} 0 & 0 & \sqrt{\alpha_{13}\tau_1\alpha_{31}\tau_3} & \sqrt{\alpha_{14}\tau_1\alpha_{41}\tau_4} \\ 0 & 0 & \sqrt{\alpha_{23}\tau_2\alpha_{32}\tau_3} & \sqrt{\alpha_{24}\tau_2\alpha_{42}\tau_4} \\ \sqrt{\alpha_{31}\tau_3\alpha_{13}\tau_1} & \sqrt{\alpha_{32}\tau_3\alpha_{23}\tau_2} & 0 & 0 \\ \sqrt{\alpha_{41}\tau_4\alpha_{14}\tau_1} & \sqrt{\alpha_{42}\tau_4\alpha_{42}\tau_2} & 0 & 0 \end{bmatrix} = \begin{bmatrix} 0_{4\times4} & M \\ M^T & 0_{4\times4} \end{bmatrix}, \quad (12)$$

where M^T is transpose of M

$$M = \begin{bmatrix} \sqrt{\alpha_{13}\tau_1\alpha_{31}\tau_3} & \sqrt{\alpha_{14}\tau_1\alpha_{41}\tau_4} \\ \sqrt{\alpha_{23}\tau_2\alpha_{32}\tau_3} & \sqrt{\alpha_{24}\tau_2\alpha_{42}\tau_4} \end{bmatrix} = \begin{bmatrix} r_{13} & r_{14} \\ r_{23} & r_{24} \end{bmatrix}, \quad (13)$$

where $r_{jk} = \sqrt{\mathbb{R}_0^{j\to k}\mathbb{R}_0^{k\to j}}$ is the geometric average of group j-to-group k and group k-to-group j reproduction numbers.

The basic reproduction number is spectral radius of $J_V^{-1}J_F$. Therefore, $\mathbb{R}_0 = \rho(A^{\frac{1}{2}}BA^{\frac{1}{2}}) = \sqrt{\rho(M^TM)}$ where

$$M^TM = \begin{bmatrix} r_{13}^2 + r_{23}^2 & r_{13}r_{14} + r_{23}r_{24} \\ r_{13}r_{14} + r_{23}r_{24} & r_{14}^2 + r_{24}^2 \end{bmatrix},$$

and

$$\mathbb{R}_0 = \frac{1}{2}((r_{13}^2 + r_{23}^2 + r_{14}^2 + r_{24}^2) + \sqrt{(r_{13}^2 + r_{23}^2 - r_{14}^2 - r_{24}^2)^2 + 4(r_{13}r_{14} + r_{23}r_{24})^2}) \quad (14)$$

[1]Let K be a hermitian matrix. We define $e^+(K)$ as the number of positive eigenvalues, $e^-(K)$ as the number of negative eigenvalues, and $e^0(K)$ as the number of zero eigenvalues. Inertia of K is a tuple $(e^+(K), e^-(K)), e^0(K)$. If A is an invertible matrix then Sylvester inertia theorem states: $inertia(K) = inertia(A^{-1}KA)$.

4 Sensitivity Analysis

We use sensitivity analysis to quantify the change in model output quantities of interest (QOIs), such as the basic reproduction number, $\mathbb{R}_0$, and endemic equilibrium point, due to variations in the model input parameters of interest (POIs), such as the average time to recovery after infection [2, 3, 5, 30].

Consider the situation where the baseline value of the input POI is p_b and generates the baseline output QOI $q_b = q(p_b)$. Sensitivity analysis is used to address what happens if p_b is changed by the fraction θ_p, $p_{new} = p_b(1 + \theta_p)$ and we want to know the resulting fractional change in the output variable $q_{new} = q_b(1 + \theta_p^q)$. That is, the normalized sensitivity index measures the relative change in the input variable p, with respect to the output variable q and can be estimated by the Taylor series

$$q_{new} = q(p_b + \theta_p p_b) \approx q_b + \theta_p p_b \left. \frac{\partial q}{\partial p} \right|_{p=p_b} = q_b(1 + \theta_p^q). \tag{15}$$

We define the normalized sensitivity index as

$$\mathbb{S}_p^q := \left. \frac{p_b}{q_b} \frac{\partial q}{\partial p} \right|_{p=p_b} = \frac{\theta_p^q}{\theta_p}. \tag{16}$$

That is, if the input p is changed by θ_p percent, then the output q will change by $\theta_p^q = \mathbb{S}_p^q \theta_p$ percent. The sign of $\mathbb{S}_p^q$ determines the direction of changes, increasing(for positive $\mathbb{S}_p^q$) and decreasing (for negative $\mathbb{S}_p^q$). Note that this local sensitivity index is valid only in a small neighborhood of the baseline values (Table 1).

4.1 *Sensitivity Indices of* $\mathbb{R}_0$

The ability of CT to become established in a population and its early growth rate is characterized by the basic reproduction number (14). Sensitivity analysis of $\mathbb{R}_0$ can quantify the relative importance of the the different social and epidemiological parameters in reducing the ability of the STI to become established in a new population.

Table 3 of the sensitivity indices of $\mathbb{R}_0$ shows that it is most sensitive to the probability of transmission per contact $\overline{\beta}$ with $\mathbb{S}_{\overline{\beta}}^{\mathbb{R}_0} = 1.95$. That is, if the probability of infection per contact decreases, say by increasing the use of condoms, by 15 % then $\theta_{\bar{\beta}} = -0.15$ and $\mathbb{R}_0$ will decrease by 29.25 % from 1.357 to 0.96

$$\mathbb{R}_{0new} = \mathbb{R}_0 \left(1 + \theta_{\bar{\beta}} \mathbb{S}_{\overline{\beta}}^{\mathbb{R}_0}\right) = 1.357(1 - 0.15 \times 1.95) = 0.96 < 1.$$

Table 3 The sensitivity indices of $\mathbb{R}_0$ with respect to parameters of the model at the baseline parameter values where $\mathbb{R}_0 = 1.357$

Parameter	Value	$\mathbb{S}_p^q$
$\bar{\beta}$	0.1100	**1.95**
C_1	0.1354	**0.76**
C_2	0.0739	0.15
C_3	0.0750	**0.71**
C_4	0.0410	0.22
d_{13}	0.7500	0.35
d_{31}	0.7500	0.58
d_{24}	0.8000	0.04
d_{42}	0.8000	0.12
$\bar{p}_1$	0.1352	0.05
$\bar{p}_2$	0.0312	−0.06
$\bar{p}_3$	0.0567	0.24
$\bar{p}_4$	0.0185	−0.07
ρ_1	0.0056	**−0.95**
ρ_2	0.0056	−0.48
ρ_3	0.0056	**−0.95**
ρ_4	0.0056	−0.48
μ	0.0003	−0.09

The most sensitive parameter is the probability of transmission per contact, $\bar{\beta}$, followed by the recovery (screening) rates of the high-risk men and women ρ_1 and ρ_3

Hence, sensitivity analysis can quantify the amount of behavior change that would be needed to keep an epidemic from becoming established in a new population.

A negative sensitivity index indicates that $\mathbb{R}_0$ is a decreasing function of correspondent parameter, while the positive ones show $\mathbb{R}_0$ increases when the parameter increases. The second most important model parameters for the early growth rate are the recovery rates of the high-risk men and women ρ_1 and ρ_3. These rates depend upon the screening recovery ρ_3, the rate that a person is identified through screening and treated. Since, $\mathbb{S}_{\rho_1}^{\mathbb{R}_0} = \mathbb{S}_{\rho_3}^{\mathbb{R}_0} = -0.95$, a 10 % increase in the screening rate would result in a 9.5 % decrease in $\mathbb{R}_0$. This supports the need to actively screen both men and women for CT infection.

The number of contacts for high-risk men, C_1, is also an important parameter for controlling the early growth of the CT. Because local-sensitivity analysis is valid in a small neighborhood of the baseline case, sometimes it is useful to plot the change in the QOI over a wide range of possible values. The sensitivity index is then the slope of the response curve at the baseline values. Figure 2 shows how $\mathbb{R}_0$ changes as these parameters are varied over a broad range.

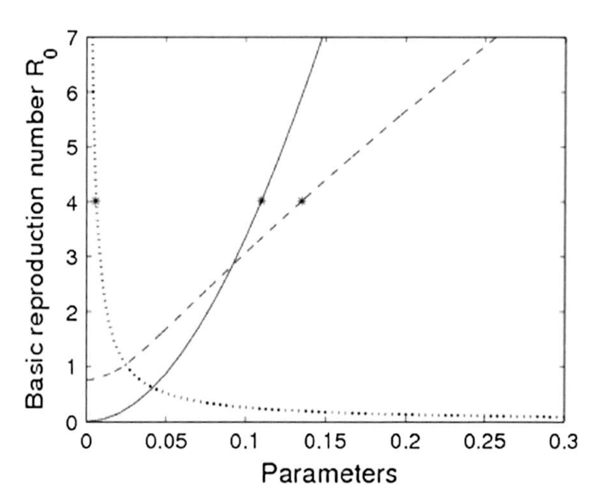

Fig. 2 The sensitivity of $\mathbb{R}_0$ with respect to $\overline{\beta}$ (*solid line*), C_1 (*dashed line*), and ρ_1 (*dotted line*). The sensitivity index is then the slope of the response curve at the baseline values, indicated by $*$. The response is approximately linear near the baseline case and, therefore, the local sensitivity analysis is actually valid over a broad range of parameters

4.2 Sensitivity Indices of Endemic Equilibriums

The current CT epidemic is established in many cities, and to evaluate the relative impact of the model parameters in bringing it under control requires that the sensitivity analysis is preformed about the current state of the system, the steady-state endemic equilibrium. We will investigate the impact of the mitigation efforts on the relative change in the number of infected people as a function of the relative change in the model parameters. This is best done in terms of the nondimensional variables defined by dividing each variable by the steady-state zero-infection equilibrium total population for each sex. That is, $i_m = I_m/N_m^o$, $i_w = I_w/N_w^o$, $n_1 = N_1/N_m^o$, $n_2 = N_2/N_m^o$, $n_3 = N_3/N_w^o$, and $n_4 = N_4/N_w^o$. Here, $N_m^o = N_1^o + N_2^o$, $N_w^o = N_3^o + N_4^o$.

Table 4 shows that the sensitivity indices for endemic (steady-state) equilibrium infected populations, i_j, as a function of the model parameters. Note that the magnitudes (relative importance) of sensitivity indices have the same order as they did for $\mathbb{R}_0$, although the magnitudes are different.

The prevalence of infection, i_j, is most sensitive to probability of transmission per contact $\bar{\beta}$, i.e. increasing $\bar{\beta}$ increases i_js more than other parameters. Then C_js and ρ_js have the second most effect on i_js in positive and negative direction, correspondingly.

Prevalence in high-risk men, i_1, is sensitive to the total number of contacts for the high-risk men C_1 and ρ_1 more than the other C_js and ρ_js for $j \neq 1$. Prevalence in high-risk women, i_3, is also sensitive to C_3 and ρ_3 more than the other C_js and ρ_js for $j \neq 3$. It means when high-risk people increase their number of contacts, regardless of what others do, the fraction of infected people among high-risk people increases, because they have lots of partners. On the other hand, when infection period for high-risk people increases, the prevalence in high-risk increases.

Table 4 Local sensitivity indices of the endemic equilibrium points

Parameter	Baseline	i_1	i_2	i_3	i_4
$\bar{\beta}$	0.1100	**2.61**	**4.05**	**2.70**	**4.02**
C_1	0.8000	**1.07**	**0.58**	**0.71**	**0.66**
C_2	0.8000	0.31	1.50	0.33	1.00
C_3	0.8000	0.65	0.56	1.13	0.53
C_4	0.8000	0.42	1.18	0.37	1.61
d_{13}	0.7500	0.36	−0.21	0.24	−0.36
d_{31}	0.7500	0.41	−0.15	0.56	0.03
d_{24}	0.8000	0.02	−0.13	0.08	−0.10
d_{42}	0.8000	0.15	−0.21	0.08	−0.33
$\bar{p}_1$	0.1352	0.04	0.17	0.08	0.23
$\bar{p}_2$	0.0312	−0.02	0.01	−0.03	−0.002
$\bar{p}_3$	0.0567	0.27	0.31	0.21	0.26
$\bar{p}_4$	0.0185	−0.05	0.03	−0.03	0.04
ρ_1	0.0056	**−1.10**	**−0.60**	**−0.73**	**−0.68**
ρ_2	0.0056	−0.35	−1.66	−0.37	−1.11
ρ_3	0.0056	−0.66	−0.56	−1.13	−0.53
ρ_4	0.0056	−0.47	−1.31	−0.41	−1.78
μ	0.0003	−0.13	−0.20	−0.13	−0.20

At this baseline $\mathbb{R}_0 \geq 1$, so this endemic point is a solution of model at steady state

For low-risk men, the prevalence, i_2, has the same sensitivity to C_2 and C_4. It means when low-risk people increase their contact, the prevalence in low-risk men increases, and we have the same story for low-risk women. It is reasonable, because low-risk people don't have too many partners, and therefore more contact for them and their partners plays an important role.

Prevalence in low-risk men, i_2, has also the same sensitivity to ρ_2 and ρ_4. It means when we decrease ρ_2 and ρ_4, infected people in low-risk men stay in infection category more and also infected women in low-risk group stay in infection category more, we see increment in the value of i_2 more than the other parameters. There is a similar analysis for low-risk group i_4: low-risk group i_4 is sensitive to ρ_2 and ρ_4 with the same magnitude and more than the other ρ_js.

Another interesting result is that the endemic equilibrium points are more sensitive, than $\mathbb{R}_0$, to most of the parameters. This result says, controlling parameters to have a low fraction of infected population is easier than adjusting the parameters to have smaller $\mathbb{R}_0$.

5 Numerical Simulations

In these numerical simulations, all the parameters are fixed with the baseline values given in Table 3, unless specifically defined otherwise.

In the first simulation, we assume that number of people who can be screened each day, ρ^s, is limited by a budget, or other factors. For example, if the budget for screening is \$10,000 per year and cost of screening is \$25 per person, then we can screen a total of $10,000/25 = 400$ people per year, or an average of $\rho^s = 1.096$ people per day. We also assume that if an infected person is screened for CT, then there is a 95 % probability that disease will be detected.

We will compare the fraction of the population that is infected as a function of the screening rate ρ_k^s people from different subgroups k. We will also optimize the ρ^s, for a fixed budget, that will minimize the number of infected people at steady state. That is, if $(I_1^*, I_2^*, I_3^*, I_4^*)$ are the number of infected people at steady state, we find the optimal screening rates that solve the optimization problem:

$$\begin{aligned} \underset{\rho_i^s}{\text{minimize}} \quad & \sum_{j=1}^{4} I_j^*(\rho_1^s, \rho_2^s, \rho_3^s, \rho_4^s), \\ \text{subject to} \quad & \sum_{j=1}^{4} \rho_j^s = \rho^s. \end{aligned}$$

Figure 3 show the result for six scenarios: (1) no screening, (2) screening high-risk men, (3) screening high-risk women, (4) screening low-risk men, (5) screening low-risk women, and (6) optimized screening for those with positive test result.

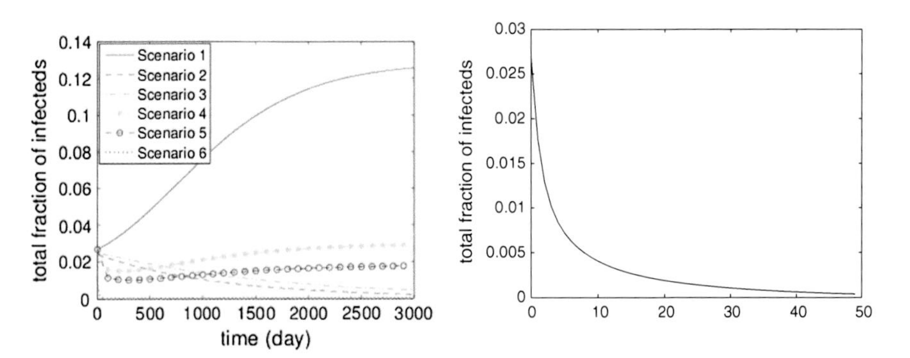

Fig. 3 *Left panel* the fraction of infected people after implementing different scenarios: no screening (*solid line*), screen 400 people per year for: high-risk men (*dash line*), high-risk women (*dash-dot line*), low-risk men (*dash-star*), low-risk women (*dash-circle*), and optimized screening (*dotted line*). *Right panel* zooms on the optimized screening, by optimized screening the disease dies out very fast

Table 5 Basic reproduction number, $\mathbb{R}_0$, for different scenarios with respect to parameters of the model at the baseline parameter values

Scenario	$\mathbb{R}_0$	Scenario	$\mathbb{R}_0$
No screening	1.3566	Screen low-risk men	1.2567
Screen high-risk men	0.8646	Screen low-risk women	1.2243
Screen high-risk women	0.9102	Optimized screening	0.1196

Implementing optimized screening decreases $\mathbb{R}_0$ to the order of -1

We observe that in case of no screening the epidemic goes up to its original endemic equilibrium point. The effectiveness of screening is seen by the dramatic reduction in the fraction of infected people. However, among all scenarios screening high-risk people and optimized screening cause that epidemic dies out and for optimal choice it dies out much faster than the two other cases.

Table 5 lists the value of $\mathbb{R}_0$ for different scenarios. Based on the Fig. 3 and Table 5, it is obvious that $\mathbb{R}_0 > 1$ implies a persistent infection, though not a macroscopic outbreak in screening cases, and when $\mathbb{R}_0 < 1$ epidemic goes to disease-free equilibrium point. Also, for the optimized scenario, which its $\mathbb{R}_0$ is the lowest one, the epidemic dies out faster than the other scenarios.

Therefore, optimized screening was the most effective scenario among all 6 cases. To push our understanding of the effect of optimized screening further, we do sensitivity analysis of equilibrium points w.r.t screening rates at their optimized values. In this case sensitivity index become a matrix like:

$$\mathbb{S} = \begin{pmatrix} I_1^* & 0 & 0 & 0 \\ 0 & I_2^* & 0 & 0 \\ 0 & 0 & I_3^* & 0 \\ 0 & 0 & 0 & I_4^* \end{pmatrix}^{-1} \times J_{I^*}(\rho^s) \times \begin{pmatrix} \rho_1^s & 0 & 0 \\ 0 & \rho_2^s & 0 \\ 0 & 0 & \rho_3^s \end{pmatrix},$$

where $J_{I^*}(\rho^s)$ is jacobian matrix. Each column k of $\mathbb{S}$ represents sensitivity indexes of equilibrium points w.r.t screening rate ρ_k^s. Therefore $(k, j)th$ element of $\mathbb{S}$ is sensitivity index of I_k^* w.r.t ρ_j^s. Table 6 lists the elements of this matrix. All the values in table are negative, it means there is a inverse pattern between equilibrium points and screening rate: when we increase screening rates the number of infected people at steady state will decrease. Among all, I_1^* is the most sensitive one, it means changing screening rates affects on the number of high-risk men more than the others.

Table 6 Sensitivity indices of equilibrium points w.r.t screening rates at optimized baseline values

Screening rates	Equilibrium points			
	$I_1^* = 0.000$	$I_2^* = 0.000$	$I_3^* = 0.000$	$I_4^* = 0.000$
$\rho_1^s = 0.0600$	-0.1294	-0.0015	-0.0065	-0.1319
$\rho_2^s = 0.2033$	-0.5576	-0.3706	-0.2728	-0.4056
$\rho_3^s = 0.0475$	-0.0805	-0.0918	-0.0946	-0.0941

The most sensitive output parameter is number of infected high-risk men

6 Summary and Conclusions

We created a two-risk sexual heterosexual SIS transmission model for the spread of CT with biased mixing partnership selection to investigate the impact that screening for the disease can have in controlling its spread. We derived the threshold conditions for the early spread of the disease and defined the basic reproductive number, $\mathbb{R}_0$, using the next generation matrix approach. The analysis of $\mathbb{R}_0$ identified a new approach to reduce the size of the next generation matrix for a heterosexual STI model with n risk groups from an $2n \times 2n$ nonsymmetric sparse matrix to an $n \times n$ symmetric full matrix. This approach can be used in similar heterosexual STI models to greatly simplify the threshold analysis.

The sensitivity analysis of $\mathbb{R}_0$ and endemic equilibrium steady-state solutions quantifies the relative effectiveness of different intervention strategies in mitigating the disease. The analysis identified the probability of transmission per contact (related to condom use) is the most sensitive parameter in controlling the epidemic. The second most effective control mechanism was the screening, and treating infections, of both high-risk men and women. Currently, most mitigation programs only target screening high-risk women, the model indicates that it is equally important to identify infections and treat high-risk men. We confirmed that in the model the higher-risk groups are driving the epidemic and that $\mathbb{R}_0$ is most sensitive to the behavior of these higher-risk people.

We implemented different screening scenarios consist of screening only high-risk men, only high-risk women, only low-risk men, only low-risk women, and optimized screening. We then solved for an optimal screening strategy for infection mitigation when there are limited resources and determined that best screening approach to minimize the endemic steady state infection prevalence. Not surprisingly, we found that this same strategy also minimizes $\mathbb{R}_0$.

Acknowledgments We thank Patricia Kissinger for her insight and guidance in determining what factors need to be considered in modeling the spread of CT. We also thank Jeremy Dewar for his assistance with the sensitivity analysis and feedback on the manuscript. This work was supported by the endowment for the Evelyn and John G. Phillips Distinguished Chair in Mathematics at Tulane University, and National Institute of General Medical Sciences of the National Institutes of Health program for Models of Infectious Disease Agent Study (MIDAS) under Award Number U01GM097658. The content is solely the responsibility of the authors and does not necessarily represent the official views of the National Institutes of Health.

References

1. Althaus, C.L., Heijne, J., Roellin, A., Low, N.: Transmission dynamics of chlamydia trachomatis affect the impact of screening programmes. Epidemics **2**(3), 123–131 (2010)
2. Arriola, L., Hyman, J.M.: Sensitivity analysis for uncertainty quantification in mathematical models. In: Mathematical and Statistical Estimation Approaches in Epidemiology, pp. 195–247. Springer, New York (2009)

3. Arriola, L.M., Hyman, J.M.: Being sensitive to uncertainty. Comput. Sci. Eng. **9**(2), 10–20 (2007)
4. Busenberg, S., Castillo-Chavez, C.: A general solution of the problem of mixing of subpopulations and its application to risk-and age-structured epidemic models for the spread of aids. Math. Med. Biol. **8**(1), 1–29 (1991)
5. Chitnis, N., Hyman, J.M., Cushing, J.M.: Determining important parameters in the spread of malaria through the sensitivity analysis of a mathematical model. Bull. Math. Biol. **70**(5), 1272–1296 (2008)
6. Clarke, J., White, K.A., Turner, K.: Exploring short-term responses to changes in the control strategy for chlamydia trachomatis. Comput. Math. Methods Med. **11**(4), 353–368 (2012)
7. Cohen, M.S.: Sexually transmitted diseases enhance HIV transmission: no longer a hypothesis. Lancet **351**, S5–S7 (1998)
8. Datta, S.D., Torrone, E., Kruszon-Moran, D., Berman, S., Johnson, R., Satterwhite, C.L., Papp, J., Weinstock, H.: Chlamydia trachomatis trends in the united states among persons 14 to 39 years of age, 1999–2008. Sex. Transm. Dis. **39**(2), 92–96 (2012)
9. Del Valle, S., Hethcote, H., Hyman, J.M., Castillo-Chavez, C.: Effects of behavioral changes in a smallpox attack model. Math. Biosci. **195**(2), 228–251 (2005)
10. Del Valle, S.Y., Hyman, J.M., Chitnis, N.: Mathematical models of contact patterns between age groups for predicting the spread of infectious diseases. Math. Biosci. Eng. MBE **10**, 1475 (2013)
11. Del Valle, S.Y., Hyman, J.M., Hethcote, H.W., Eubank, S.G.: Mixing patterns between age groups in social networks. Soc. Netw. **29**(4), 539–554 (2007)
12. Eaton, D.K., Kann, L., Kinchen, S., Shanklin, S., Ross, J., Hawkins, J., Harris, W.A., Lowry, R., McManus, T., Chyen, D., et al.: Youth risk behavior surveillance-united states, 2009. Morb. Mortal. Wkly. Rep. Surveill. Summ. (Washington, DC: 2002), **59**(5), 1–142 (2010)
13. Golden, M.R., Hogben, M., Handsfield, H.H., St Lawrence, J.S., Potterat, J.J., Holmes, K.K.: Partner notification for HIV and STD in the united states: low coverage for gonorrhea, chlamydial infection, and HIV. Sex. Transm. Dis. **30**(6), 490–496 (2003)
14. Gottlieb, S.L., Brunham, R.C., Byrne, G.I., Martin, D.H., Xu, F., Berman, S.M.: Introduction: the natural history and immunobiology of chlamydia trachomatis genital infection and implications for chlamydia control. J. Infect. Dis. **201**(Supplement 2), S85–S87 (2010)
15. Gottlieb, L.S., Martin, D.H., Xu, F., Byrne, G.I., Brunham, R.C.: Summary: the natural history and immunobiology of chlamydia trachomatis genital infection and implications for chlamydia control. J. Infect. Dis. **201**(Supplement 2), S190–S204 (2010)
16. Heffernan, J.M., Smith, R.J., Wahl, L.M.: Perspectives on the basic reproductive ratio. J. R. Soc. Interface **2**(4), 281–293 (2005)
17. Hillis, S.D., Wasserheit, J.N.: Screening for chlamydia: a key to the prevention of pelvic inflammatory disease. N. Engl. J. Med. **334**(21), 1399–1401 (1996)
18. Hyman, J.M., Li, J.: Behavior changes in SIS STD models with selective mixing. SIAM J. Appl. Math. **57**(4), 1082–1094 (1997)
19. Hyman, J.M., Li, J.: Disease transmission models with biased partnership selection. Appl. Numer. Math. **24**(2), 379–392 (1997)
20. Hyman, J.M., Li, J., Stanley, E.A.: The differential infectivity and staged progression models for the transmission of HIV. Math. Biosci. **155**(2), 77–109 (1999)
21. Hyman, J.M., Li, J., Stanley, E.A.: The initialization and sensitivity of multigroup models for the transmission of HIV. J. Theor. Biol. **208**(2), 227–249 (2001)
22. Hyman, J.M., Li, J., Stanley, E.A.: Modeling the impact of random screening and contact tracing in reducing the spread of HIV. Math. Biosci. **181**(1), 17–54 (2003)
23. Hyman, J.M., Stanley, E.A.: Using mathematical models to understand the AIDS epidemic. Math. Biosci. **90**(1), 415–473 (1988)
24. Hyman, J.M., Stanley, E.A.: The effect of social mixing patterns on the spread of AIDS. In: Castillo-Chavez, C.C., Levin, S.A., Shoemaker, C.A. (eds.) Mathematical Approaches to Problems in Resource Management and Epidemiolog, pp. 190–219. Springer, Berlin (1989)

25. Hyman, J.M., Stanley, E.A.: A risk-based heterosexual model for the AIDS epidemic with biased sexual partner selection. In: Kaplan, E.E., Brandeau, M. (eds.) Modeling the AIDS Epidemic, pp. 331–364. Raven Press, New York (1994)
26. Kretzschmar, M., van Duynhoven, Y.T.H.P., Severijnen, A.J.: Modeling prevention strategies for gonorrhea and chlamydia using stochastic network simulations. Am. J. Epidemiol. **144**(3), 306–317 (1996)
27. Kretzschmar, M., Welte, R., Van den Hoek, A., Postma, M.J.: Comparative model-based analysis of screening programs for chlamydia trachomatis infections. Am. J. Epidemiol. **153**(1), 90–101 (2001)
28. Lan, J., van den Brule, A.J., Hemrika, D.J., Risse, E.K., Walboomers, J.M., Schipper, M.E., Meijer, C.J.: Chlamydia trachomatis and ectopic pregnancy: retrospective analysis of salpingectomy specimens, endometrial biopsies, and cervical smears. J. Clin. Pathol. **48**(9), 815–819 (1995)
29. Low, N., McCarthy, A., Macleod, J., Salisbury, C., Campbell, R., Roberts, T.E., Horner, P., Skidmore, S., Sterne, J.A., Sanford, E., et al.: Epidemiological, social, diagnostic and economic evaluation of population screening for genital chlamydial infection. Health Technol. Assess. (Winchester, England), **11**(8):iii–iv (2007)
30. Manore, C.A., Hickmann, K.S., Xu, S., Wearing, H.J., Hyman, J.M.: Comparing dengue and chikungunya emergence and endemic transmission in A. aegypti and A. albopictus. J. Theor. Biol. **356**, 174–191 (2014)
31. Niccolai, L.M., Livingston, K.A., Laufer, A.S., Pettigrew, M.M.: Behavioural sources of repeat chlamydia trachomatis infections: importance of different sex partners. Sex. Transm. Infect. **87**(3), 248–253 (2011)
32. Pearlman, M.D., Mcneeley, S.G.: A review of the microbiology, immunology, and clinical implications of chlamydia trachomatis infections. Obstet. Gynecol. Surv. **47**(7), 448–461 (1992)
33. Schwebke, J.R., Rompalo, A., Taylor, S., Sena, A.C., Martin, D.H., Lopez, L.M., Lensing, S., Lee, J.Y.: Re-evaluating the treatment of nongonococcal urethritis: emphasizing emerging pathogens-a randomized clinical trial. Clin. Infect. Dis. **52**(2), 163–170 (2011)
34. Sylvester, J.J.: Xix. a demonstration of the theorem that every homogeneous quadratic polynomial is reducible by real orthogonal substitutions to the form of a sum of positive and negative squares. Lond. Edinb. Dublin Philos. Mag. J. Sci. **4**(23), 138–142 (1852)
35. Torrone, E., Papp, J., Weinstock, H.: Prevalence of chlamydia trachomatis genital infection among persons aged 14–39 years-united states, 2007–2012. MMWR Morb. Mortal. Wkly. Rep. **63**(38), 834–838 (2014)
36. Turner, K.M.E., Adams, E.J., LaMontagne, D.S., Emmett, L., Baster, K., Edmunds, W.J.: Modelling the effectiveness of chlamydia screening in England. Sex. Transm. Infect. **82**(6), 496–502 (2006)
37. Van den Driessche, P., Watmough, J.: Reproduction numbers and sub-threshold endemic equilibria for compartmental models of disease transmission. Math. Biosci. **180**(1), 29–48 (2002)
38. Walker, J., Tabrizi, S.N., Fairley, C.K., Chen, M.Y., Bradshaw, C.S., Twin, J., Taylor, N., Donovan, B., Kaldor, J.M., McNamee, K., et al.: Chlamydia trachomatis incidence and re-infection among young women-behavioural and microbiological characteristics. PLoS One **7**(5), e37778 (2012)
39. Ward, H., Rönn, M.: The contribution of STIs to the sexual transmission of HIV. Curr. Opin. HIV AIDS **5**(4), 305 (2010)
40. Westrom, L.: Effect of pelvic inflammatory disease on fertility. Venereol. Off. Publ. Natl. Venereol. Counc. Aust. **8**(4), 219–222 (1995)
41. Weström, L.V.: Sexually transmitted diseases and infertility. Sex. Transm. Dis. **21**(2 Suppl), S32–S37 (1993)

The 1997 Measles Outbreak in Metropolitan São Paulo, Brazil: Strategic Implications of Increasing Urbanization

José Cassio de Moraes, Maria Claudia Corrêa Camargo, Maria Lúcia Rocha de Mello, Bradley S. Hersh and John W. Glasser

The findings and conclusions in this report are those of the authors and do not necessarily represent the official position of the Centers for Disease Control and Prevention or other institutions with which they are affiliated.

Abstract *Background*: Despite a routine two-dose measles vaccination program, mass campaigns in 1987 and 1992 and low subsequent incidence, São Paulo experienced an outbreak between May and October of 1997 with over 42,000 confirmed cases, mostly young adults, and 42 measles-associated deaths, mostly infants. To eliminate measles, the Pan American Health Organization (PAHO) recommended supplementing routine childhood vaccination (keep-up) via mass campaigns, initially to reduce (catch-up) and periodically to maintain (follow-up) susceptible numbers below the epidemic threshold. *Methods*: To determine if a follow-up campaign during 1996, when due in São Paulo State, might have prevented or mitigated this outbreak, we modeled measles in metropolitan São Paulo. We also evaluated the actual impact of emergency outbreak-control efforts and hypothetical impact of vaccinating adolescent and young adult immigrants. *Results*: A mass campaign targeting children aged 6–59 months reduced cases as much as 77 %, but a follow-up campaign among children aged 1–4 years during 1996 might have been even more effective. Susceptible adolescents would have escaped, however, setting the stage for future outbreaks. Vaccinating people in the immigrant age range mitigated this potential. *Conclusions*: As the immunity required to prevent outbreaks depends on population density, rural

J.C. de Moraes · M.C.C. Camargo · M.L.R. de Mello
Centro de Vigilancia Epidemiologica, Estado de São Paulo, São Paulo, Brazil
e-mail: jcassiom@uol.com.br

B.S. Hersh
Joint United Nations Programme on HIV/AIDS, Geneva, Switzerland
e-mail: hershb@unaids.org

J.W. Glasser (✉)
National Center for Immunization and Respiratory Diseases, Atlanta, GA, USA
e-mail: jglasser@cdc.gov

G. Chowell and J.M. Hyman (eds.), *Mathematical and Statistical Modeling for Emerging and Re-emerging Infectious Diseases*,
DOI 10.1007/978-3-319-40413-4_16

people are less likely to be immune than urban ones the same age. Thus, when there is rural-urban migration, births are not the sole demographic process eroding urban population immunity. Vaccinating immigrants in bus stations, peripheral shanty-towns, or sites of employment for unskilled laborers is more efficient than increasing rural immunity.

Keywords Measles · Epidemic model · Vaccination · Brazil · Mass campaign · Immunity · Vaccination strategies

1 Introduction

In 1994, countries in the Americas adopted the goal of measles elimination by 2000 (Resolution XVI of the XXIV Pan American Sanitary Conference). In São Paulo State, Brazil, more than 42,000 measles cases were confirmed from December 1996 through October 1997, 42 people died of complications, and disease spread to other Latin American countries. This setback raised important questions: Are outbreak-prevention strategies being implemented as recommended? And if so, do they suffice for the task?

1.1 Background

Following measles vaccine licensure in 1973, the primary prevention strategy in Brazil was infant vaccination. Public health authorities initially recommended a dose of single-antigen measles vaccine at 9 months of age. In 1979, to protect younger infants without compromising lifetime protection, officials in São Paulo State replaced this schedule with 7- and 15-month doses, for the second of which measles and rubella vaccine was used. However, because vaccine efficacy is less than 80 % among infants younger than 10 months (Brazilian, Chilean, Costa Rican, and Ecuadorian Ministries of Health and PAHO [3]), many first-dose recipients remained susceptible. And, because second-dose coverage remained low, 1,636 measles cases occurred per 10^5 children aged less than 15 years during 1986 despite 84 % of infants being vaccinated. To interrupt the 2–4 year outbreak cycle [15], the Department of Health restored the 9 month age at first dose and conducted a mass vaccination campaign throughout São Paulo State during May of 1987. Authorities estimate that 86 % of residents aged 9 months to 14 years were vaccinated [29]. During June of 1992, a second campaign targeted children aged 1–10 years for measles, mumps and rubella vaccination.

Together with single-dose routine vaccination programs, periodic mass campaigns comprised PAHO's tripartite strategy for eliminating measles in Latin America [11]. *Catch-up* campaigns were designed to increase immunity among those 9 months through 14 years of age, reducing younger infants' risk of infection, permitting delayed first doses and increasing vaccine efficacy. The immunity maintained via routine *keep-up* efforts determines how frequently *follow-up* campaigns are required to prevent susceptible children from exceeding the threshold above which infectious people would on average infect more than one susceptible person, causing outbreaks. Measles is endemic in populations of 300,000 or more absent vaccination [2], with alternating years of higher and lower incidence. In the belief that births alone could exceed urban population-immunity thresholds, strategists reasoned that, once vaccination began, uptake among resident children and efficacy together would determine the period required to attain critical levels of susceptibility. In diverse Latin American and Caribbean countries, 3–5 years was both the typical interval between successive *follow-up* campaigns and upper age. As this strategy proved effective [6], the international health community adopted it [5].

1.2 Outbreak Control in São Paulo

Only sporadic cases were reported to the Department of Health, São Paulo State, until early 1997 [4]. Of the 65,540 suspected cases of measles reported that year, 23,907 (37.0 %) were either confirmed via detection of measles-specific IgM antibodies in blood specimens via enzyme immunoassay (EIA) or linked via contact with laboratory-confirmed measles cases, 18,148 (28.1 %) were confirmed on clinical grounds alone without laboratory investigation, and 23,485 (35.8 %) were discarded. Of the 42,055 confirmed cases, 36,803 (87.5 %) occurred among residents of metropolitan São Paulo and 29,916 (56.8 %) among adults aged 20 years or older. The greatest incidence was observed in São Paulo County (246 cases per 10^5 people), followed by suburban São Paulo (181 cases per 10^5 people) and the interior of São Paulo State (30 cases per 10^5 people). The greatest age-specific incidence occurred among infants (1,577 cases per 10^5 people), adults 20–29 years of age (539 cases per 10^5 people) and children 1–4 years of age (205 cases per 10^5 people).

Despite a selective vaccination campaign mid-June, the outbreak continued seemingly unabated. So a mass campaign targeting children aged 6–59 months was conducted mid-August; the outbreak ended several weeks later. Here we present a synthesis of relevant surveys and results from experiments with a mathematical model designed to assess the effectiveness of prevention and control strategies employed in São Paulo. We also assess the potential impact of more frequent *follow-up* campaigns and supplemental adolescent and young adult vaccination.

2 Methods

We assembled measles case reports, vaccination and serological surveys, and internal migration surveys. Scrutiny of this information led us to attribute the unusual age-distribution of cases during the 1997 outbreak to (1) the aging of unvaccinated children who had been protected by the vaccination of others and (2) an unusual influx, following a protracted drought and resulting crop failures [8], of adolescents and young adults from rural areas with lower population immunity. Next, using an age-structured model of the metropolitan São Paulo population, including immigration from and emigration to its environs, we reproduced the outbreak. Then we experimented with our model to evaluate control efforts and to determine if timely implementation of the *follow-up* portion of PAHO's strategy could have prevented or mitigated this outbreak and if not, to evaluate other measures, such as supplemental vaccination of adolescents and young adults, particularly immigrants from rural areas. The tables to which we refer in this section are in the Appendix.

2.1 Descriptive Modeling

We synthesized information from five serological surveys conducted during 1987–1998 (Table A.2) via multivariate logistic regression in which both age and time are represented as polynomials. As these variables are related biologically (i.e., people aged x in year y are aged $x + 1$ in year $y + 1$), our regression model includes all un-aliased interaction terms. We used GLIM4 [17], which eliminates parameter combinations that are aliased. We also calculated age-specific immigration and emigration rates from the age-distribution of migrants and overall migration rates during 1988-95 from the Brazilian Institute of Geography and Statistics (http://www.ibge.gov.br/english/).

In our transmission model, newborns are protected or susceptible, depending on their mother's immune status, but passively acquired maternal antibodies decay, after which children may be infected, transiting latent and infectious states, or vaccinated, alternative routes to lifelong immunity. The age-specific proportions of residents who were susceptible on 1 January 1995, when simulations began, are complements of a cross-section through our synthesis of serological surveys. Similarly, we estimated the age-specific rates of infection among susceptible people by fitting a catalytic model [13] to the 1 January 1985 cross-section. Then we calculated the corresponding attack rates and, using the mixing model of Jacquez et al. [22], age-specific probabilities of infection on contact and, finally, infection rates.

We estimated proportions protected via passively-acquired maternal antibodies by fitting a logistic regression to published results from a serological survey during 1987 [29]. Our vaccination rates were calculated from overall coverage and Gamma distributed age-specific proportions via the relationship between rates and proportions, proportion $= 1 - \exp(-\text{rate} \times \text{time})$. The Gamma distribution's parameters were (a) estimated from a composite of cluster vaccination surveys of children born in 1996 who resided in 8 neighborhoods differing in socio-economic status during October of 1998 [10], (b) calculated via the method of moments from the age ranges targeted in *follow-up* and emergency outbreak-control campaigns or (c) fitted to the age distribution of immigrants. Our measles mortality rates were quotients of deaths attributed to measles and laboratory-confirmed cases.

As individuals simultaneously age through ten classes (<1, 1–4, 5–9, ..., 30–39, 40–49, 50+ years), they risk dying of other causes, emigrating, and if female, giving birth, all at age-specific rates. Individuals from rural areas immigrate at rates calculated from the average age-distribution from 1988–1995 immigration surveys and average annual immigration rate from 1992–1995. Age-specific proportions immune (and susceptible, their complements) were calculated by multiplying those from the above-mentioned 1995 cross-section through our synthesis of serological surveys by age-specific ratios of proportions immune in rural and urban Maryland early in the 20th Century [12]. Individuals also emigrate at rates that we calculated similarly.

2.2 Mechanistic Modeling

Our model system comprises equations for metropolitan residents who are protected by maternal antibodies, $V_i(t)$; susceptible, $W_i(t)$; harboring latent infections (i.e., infected, but not yet infectious), $X_i(t)$; infectious, $Y_i(t)$; and immune following disease or vaccination, $Z_i(t)$. Our equations describe the rates at which persons in age group i (<1, 1–4, 5–9, ..., 30–39, 40–49 and 50+ years) transit these 5 epidemiological states at time t.

$$\frac{dV_1}{dt} = V_0(t) - [\sigma + \mu_1 + o_1 - \iota_1(1 - \varphi_1) - \theta_1]\, V_1(t)$$

$$\frac{dV_k}{dt} = V_{k-1}\theta_{k-1} - \left[\sigma + \mu_k + o_k - \iota_k(1 - \varphi_k) - \theta_i\right] V_k(t), \quad 1 < k < n$$

$$\frac{dV_n}{dt} = V_{n-1}\theta_{n-1} - [\sigma + \mu_n + o_n - \iota_n(1 - \varphi_n)]\, V_n(t)$$

$$\frac{dW_1}{dt} = W_0(t) + \sigma V_1(t) - (\alpha\nu_1 + \lambda_1(t) + \mu_1 + o_1 - \iota_1\varphi_1 - \theta_1)\, W_1(t)$$

$$\frac{dW_k}{dt} = W_{k-1}\theta_{k-1} + \sigma V_k(t) - (\alpha\nu_k + \lambda_k(t) + \mu_k + o_k - \iota_k\varphi_k - \theta_i)\, W_k(t), \quad 1 < k < n$$

$$\frac{dW_n}{dt} = W_{n-1}\theta_{n-1} + \sigma V_n(t) - (\alpha\nu_n + \lambda_n(t) + \mu_n + o_n - \iota_n\varphi_n)\, W_n(t)$$

$$\frac{dX_1}{dt} = \lambda_1(t) W_1(t) - (\gamma + \mu_1 + o_1 - \iota_1\varphi_1 - \theta_1)\, X_1(t)$$

$$\frac{dX_k}{dt} = X_{k-1}\theta_{k-1} + \lambda_k(t) W_k(t) - (\gamma + \mu_k + o_k - \iota_k\varphi_k - \theta_i)\, X_k(t), \quad 1 < k < n$$

$$\frac{dX_n}{dt} = X_{n-1}\theta_{n-1} + \lambda_n(t) W_n(t) - (\gamma + \mu_n + o_n - \iota_n\varphi_n)\, X_n(t)$$

$$\frac{dY_1}{dt} = \gamma X_1(t) - (\rho + \delta_1\mu_1 + o_1 - \iota_1\varphi_1 - \theta_1)\, Y_1(t)$$

$$\frac{dY_k}{dt} = Y_{k-1}\theta_{k-1} + \gamma X_k(t) - (\rho + \delta_k\mu_k + o_k - \iota_k\varphi_k - \theta_i)\, Y_k(t), \quad 1 < k < n$$

$$\frac{dY_n}{dt} = Y_{n-1}\theta_{n-1} + \gamma X_n(t) - (\rho + \delta_n\mu_n + o_n - \iota_n\varphi_n)\, Y_n(t)$$

$$\frac{dZ_1}{dt} = \alpha\nu_1 W_1(t) + \rho Y_1(t) - [\mu_1 + o_1 - \iota_1(1 - \varphi_1) - \theta_1]\, Z_1(t)$$

$$\frac{dZ_k}{dt} = Z_{k-1}\theta_{k-1} + \alpha\nu_k W_k(t) + \rho Y_k(t) - \left[\mu_k + o_k - \iota_k(1 - \varphi_k) - \theta_i\right] Z_k(t), \quad 1 < k < n$$

$$\frac{dZ_n}{dt} = Z_{n-1}\theta_{n-1} + \alpha\nu_n W_n(t) + \rho Y_n(t) - [\mu_n + o_n - \iota_n(1 - \varphi_n)]\, Z_n(t)$$

The transition processes and their respective *per capita* rates are vaccination, ν_i, whose efficacy is α; infection, $\lambda_i(t)$; becoming infectious, γ; and recovering, ρ. The reciprocals of γ and ρ are the latent and infectious periods, 6–9 and 6–7 days, respectively [1]. Newborns with immune mothers are protected via passively acquired antibodies that decay at rate σ; others are susceptible. Individuals immigrate and emigrate at per capita rates ι_i and o_i, respectively, with probabilities φ_i of being susceptible and $1-\varphi_i$ immune, and die at per capita rates μ_i, which disease increases by factors δ_i. The forces (or hazard rates) of infection,

$$\lambda_i(t) = a_i\beta_i \sum\nolimits_j c_{ij}\left[\frac{Y_j(t)}{N_j(t)}\right], \quad 1 \le i, j \le n$$

$$N_i(t) = V_i(t) + W_i(t) + X_i(t) + Y_i(t) + Z_i(t),$$

where a_i are *per capita* rates of contact, called activities, β_i are probabilities of infection on contact and c_{ij} are proportions of their contacts that members of group i have with members of group j [9]. We formulate c_{ij} as follows: If a proportion ε_i of i-group contacts is reserved for others in group i, called preferences, and the complement $(1-\varepsilon_i)$ is distributed among all groups, including i, via the proportionate mixing formula, f_j, then

$$c_{ij} = \varepsilon_i\delta_{ij} + (1-\varepsilon_i)f_j, \text{ where } f_j = \frac{\left(1-\varepsilon_j\right)a_jN_j}{\sum_k (1-\varepsilon_k)\,a_kN_k},$$

where δ_{ij} is the Kronecker delta (i.e., $\delta_{ij} = 1$ if $i = j$ and 0 otherwise). Glasser et al. [18] derive this expression, which Jacquez et al. [22] obtained by allowing preference, ε in Nold's [27] preferred mixing model, to vary among groups. Hethcote's [19] Eq. (4.14) is equivalent to hers with epsilon and its complement reversed.

We chose $\varepsilon_i = 0.2\forall i$, meaning that 20 % of contacts were reserved for others in the same age group and the complement was distributed randomly among all groups. Then we estimated the $a_i \times \beta_i$ required to yield pre-vaccination λ_i that we obtained by fitting $F(\alpha) = 1 - e^{-\int_0^\alpha \lambda(u)du}$, where $\lambda(\alpha) = (w\alpha - y)e^{-x\alpha} + z$, α is age and w, x, y, and z are fitted parameters [13], to the 1 January 1985 cross-section through our synthesis of serological surveys. We analyzed histories of measles in Baltimore and rural Maryland recorded early in the 20th Century similarly to learn how rural and urban immune profiles differed.

2.3 Parameters and Initial Conditions

As demographic processes may affect disease dynamics (cf. [23]), we also modeled metropolitan São Paulo's population dynamics (i.e., via its age and gender distributions and vital statistics, Table A.3). Protected and susceptible children are born at rates $V_0(t) = \sum_i f_i \times \Pr(i, ♀) \times Z_i(t)$ and $W_0(t) = \sum_i f_i \times \Pr(i, ♀) \times S_i(t)$, respectively, with *per capita* rate f_i, proportions female $\Pr(i, ♀)$, and susceptible populations, $S_i(t) = W_i(t) + X_i(t) + Y_i(t)$.

We represent the age-distribution of vaccination via Gamma distributions whose parameters we estimated or calculated via the method of moments from recent surveys or age ranges targeted in various campaigns, respectively. And we formulate aging after Ferguson, Nokes and Anderson [14], whose per capita rates θ are reciprocals of age class widths, which is accurate only when widths are small.

Proportions of the resident population that were susceptible and immune by age group were obtained from the 1 January1995 cross-section through our synthesis of serological surveys. Proportions immune among members of the rural population who immigrated to metropolitan São Paulo were estimated by multiplying the proportions in São Paulo by age-specific ratios of cumulative incidences in rural and urban Maryland. This is tantamount to assuming that vaccination affected the immune profiles of São Paulo and its environs similarly.

The *per capita* immigration and emigration rates were quotients of the estimated annual numbers of immigrants and emigrants and the metropolitan São Paulo population (Tables A.3 and A.4). Expressing immigration rates as functions of source populations would have been preferable, but that information was not available at the time. Immigrants have the immune profile calculated as described above, whereas emigrants have that of the metropolitan Sao Paulo population. Because greater proportions of immigrants were susceptible than residents in any age group, there was an influx of susceptible people even in the age groups with negative net migration.

2.4 Experimental Design

To assess the effectiveness of outbreak-control efforts in São Paulo and determine if this epidemic could have been mitigated if not prevented, we simulated the actual scenario, a routine two-dose vaccination program and emergency mass campaign. Parameters that we could not estimate from observations in contemporary São Paulo were adjusted to reduce disparities between predicted and observed case reports. Then we simulated three scenarios: 1) routine vaccination only (i.e., with routine 2-dose vaccination, but not the emergency campaign); 2) plus the recommended 1996 *follow-up* campaign (i.e., routine vaccination plus a hypothetical mass campaign among children aged 6 to 59 months during the week of 15 June 1996); and 3) plus adolescent and young adult vaccination (i.e., routine vaccination, the hypothetical 1996 campaign and supplemental vaccination having the age distribution of immigrants).

Because these hypothetical scenarios are nested, we can evaluate individual interventions: The difference between actual (i.e., routine doses at 9 and 15 months, plus mass campaign among children aged 6–59 months during the week of 16 August 1997) and hypothetical scenario 1 estimates the impact of outbreak-control efforts. Similarly, the difference between scenarios 1 and 2 estimates the hypothetical *follow-up* campaign's impact. And finally, the difference between scenarios 2 and 3 estimates the impact of targeted adolescent and adult vaccination. All comparisons are conditional on routine vaccination, and the last also is conditional on periodic *follow-up* campaigns.

3 Results

We present descriptive results suggesting the cause of the 1997 measles outbreak in São Paulo and modeling results to evaluate that hypothesis and possible remedies separately.

3.1 Descriptive Epidemiology

Figures 1 and 2a describe proportions of the metropolitan São Paulo populace who were immune by age and time from the early 1980s through mid-90s. In the table

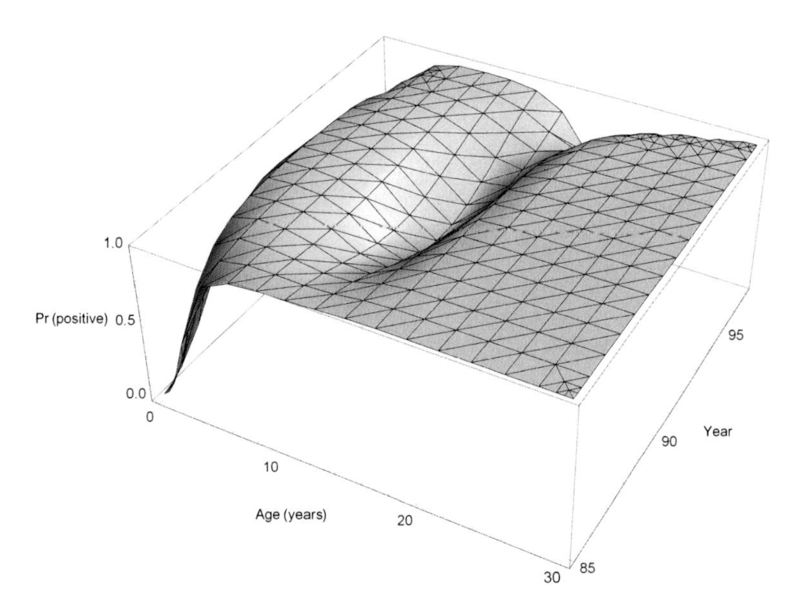

Fig. 1 Synthesis of five serological surveys during 1987–1998 (Pannuti et al. [29] and Table A.2) via bivariate logistic regression: a cubic polynomial in age, quadratic polynomial in time and, because people age in time, all interactions

below, selected GLIM4 output from our logistic regression modeling of historical published [29] and unpublished (Table A.2) serological surveys in metropolitan São Paulo, A denotes age, Y year, and 1 is the intercept:

```
scaled deviance = 422.31
residual degrees of freedom = 46
number of observations: 58
linear model: 1+A+A2+A3+Y+Y2+A.Y+A2.Y+A3.Y+A.Y2+A2.Y2
+A3.Y2
```

Estimate	Standard Error	Parameter
−1308.	426.9	1
159.9	138.5	A
14.42	14.85	A2
−1.131	0.5699	A3
28.85	9.445	Y
−0.1589	0.05217	Y2
−3.524	3.050	A.Y
−0.3213	0.3241	A2.Y
0.02525	0.01236	A3.Y
0.01961	0.01675	A.Y2
0.001757	0.001765	A2.Y2
−0.0001396	0.00006687	A3.Y2

```
scale parameter: 1.000
```

The data are numbers of sera containing measles-specific IgM antibodies and numbers tested, the link is logit, and the probability distribution is binomial. The trough that develops when vaccination intensified during the mid-80s represents children who either were not vaccinated or who failed to respond immunologically. By virtue of others being vaccinated, some also escaped infection, and had become adolescents by 1997.

Immigration rates varied year to year, but their age distributions were remarkably similar (Fig. 2b). Almost half of São Paulo's residents originated elsewhere, with 2.6 % having resided in the metropolitan area for less than a year, but net migration was −7.5 per 10^4 people per year (i.e., emigration exceeded immigration) during the most recent period available, 1992–1995 (Brazilian Institute of Geography and Statistics). Because of drought and resulting crop failures in the northeast, immigration accelerated during 1997 [8]. We attribute the deepening and faster movement of the trough along the age axis of Fig. 1 than before—which Fig. 2a emphasizes via several recent cross-sections—to the confluence of these factors.

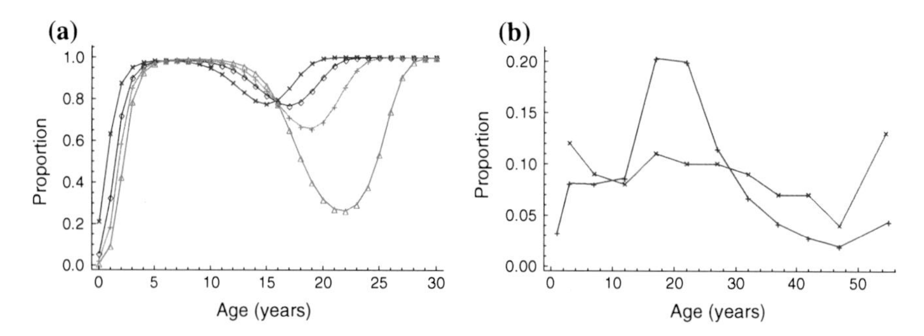

Fig. 2 **a** Cross-sections through the surface illustrated in Fig. 1 at 1 January 1995 (*blue* × symbols), 1996 (*pink* ◇ symbols), and 1997 (*green* Δ symbols) and 1 July 1996 (*gold* + symbols) and **b** Ages of immigrants to (*blue* + symbols) and emigrants from (*red* × symbols) metropolitan São Paulo in 1991 and 1994, respectively (Fundação Seade, State Data Analysis System Foundation)

Figure 3 is a diagram of our transmission model and Fig. 4a, b are fits of Farrington's [13] catalytic model to the 1995 cross section through our serological surface and estimates of the age-specific forces (or hazard rates) of infection, respectively. Analysis of information presented by Fales [12] suggests that immunity among children aged 0–4, 5–9, 10–14, 15–19 years in rural Maryland was roughly 0.63, 0.69, 0.72, 0.74, respectively, of that among similarly-aged children in Baltimore (Fig. 4c, d), suggesting that immunity increased more slowly with age in rural than urban Maryland and ultimately attained only about three-quarters of the urban level. These population-immunities are consistent with rural and urban $\Re_0$ (the average number of effective contacts while infectious, where effective contacts suffice for infection if susceptible) during this period (5–6 in Kansas and 11–12 in Ontario, Table 4.1 of Anderson and May [1]). Because contact rates are in the numerator of expressions for $\Re_0$, these observations also are consistent with Hethcote's and van Ark's [20] belief that contact rates in urban areas are at most twice those in rural ones.

3.2 *Mechanistic Modeling*

The sum of squared differences between predictions of our optimized model and laboratory-confirmed case reports, $R^2 \approx 0.67$ (Fig. 5). Modeled and observed outbreaks are roughly concordant, with disease spreading from young adults to children (and thence other ages). But incidence among older people is less accurately predicted than among younger ones, and the observed outbreak was more explosive than predicted. These disparities may be due to our stratification on age alone and use

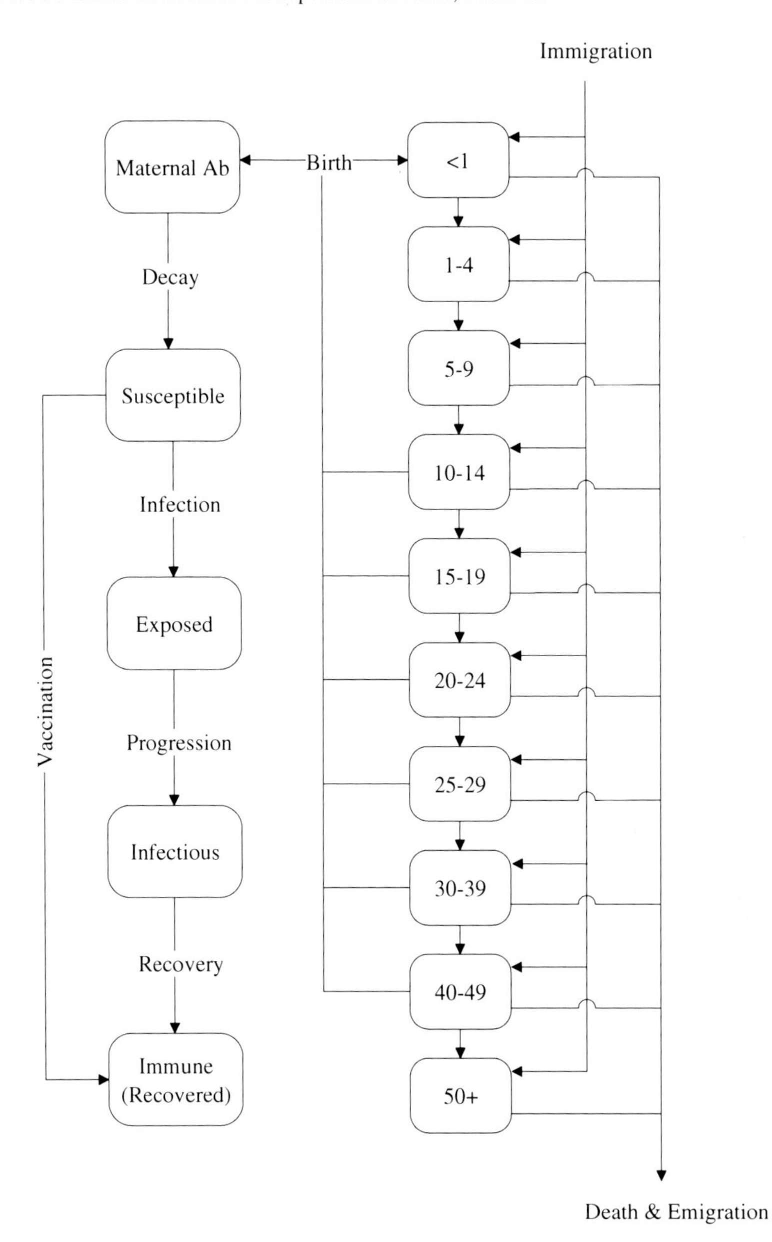

Fig. 3 Five epidemiological and 10 demographic states and processes by which individuals move among them simultaneously at constant or age-specific rates that are conventional medical wisdom [21] or were estimated from observations in São Paulo, Brazil, or fitted to reported laboratory-confirmed cases

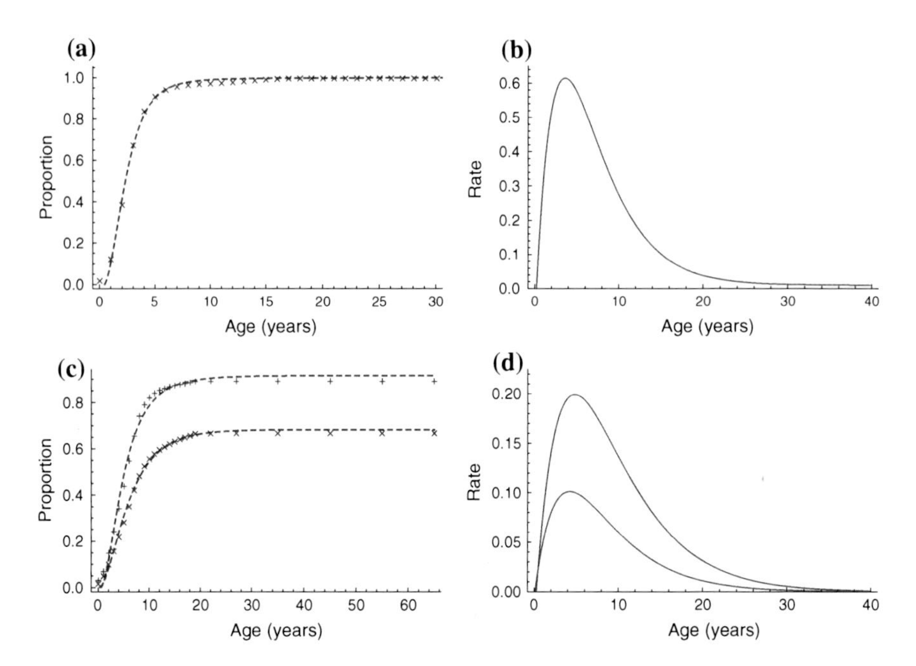

Fig. 4 **a** 1 January 1985 cross-section through Fig. 1 and **b** risks of infection deduced from Farrington's [13] catalytic model with $w = 0.52$, $x = 0.29$, $y = 0.12$, and $z = 0.01$. Figures **c** and **d** illustrate risks of infection estimated similarly from histories of measles in Baltimore and rural Maryland from 1908–1917 [12]. In these models, $z \approx 0$; other parameters are $w = 0.13$, $x = 0.22$, and $y = 0.03$ in Baltimore and $w = 0.07$, $x = 0.24$, and $y = 0.01$ in rural Maryland

of constant versus time-varying immigration rates. Compared to residents, recent immigrants of any age are more likely to be concentrated via crowded housing, public transportation, or limited sites of employment for unskilled and semi-skilled workers. However, these differences could not be quantified with resources available immediately after this outbreak.

With routine age-appropriate vaccination, but without an emergency campaign reaching 80 % of 1–4 year old children, our age-stratified model with constant rates predicts 77 % more cases than reported (Fig. 6a and Table 1). With a hypothetical 1996 *follow-up* campaign, it predicts 98 % fewer cases (Fig. 6c and Table 1), not however including adolescents 10–14 years and older who might have seeded future outbreaks. Finally, our model predicts that vaccinating 70 % of adolescents and young adults via the immigrant age-distribution would have prevented 92 % of the remaining cases (Fig. 6d and Table 1), whereupon the predicted outbreak would have been barely perceptible. Thus, together with PAHO's tripartite *keep-up*, *catch-up* and *follow-up* strategy, supplemental vaccination of immigrants would prevent future outbreaks.

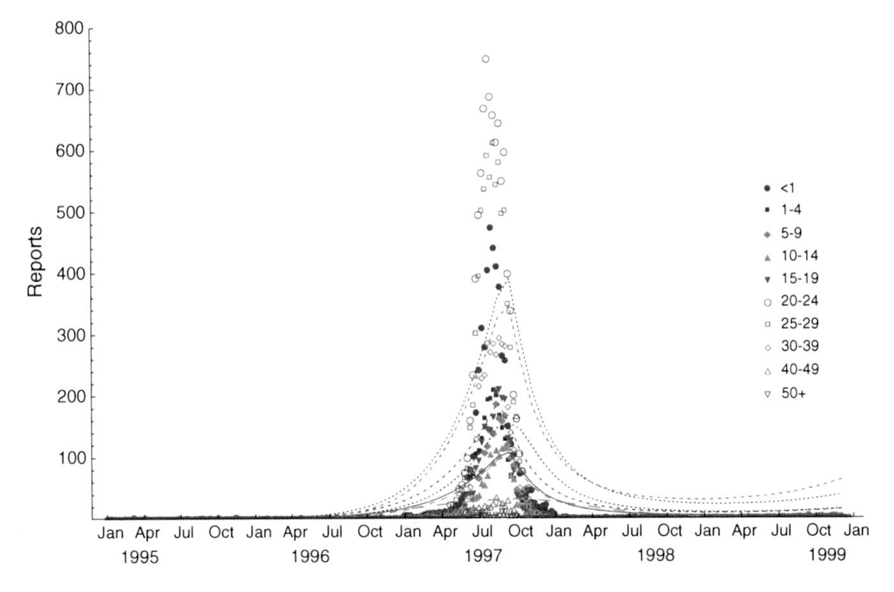

Fig. 5 Observed (*symbols*) and predicted (*lines*) measles cases among infants, 1–4, 5–9, 10–14, 15–19, 20–24, 25–29, 30–39, 40–49 and 50+ year old individuals from the first week of 1995 through last week of 1998 in São Paulo, Brazil, given a routine two-dose vaccination program and emergency mass campaign. *Line* and *symbol colors* correspond

4 Discussion

Based on historical serological and migration surveys, together with a contemporary drought and crop failures in the northeast, we hypothesized that the 1997 outbreak of measles in São Paulo resulted from the confluence of two processes—accumulation of susceptible children and influx of susceptible adolescent and young adult immigrants—only the first anticipated by current vaccination policy. We made a mathematical model capable of reproducing this phenomenon and experimented with it to deduce the impact of actual and hypothetical interventions.

4.1 Policy Implications

Our model explains roughly two-thirds of the temporal variation in case reports, particularly among younger people, with predicted and observed epidemics differing notably in explosiveness (Fig. 5). We attribute this disparity to the differential concentration of recent immigrants in favelas (i.e., peripheral shantytowns), unskilled

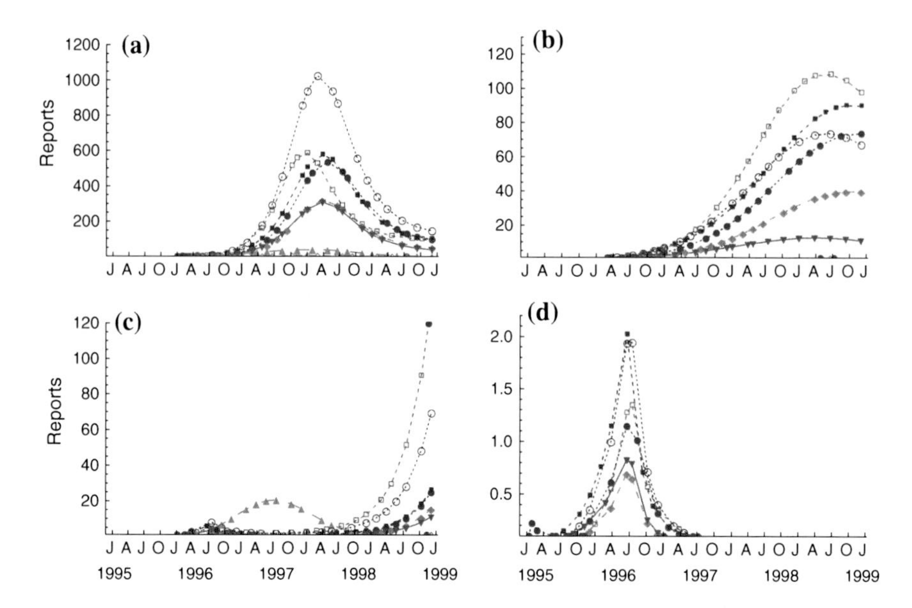

Fig. 6 Predicted cases under four hypothetical scenarios, *left* to *right* and *top* to *bottom*: **a** with routine age-appropriate vaccination alone; **b** averted by outbreak control efforts (i.e., difference between routine vaccination with and without outbreak control efforts); **c** would not have been averted by follow-up of children aged 1–4 years during 1996 (i.e., difference between routine vaccination with and without follow-up); **d** would not have been averted by a supplemental program having the age distribution of recent immigrants (i.e., difference between routine and follow-up with and without supplemental immunization). Ordinates differ markedly. Symbols as in Fig. 5

and semiskilled occupations (e.g., agriculture and construction, respectively), and on public transportation. Modeling migration among, and differential concentration within rural, urban and recent immigrant sub-populations, phenomena whose relevance this outbreak indicates (see Chap. 12), would have required information that was not available.

Our model indicates that the emergency mass campaign effectively controlled the 1997 measles outbreak in São Paulo, which the recommended *follow-up* campaign would have even more effectively mitigated, but not prevented (Table 1). This may be counter-intuitive insofar as these interventions were and would have been, respectively, directed at children 6–59 months of age, whereas roughly half of the cases occurred among adults 20–29 years old. Children are more active than adults, and school-aged ones have more contacts, particularly with classmates, but also siblings [18]. Moreover, children have relatively poor personal hygiene (e.g., are more likely to wipe their noses on their hands and cough in each other's faces than adults).

Table 1 Simulated scenarios, cases of measles in São Paulo, 1995–1999

Scenario	Age groups										Cases
	<1	1–4	5–9	10–14	15–19	20–24	25–29	30–39	40–49	50+	
Actual	6,161	6,303	3,448	2,261	3,759	13,433	12,306	114	0	0	47,786
Routine	32,506	35,467	19,262	3,404	18,900	62,156	34,509	318	1	0	206,522
Plus campaigns	247	281	136	1,501	184	542	581	5	0	0	3,477
Plus supplemental	2,732	3,744	1,565	24	835	3,834	5,093	46	0	0	17,874
Plus both	49	66	24	2	30	67	47	0	0	0	285

Actual: routine plus outbreak-control campaign
Routine: doses at 9 and 15 months
Campaigns: children aged 6–59 months
Supplemental: people having the age-distribution of immigrants (Fig. 2b)

Because the number and intimacy of contacts affect disease transmission, children are super-spreaders [24]. These interventions were and would have been effective, respectively, because they reduced, and might even have eliminated this source.

Were most susceptible adolescents and young adults longtime residents, increased second dose coverage or extension of the upper age of *follow-up* campaigns (as in 1992, albeit to *catch-up* older children for the inclusion of rubella among routine vaccinations) would be indicated. If immigrants, the immunity of rural children must be increased or adolescents and young adults must be vaccinated upon arrival. The latter approach has proven effective in São Paulo; for example, health authorities prevented urban yellow fever, epidemic in rural areas, by vaccinating in bus stations and airports. Many immigrants lack technical skills, narrowing the scope of their economic opportunities, but facilitating access to them for vaccination in workplaces. Similarly, the concentration of immigrant families in favelas also facilitates access via community outreach.

Neither of the processes that produced the susceptible adolescents and young adults in this outbreak is unique to São Paulo in 1997. Vaccination not only protects recipients, but others whom they might have infected had they become infectious, an indirect effect popularly called herd immunity [16]. Unvaccinated people who escape infection, at least temporarily, accompany all vaccination programs with gradually increasing coverage, and may cause future problems (e.g., congenital rubella syndrome). Internal migration is another potential source of susceptible people. Its magnitude depends on characteristics of urban centers and their rural environs, between which economic disparities are increasing, especially where measles remains a major source of morbidity and mortality.

4.2 Reflections

PAHO's *keep-up* and *follow-up* strategies may have been successful in part because routine age-appropriate vaccination and mass campaigns are complementary. Campaigns reach children who are not receiving routine care or whose immune systems did not respond to vaccination. But PAHO's *catch-up* campaigns are designed to reach children who are too old to have been vaccinated, but who escaped infection by virtue of the immunization of others. Their target does not include the older adolescents, much less the young adults who immigrated to São Paulo during 1997.

The 1997 measles outbreak in São Paulo identified a source of susceptible people that is not unique to that time or place. Internal migration must be considered in designing regional vaccination strategies to ensure that the ever increasing urbanization of the developing world does not impede measles eradication.

Because of rural-urban migration, this was not a prototypical post-honeymoon outbreak [7, 26]. Under these circumstances, the optimum strategy for urban policy-makers depends on socio-demographic and epidemiological characteristics of rural populations (and, possibly, vice versa). Health authorities in São Paulo State could vaccinate migrants or rural inhabitants. Should migrants contribute to outbreaks elsewhere in Latin America (see, e.g., PAHO [28]), not to mention the increasingly urbanized developing world, successful measles eradication will depend on policy-makers adopting such regional versus local perspectives.

4.3 Further Modeling

We attribute the explosiveness of this outbreak to the concentration of recent immigrants, via residing in favelas and traveling to and from common workplaces in crowded conveyances for examples, but modeled none of those phenomena. A model of São Paulo State as loosely coupled rural, urban and possibly recent immigrant subsystems beginning in the mid-1980s would improve our understanding of movement among and differential concentration within populations differing in other relevant characteristics (see Chap. 12).

The utility of supplemental immunization activities is better appreciated nowadays. Rural adolescents and young adults will migrate to urban areas in search of greater economic opportunities, particularly during droughts, and be concentrated via marginal housing, public transportation and limited occupations for unskilled and semi-skilled workers, not just in Latin America. Together, these phenomena can lead to outbreaks of vaccine-preventable diseases that may be best averted by vaccinating immigrants.

To ensure that the ever increasing urbanization of the developing world does not impede measles eradication, the development of more realistic models with which to explore regional vaccination strategies is warranted.

Acknowledgments We are grateful to Betsy Cadwell, Mary McCauley, Ciro de Quadros, Peter Strebel and Jacco Wallinga for discussions of this work and to Jim Alexander, Jim Goodson, Chris Gregory and Aaron Curns for comments on earlier drafts of this manuscript.

Appendix

Table A.2 Unpublished metropolitan São Paulo serological surveys included, together with that reported by Pannuti et al. [29], in the synthesis illustrated in Fig. 1

Age	1992		1993		1994		1998	
	Sera	N(+)	Sera	N(+)	Sera	N(+)	Sera	N(+)
0					63	36		
1	200	196	165	164	171	166		
2	197	193	220	219	160	158		
3	219	214	205	199	148	148		
4	223	218	152	151	80	79		
5	192	190	248	244	176	172		
6	209	205	155	155	143	140		
7	209	201	137	134	50	50		
8	207	201						
9	217	213						
10	186	181						
11			188	168	166	164		
12			202	192	195	193		
13			180	172	193	190		
14			161	157	123	123		
15							15	15
16							21	20
17							22	22
18							24	23
19							19	18
20							17	17
21							30	29
22							64	59
23							50	49
24							38	37
25							30	29
26							46	43
27							43	41
28							47	46
29							42	41
Totals	2059		2013		1668		508	

Massad et al. [25] describe the methodology for the 1992 and 1993 surveys. In 1994, the 50 individuals in the 7-year row were 7–10 years of age. The 1998 survey was among controls in the study conducted during the outbreak to determine risk factors for disease [4], explaining the apparent lack of susceptible adults

Table A.3 Initial conditions ($t = 0$ is 1 January 1995) and parameters estimated from observations in São Paulo, Brazil, via standard demographic methods

Age	$N_i(0)$	$S_i(0)$	$Pr(i, ♀)$	f_i	μ_i	δ_i
<1	300,240	174,889	0.4806	0	0.01969	3.089
1–4	1,193,592	89,723	0.4849	0	0.00089	26.395
5–9	1,545,968	27,996	0.4901	0	0.00033	24.439
10–14	1,584,251	196,327	0.496	0.00239	0.0005	8.536
15–19	1,593,181	238,337	0.5055	0.07978	0.00172	2.541
20–24	1,553,289	152	0.5088	0.13509	0.00265	1.984
25–29	1,481,538	0	0.5095	0.12486	0.00285	2.171
30–39	2,664,412	0	0.5006	0.06405	0.00346	2.973
40–49	1,947,447	0	0.5206	0.00613	0.00538	5.444
50+	2,755,566	0	0.5476	0	0.04746	3.177

Age-specific population numbers, $N_i(0)$, were back calculated from the 1997 census, children per mother, f_i, and overall death rates, μ_i, that year. Susceptible numbers, $S_i(0)$, were derived from them and proportions susceptible (Fig. 1). Factors by which disease transiently increases the death rates, δ_i, were derived from age-specific probabilities of dying from measles and all causes, estimated from μ_i via a conventional abridged life table. All-cause probabilities were adjusted to 30 days, the period during which deaths were attributed to measles, assuming constancy within age classes

Table A.4 Estimated average annual numbers of immigrants and emigrants by age, 1992–1995, from which the age-specific *per capita* immigration, ι_i, and emigration rates, o_i, were derived (Brazilian Institute of Geography and Statistics)

Age group	Immigrants	Emigrants	Net
<1	13,997	20,237	−6,240
1–4	49,914	48,326	1,587
5–9	78,194	66,608	11,586
10–14	80,639	69,295	11,343
15–20	68,195	63,083	5,112
20–24	51,341	53,106	−1,766
25–29	35,805	42,464	−6,660
30–39	23,653	32,739	−9,086
40–49	15,006	24,564	−9,558
50+	9,227	18,047	−8,819
Totals	425,970	438,470	−12,500

References

1. Anderson, R.M., May, R.M.: Infectious Diseases of Humans, Dynamics and Control. Oxford Univ Press, Oxford (1991)
2. Bartlett, M.S.: Measles periodicity and community size. J. R. Stat. Assoc. **A120**, 48–70 (1957)
3. Brazilian, Chilean, Costa Rican, and Ecuadorian Ministries of Health and Pan American Health Organization. Seroconversion rates and measles antibody titers induced by measles vaccine in Latin American children 6–12 months of age. Bull World Health Organ **16**, 272–285 (1982)
4. Camargo, M.C.C., de Moraes, J.C., Souza, V.A.U.F., Matos, M.R., Pannuti, C.S.: Predictors related to the occurrence of a measles epidemic in the city of São Paulo in 1997. Rev. Panam. Salud Publica **7**, 359–365 (2000)
5. Castillo-Solorzano, C.C., Matus, C.R., Flannery, B., Marsigli, C., Tambini, G., Andrus, J.K.: The Americas: paving the road toward global measles eradication. J. Infect. Dis. **204**(Suppl 1), S270–S278 (2011)
6. Centers for Disease Control and Prevention. Progress toward elimination of measles from the Americas. MMWR Morb. Mortal. Wkly. Rep. **47**, 189–193 (1998)
7. Chen, R.T., Weierbach, R., Bisoffi, Z., Cutts, F., Rhodes, P., Ramaroson, S., Ntembagara, C., Bizimana, F.: A 'post-honeymoon period' measles outbreak in Muyinga sector. Burundi. Int. J. Epidemiol. **23**, 185–193 (1994)
8. Dedecca, C.S., Pinto da Cunha, J.M.: Migration, employment and income in the 90s: the case of the metropolitan region of São Paulo. R. Bras. Est. Pop. Campinas **21**, 49–66 (2004)
9. de Jong, M.C.M., Diekmann, O., Heesterbeek, H.: How does transmission of infection depend on population size? In: Mollison, D. (ed.) Epidemic Models, their Structure and Relation to Data, pp. 84–94. Cambridge Univ Press, Cambridge (1995)
10. de Moraes, J.C., Barata, R.C.B., Ribeiro, M.C.S.A., de Castro, P.C.: Immunization coverage in the first year of life in four cities of the State of São Paulo. Brazil. Rev. Panam. Salud Publica **8**, 332–341 (2000)
11. de Quadros, C.A., Olive, J.-M., Hersh, B.S., Strassburg, M.A., Henderson, D.A., Brandling-Bennett, D., Alleyne, G.A.O.: Measles elimination in the Americas; evolving strategies. JAMA **275**, 224–29 (1996)
12. Fales, W.T.: The age-distribution of whooping cough, measles, chicken-pox, scarlet fever, and diphtheria in various areas of the United States. Am. J. Hyg. Public Health **8**, 759–799 (1928)
13. Farrington, C.P.: Modeling risks of infection for measles, mumps and rubella. Stat. Med. **9**, 953–967 (1990)
14. Ferguson, N.M., Nokes, D.J., Anderson, R.M.: Dynamical complexity in age structured models of the transmission of the measles virus: epidemiological implications at high levels of vaccine uptake. Math. Biosci. **138**, 101–130 (1996)
15. Fine, P.E., Clarkson, J.A.: Measles in England and Wales I: an analysis of factors underlying seasonal patterns. Int. J. Epidemiol. **11**, 5–14 (1982)
16. Fine, P., Eames, K., Heymann, D.L.: "Herd Immunity": a rough guide. Clin. Infect. Dis. **52**, 911–916 (2011)
17. Francis, B., Green, M., Payne, C.: The GLIM System: Generalized Interactive Linear Modeling. Oxford Univ Press, Oxford (1993)
18. Glasser, J.W., Feng, Z., Moylan, A., Del Valle, S., Castillo-Chavez, C.C.: Mixing in cross-classified population models of infectious diseases. Math. Biosci. **235**, 1–7 (2012)
19. Hethcote, H.W.: Modeling heterogeneous mixing in infectious disease dynamics. In: Isham, V., Medley, G. (eds.) Models for Infectious Human Diseases, their Structure and Relation to Data, pp. 215–237. Cambridge Univ Press, Cambridge (1996)
20. Hethcote, H.W., van Ark, J.W.: Epidemiological models for heterogeneous populations: proportionate mixing, parameter estimation and immunization programs. Math. Biosci. **84**, 85–118 (1987)
21. Heymann, D.L.: Control of Communicable Diseases Manual, 20th edn. American Public Health Association, Washington, DC (2014)

22. Jacquez, J.A., Simon, C.P., Koopman, J., Sattenspiel, L., Perry, T.: Modeling and analyzing HIV transmission: the effect of contact patterns. Math. Biosci. **92**, 119–199 (1988)
23. John, A.M.: Transmission and control of childhood infectious diseases: does demography matter? Popul. Stud. **44**, 195–215 (1990)
24. Lloyd-Smith, J.O., Schreiber, S.J., Kopp, P.E., Getz, W.M.: Superspreading and the effect of individual variation on disease emergence. Nature **438**, 355–59 (2005)
25. Massad, E., Azevedo Neto, R.S., Burattini, M.N., Zanetta, D.M.T., Coutinho, F.A.B., Yang, H.M., Moraes, J.C., Pannutti, C.S., Souza, V.A.U.F., Silveira, A.S.B., Struchiner, C.J., Oselka, G.W., Camargo, M.C.C., Omoto, T.M., Passos, S.D.: Assessing the efficacy of a mixed vaccination strategy against rubella in São Paulo, Brazil. Int. J. Epidemiol. **24**, 842–850 (1995)
26. Mulholland, K.: Measles and pertussis in developing countries with good vaccine coverage. Lancet **345**, 305–7 (1995)
27. Nold, A.: Heterogeneity in disease transmission modeling. Math. Biosci. **124**, 59–82 (1980)
28. PAHO: Update: measles outbreak in Bolivia. EPI Newsl. 21, 1–3 (1999)
29. Pannuti, C.S., Moraes, J.C., Souza, V.A.U.F., Camargo, M.C.C., Hidalgo, N.T.R., Brito, G.S., Almeida, M.M., Vilela, M.F.G., Paula, M.C.M.G., Cristiano, E.L.V.C., Stefano, I.C.A., Sato, H.K.: Measles antibody prevalence after mass vaccination in São Paulo. Brazil. Bull. World Health Organ. **69**, 557–560 (1991)

Methods to Determine the End of an Infectious Disease Epidemic: A Short Review

Hiroshi Nishiura

Abstract Deciding the end of an epidemic is frequently associated with forthcoming changes in infectious disease control activities, including downgrading alert level in surveillance and restoring healthcare workers' working shift back to normal. Despite the practical importance, there have been little epidemiological and laboratory methods that were proposed to determine the end of an epidemic. This short review was aimed to systematically discuss methodological principles of a small number of existing techniques and understand their advantages and disadvantages. Existing epidemiological methods have been mostly limited to a single-and-brief exposure setting, while the application to human-to-human transmissible disease epidemic with stochastic dependence structure in the observed case data has remained to be a statistical challenge. In veterinary applications, a large-scale sampling for laboratory testing has been commonly adapted to substantiate a freedom from disease, but such study has only accounted for binomial sampling process in estimating the error probability of elimination. Surveillance and mathematical modeling are two complementary instruments in the toolbox of epidemiologists. Combining their strengths would be highly beneficial to better define the end of an epidemic.

Keywords Epidemic · Ebola · Epidemic elimination · Incubation period · Exposure · Polio · Heuristic method

1 Prologue

Rather than declaring the start of an epidemic, it has been harder to determine the end of the epidemic. Erroneous declaration of the start might be understood as part of errors in risk assessment practice, and such an occasional error might not impose serious irreversible damage to our society. However, deciding the end of an

H. Nishiura (✉)
Hokkaido University, Kita 15 Jo Nishi 7 Chome,
Hokkaido, Kita-ku Sapporo-shi 060-8638, Japan
e-mail: nishiurah@gmail.com

G. Chowell and J.M. Hyman (eds.), *Mathematical and Statistical Modeling for Emerging and Re-emerging Infectious Diseases*,
DOI 10.1007/978-3-319-40413-4_17

epidemic is frequently associated with forthcoming changes in infectious disease control activities, and its decision imposes a pressure to epidemiologists to a certain extent. Declaring the end of an epidemic, the alert level in surveillance system may be downgraded, and working shift of medical and public health experts in charge of control practice (e.g. contact tracing effort) may also be restored [1]. In the case of the end of a vaccine preventable disease, the declaration would always lead to a discussion over the cessation of routine immunization [2]. The impact of the end of an epidemic is not limited to healthcare settings. Reduced volume of travelers may be recovered to normal due to declaration of the end of an outbreak, and thus, the declaration of safety would involve a pressure from tourism industry and have substantial impact on associated economics. In the case of an epizootic event of a veterinary disease, especially among livestock animals, the freedom from the epizootic disease indicates a permission to restart international transportation or trade of specific animals [3]. Getting along with these social and political interests, the end of an epidemic must be determined without serious errors and the announcement should be made carefully and appropriately.

Despite the importance of the determination of the end of an epidemic, there have been little available methods to explicitly judge the end of an epidemic [4]. In particular, published studies have been mostly limited to a setting with single and brief exposure, e.g. a point source outbreak of food-borne disease. While methods are scarce, there have been multiple practical events on the ground that did require explicit methodological assistance in deciding the end of an epidemic. Nevertheless, it is also true that practical side has involved a number of complications that cannot be immediately addressed by epidemiological modeling only. For instance, many epidemics have involved a substantial number of asymptomatic infections, ascertainment biases and underreporting issues. In passive surveillance, diagnosed cases are notified to the public health authority. In addition to passive information, there might be datasets based on active surveillance (e.g. case finding effort through outbreak investigation) or laboratory testing of (a part of) possible exposed individuals, but their utilities have not been taken into account in the determination of the end of an epidemic. Moreover, one may ultimately wish to judge the end of an epidemic, not using notified case data but using other informative resources such as event-based or syndromic surveillance data.

Facing these complexities in empirical observation, what can epidemiological modelers offer to the society? The purpose of this short review is to understand methodological principles of available criteria of the end of an epidemic, identifying their advantages and disadvantages. This exercise will shed light on future path of the objective judgment of the end of infectious disease epidemics.

2 Classical WHO Approach

The most stimulating practice has been seen in the adoption of classical criteria by the World Health Organization (WHO) on its definition of zero Ebola cases from 2013-15 [6]. In that criteria, the outbreak of EVD is considered ended in any one of affected

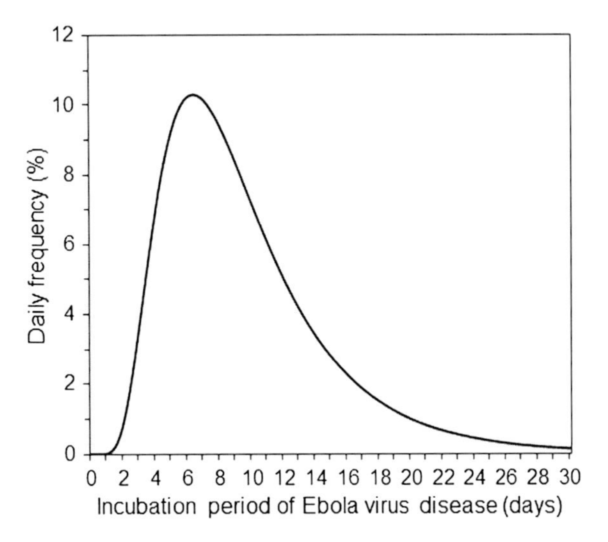

Fig. 1 *Probability density function of the incubation period of Ebola virus disease (EVD)*. The daily frequency of the incubation period, the time from infection to illness onset, for EVD is shown [5]. The mean and variance of the incubation period were assumed at 9.7 and 30.3 days^2, respectively. A lognormal distribution was employed, and parameters μ and σ were thus 2.13 and 0.53, respectively

countries (e.g. Guinea, Liberia and Sierra Leone) after 42 days have passed since the last confirmed case has tested negative twice for the virus on blood samples. Along with this criterion, it has been also suggested that, after the 42-day period has elapsed, each country should maintain a system of heightened surveillance for a further 90 days, and ensure that ongoing EVD surveillance and notification thereafter will be conducted. Moreover, it is determined that the end of the EVD outbreak in the West African sub-region will be declared when the 42-day period has elapsed in the last affected country.

The choice of 42 days stems from the right tail of the incubation period. Figure 1 shows the probability density function of the incubation period of EVD [5]. Empirically observed certain maximum of the incubation period has been 21 days. Taking a double of this empirical maximum value, 42-day waiting period has been determined. Unfortunately, there has been no additional justification of using the incubation period and taking twice the empirical maximum, but the choice of a fixed length has been very transparent to public health societies and the criteria were made easy to follow for those working on the ground in West African countries.

Incubation period is the time from infection to illness onset [7]. As long as the time of potential exposure among traced contacts is known, the incubation period could indicate the length of time to be waited to ensure that no more symptomatic case exists. Even provided that the time of potential exposure is not directly observed, the use of the latest time at which an exposure could have occurred (e.g. the last date of PCR positive outcome in the last confirmed case) as "clock zero" point would offer a conservative suggestion to ascertain the absence of additional symptomatic infections [8].

Nevertheless, despite the simple and transparent fixed length, the classical approach suffers from a number of technical problems. First, the use of empirically observed maximum would be vulnerable to sample size of the incubation period.

Namely, the greater the sample size, the greater the observed value of maximum would be [9]. Second, it is evident that the use of the incubation period is not justified for diseases that involve substantial number of asymptomatic infections [10]. There could be unrecognized chains of transmission among asymptomatic cases. Third, due to the shortage of objectiveness, the waiting period does not directly measure the probability of the end of an epidemic. For instance, it appeared that viable Ebola virus could be maintained in semen of infected males even after recovery from convalescent phase. A number of sexual transmission events have been reported to have fueled local reemergence of EVD, but such event has never been captured by the right tail of the incubation period. As a consequence, several erroneous declarations of the end of Ebola epidemic were unfortunately observed in West Africa.

3 Single Exposure Approach

Food-borne outbreak is frequently referred to as the common source outbreak, because the causative food is mostly shared among exposed individuals. The point source outbreak is a special case of common source outbreak in that the exposure is very brief in time (e.g. sharing an identical party lunch menu on the same day). The point source outbreak has been well studied by statisticians, because the resulting epidemic curve can be assumed as identical to the density function of the incubation period (Fig. 2), permitting us to estimate the time of exposure and analyze a variety of statistical features of that distribution.

Determination of the end of point source outbreak is perhaps the most well studied statistical subject in the context of the end of outbreak. Figure 2 shows the typical

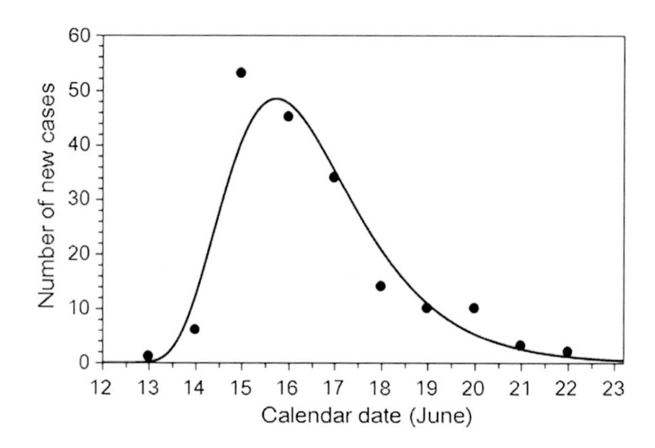

Fig. 2 *Fitting a three-parameter log-normal distribution to the epidemic curve of Salmonellosis in Gifu prefecture, Japan, 2003.* An outbreak of food-borne Salmonellosis was observed in Gifu prefecture involving a total of 178 cases [7]. A three-parameter log-normal distribution includes not only μ and σ but a threshold parameter that determines the time at which an exposure occurred

epidemic curve of food-borne outbreak, caused by Salmonellosis in Gifu, Japan, 2003. To capture the epidemic pattern, one can fit the following three-parameter log-normal distribution:

$$f(t;\gamma,\mu,\sigma^2)=\frac{1}{(t-\gamma)\sigma\sqrt{2\pi}}\exp\left(\frac{-(\ln(t-\gamma)-\mu)^2}{2\sigma^2}\right), \tag{1}$$

for $t-\gamma>0$, where t is the calendar time and γ is the so-called threshold parameter indicating the time at which an exposure occurred. In the Gifu outbreak example, the maximum likelihood estimate of γ was 11.7 on the calendar time scale in June 2003, indicating that the most likely brief exposure may have happened at lunch or dinner on 11 June. In many food-borne outbreaks, food traceback effort during the outbreak investigation involves a serious problem of recall bias. However, employing the model (1), one could dramatically narrow down the scope of food menus to be recalled [7].

In addition to estimating the time of exposure, one can subsequently assess the right tail in detail, because the percentile of the incubation period distribution directly indicates the proportion of cases that we have already observed by a given calendar time. Brookmeyer and You [4] have exploited this knowledge to develop a hypothesis testing method. Suppose that the total outbreak size is N among which we have already observed n cases. We have the ordered calendar time of disease onset of cases, $y_1,\ldots,y_n$ and suppose that T days have passed since the last case (y_n) occurred. The hypotheses are $H_0: N>n$ versus $H_1: N=n$.

For the hypothesis testing, we consider the jth spacing $s_j=y_{j+1}-y_j$. Assuming that the incubation period follows a two-parameter exponential model with a guarantee time G, i.e., $f(u)=\lambda\exp(-\lambda(u-G))$ for $u>G$ and 0 for $u<G$, jth spacing arising from a sample size of N from the two parameter exponential model also has an exponential distribution with parameter $\lambda(N-j)$, and thus, the density function of the spacing is

$$f(s_j)=\lambda(N-j)\exp(-\lambda(N-j)s_j). \tag{2}$$

The probability that the nth spacing is greater than t days is

$$\Pr(s_n>t)=\exp(-\lambda(N-n)t) \tag{3}$$

Let α be the level of significance test. The length of waiting time t is set such that the Eq. (3) is equal to α at the particular null hypothesis when $N=n+1$. Then, we obtain

$$T\geq-\frac{1}{\lambda}\ln(\alpha) \tag{4}$$

In general for any $N>n$, the probability of rejecting H_0 is

$$\Pr\left(s_n \geq -\frac{1}{\lambda}\ln(\alpha)\right) = \alpha^{(N-n)} \tag{5}$$

While the method is statistically very solid, the range of direct application is unfortunately limited to the point source outbreak. Moreover, the application is justified only when all of infected individuals develop symptoms and all cases are reported. Despite these problems, the proposed method is maintained very simple and can be implemented in some other settings with a little extensions, especially when the spacing of a single distribution can be applied.

4 Laboratory Testing to Ensure the Absence of Cases

In veterinary epidemiological practice, a mass laboratory testing may be more easily implemented than in human population. Due to economic interest to urge the government to be acknowledged as being free from a specific disease and resume trade, the cost that is required for laboratory testing may be justified well. Obtaining laboratory samples even from a part of the population, the following assessment would be feasible.

Suppose that we have a perfect laboratory test and we handle infinitely large population of animals. The probability of selecting a given number of positives when randomly selecting n animals from a population with disease prevalence p is given by the binomial distribution [11]:

$$\Pr(X = x) = \binom{n}{x} p^x (1 - p)^{(n-x)} \tag{6}$$

Using the perfect test (i.e. with 100 % sensitivity and 100 % specificity), an epidemiological survey to substantiate freedom from disease requires that no positives are found. When $x = 0$, the Eq. (6) simplifies to:

$$\Pr(X = 0) = (1 - p)^n \tag{7}$$

Even in the case that we should consider imperfect laboratory testing, the abovementioned scheme can be easily extended [11]. The probability of observing x positive animals when testing n animals from an infinite population is given by the binomial distribution:

$$\Pr(X = x) = \binom{n}{x} (p\mathrm{Se} + (1 - p)(1 - \mathrm{Sp}))^x \, (p(1 - \mathrm{Se}) + (1 - p)\mathrm{Sp})^{(n-x)}, \tag{8}$$

Of course, the Eq. (8) is followed by the same argument in (7) to calculate the probability that substantiates freedom from disease. That equation or the Eq. (7)

would help veterinary epidemiologist to determine the minimum sample size of laboratory testing.

The abovementioned model is kept very simple. However, the method heavily relies on laboratory testing performance and sampling effort. As an important remark about the sampling, considering that clustering is common for directly transmitted infectious diseases, it is hard to truly achieve a random sampling. Another technical issue is that the prevalence is assumed to be a constant, and thus, the stationarity is inherently assumed. For the similar reason, it is quite unfortunate that the error probability of elimination is only based on binomial sampling error (without accounting for stochastic dependence structure in empirical data of cases). Despite these problems, it is worth noting that the use of laboratory testing can overcome the problem of involving asymptomatic infections.

5 An Explicit Method for Multiple Exposure Setting

Epidemiological methods to determine the end of an epidemic in the presence of multiple exposures (and thus, involving stochastic dependence structure) are very scarce. This might be attributable to a difficulty in capturing the complex epidemic dynamics using simple equations in the presence of human-to-human transmissions.

An exceptionally careful pioneering study in this context was conducted by Eichner and Dietz [12] on poliomyelitis. Polio virus infection involves a substantial number of asymptomatic infections, and it is believed that only one paralytic case would occur among a total of 200 infections in naive host. Besides, because polio eradication program is underway due to effective vaccines and routine immunization programs, the so-called endgame of polio has called for a solid method to determine the local elimination of polio.

In principle, a stochastic compartmental model was employed for simulations, and Eichner and Dietz examined the probability that silent infections are underway as a function of time since the observation of last paralytic case [12]. Using the Markov jump process and simulating from the endemic equilibrium, the probability of silent infections as a function of the time since the last paralytic case, as shown in Fig. 3, was obtained. Examining realistic range of the frequency of paralytic case, ranging from one among 300 infections to 100 infections, Fig. 3 indicated that the probability of silent infections would be less than 1 % if 5 years is secured as the waiting time since the last paralytic case.

Fitting the stochastic model to empirically observed epidemiological data would be perhaps the most straightforward method to estimate the probability of extinction (and thus, the probability that the epidemic is still going on). Such model could also have a potential to be fitted to the dataset both with and without case finding efforts on the ground. Nevertheless, in practice, it is extremely difficult to fit such a stochastic model to a portion of epidemic data. That is, fitting to the latest data only would force us to focus on a chopped epidemic curve (with unknown infection-age structure) and the determination of the end of epidemic without fully realizing the

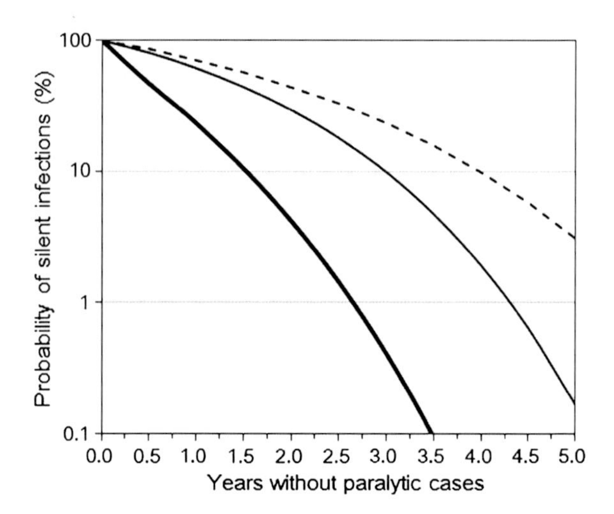

Fig. 3 *Probability of silent infection as a function of time since the last paralytic polio case.* Probability that silent infections still occur when no paralytic polio cases have been observed for a given period of time is shown [12]. The figure was reproduced by the author with reference to methods of Eichner and Dietz [12] for the scenario in which IPV (inactivated polio vaccine) was employed with the 80 % vaccination coverage. One case per 100 infections (*bold line*), one case per 200 infections (*solid line*), and one case per 300 infections (*dashed line*) were assumed

epidemiological dynamics might be too challenging. In fact, Fig. 3 is the result from simulations starting with a boundary condition and is not the time from the actual latest observation.

6 A Heuristic Method for Multiple Exposure Setting

The last approach to be reviewed is a heuristic approach in the presence of stochastic dependence structure with an application to the Middle East respiratory syndrome (MERS) in the Republic of Korea [1]. Not involving any additional cases of MERS for several weeks in the South Korea, the government and the WHO discussed an appropriate timing to declare the end of the outbreak. As discussed in the second section, a widely acknowledged criteria of the WHO to decide the end of an epidemic has been to ensure no further report of cases, setting twice the long incubation period (i.e. 14 days for MERS) as the standard waiting period since the latest date of diagnosis or recovery. Adopting 28 days as the waiting time and count days from 4 July, the date on which the latest case was diagnosed, the earliest date that Korean government could have declared the end of outbreak was 2 August adhering to the WHO criteria. If we count the days from the last PCR positive date, the date of declaration would even have been in late December 2015. Nevertheless, to emphasize the safety to the nation as well as forthcoming international travelers at an earlier time, the Korean government made an original decision to announce the end of MERS outbreak on 27 July due to the fact that the last quarantined case was freed from movement restriction. To judge the appropriateness of these decisions, the probability of observing additional cases as a function of calendar time was explicitly calculated and such objective judgment was compared against that based on the WHO criteria.

The probability of observing additional cases was derived, using the serial interval, i.e. the time from illness onset in a primary case to illness onset in the secondary case, and the transmissibility of MERS. Let $F(t)$ be the cumulative distribution function of the serial interval. If time t is elapsed since the last case and provided that the last case were able to produce only one secondary case, the probability that at least one additional case is observed at time t since the illness onset of last case would be $1 - F(t)$. To address the potential of observing multiple secondary transmissions produced by a single primary case, we use the offspring distribution $p_y = \Pr(Y = y)$. Then, the risk of observing at least one additional case at time t since the illness onset of primary case is

$$\Pr(X \geq 1) = 1 - \sum_{y=0}^{\infty} p_y F(t)^y \tag{9}$$

Using the dataset of t_i, the calendar date of illness onset of diagnosed cases i ($i = 0, 1, \ldots, 185$), the probability of observing additional cases in future at calendar date t is calculated as

$$\Pr(X \geq 1) = 1 - \prod_{i=1}^{185} \sum_{y=0}^{\infty} p_y F(t - t_i)^y \tag{10}$$

It should be noted that the Eq. (10) does not manually subtract all existing secondary transmissions from the model, despite the fact that the observed cases have already generated a part of secondary cases that they have been supposed to cause. For that reason, the probability that is derived from the Eq. (10) may be slightly an overestimate.

As practiced in the determination of the length of quarantine [8, 10], one can declare the end of outbreak if that probability is smaller than 5 %, a threshold value. Our analysis showed that the first date on which the posterior median probability decreased to less than 5 % was 21 July (Fig. 4). The first date on which the posterior median lowered 1 % was 23 July. Namely, compared with 2 August as calculated from the WHO criteria, the declaration date of the end of outbreak could have been 11 and 9 days earlier, respectively.

The calculated probability is interpreted as the risk of observing at least one more case on or after a specified date and has a good potential to assist objective determination of the end of outbreak. The model efficiently addressed three practical problems in objectively calculating the probability that an outbreak leads to the end: (i) multiple cases on the same date, (ii) several recent cases with different illness

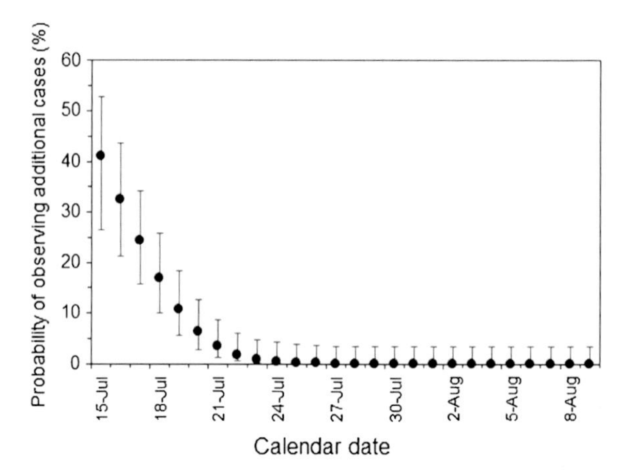

Fig. 4 *Estimated probability of observing additional cases of the Middle East respiratory syndrome coronavirus infection in the Republic of Korea, 2015.* Probability of observing additional cases on each calendar date, given no illness onset has been observed, is calculated [1]. *Circles* represent posterior median values that were calculated from resampled parameters governing the offspring distribution and serial interval. Whiskers extend to upper and lower 95 % credible intervals

onset dates, and (iii) variations in the number of secondary cases generated by a single primary case.

Of course, missing undiagnosed or mild cases is not taken into account in this method, and under-diagnosis would considerably extend the time to declare the end of outbreak (and thus, the proposed method is not directly applicable to EVD in West Africa to which we are presently developing an alternative method), all possible contact of diagnosed cases in the late phase of MERS outbreak in Korea were all traced, and thus, it was appropriate to ignore ascertainment bias in this specific setting. Important limitations include (i) the absence of dependence between serial interval and offspring distribution (as long as the two were estimated separately from independent datasets) and (ii) need to infer the offspring distribution precisely, perhaps requiring us to analyze contact tracing data or outbreak size distribution.

7 Conclusions

Epidemiological and laboratory methods of ascertaining the end of an epidemic were reviewed. To declare the end of an epidemic, it has been shown that multitude of methods might be used in combination with or without case finding efforts and biological samples for laboratory testing. To achieve this task, it is evident that surveillance and mathematical modeling are two complementary instruments in the toolbox of epidemiologists. Combining their strengths would be highly beneficial to better define the end of an epidemic so that necessary public health actions can be taken properly.

Lastly, it is inevitable that the decision for declaring the end of an epidemic is highly politicized, and thus, the final decision must not solely be based on mathematical modeling results alone. Nevertheless, offering scientific evidence would make a big difference in epidemiological capacity and definitely ease the decision by policymakers. Ideally, there should be regular opportunity for modeling experts and policymakers to sit together to work on and discuss this matter.

Acknowledgments HN received funding support from the Japan Society for the Promotion of Science (JSPS) KAKENHI Grant Numbers 16K15356 and 26700028, Japan Agency for Medical Research and Development, the Japan Science and Technology Agency (JST) CREST program and RISTEX program for Science of Science, Technology and Innovation Policy. The funders had no role in study design, data collection and analysis, decision to publish, or preparation of the manuscript.

References

1. Nishiura, H., Miyamatsu, Y., Mizumoto, K.: Objective determination of end of MERS outbreak, South Korea, 2015. Emerg. Infect. Dis. **22**, 146–148 (2016)
2. Arita, I., Wickett, J., Nakane, M.: Eradication of infectious diseases: its concept, then and now. Jpn. J. Infect. Dis. **57**, 1–6 (2004)
3. Greiner, M., Dekker, A.: On the surveillance for animal diseases in small herds. Prev. Vet. Med. **70**, 223–234 (2005)
4. Brookmeyer, R., You, X.: A hypothesis test for the end of a common source outbreak. Biometrics **62**, 61–65 (2006)
5. Ebola virus disease in West Africa: The first 9 months of the epidemic and forward projections. N. Engl. J. Med. **371**, 1481–1495 (2014)
6. World Health Organization: Definition of zero Ebola cases, World Health Organization: Geneva (2014). http://www.who.int/csr/disease/ebola/declaration-ebola-end/en/
7. Nishiura, H.: Early efforts in modeling the incubation period of infectious diseases with an acute course of illness. Emerg. Themes. Epidemiol. **4**, 2 (2007)
8. Nishiura, H.: Determination of the appropriate quarantine period following smallpox exposure: an objective approach using the incubation period distribution. Int. J. Hyg. Environ. Health. **212**, 97–104 (2009)
9. Farewell, V.T., Herzberg, A.M., James, K.W., Ho, L.M., Leung, M.: SARS incubation and quarantine times: when is an exposed individual known to be disease free? Stat. Med. **24**, 3431–3445 (2005)
10. Nishiura, H., Wilson, N., Baker, M.G.: Quarantine for pandemic influenza control at the borders of small island nations. BMC Infect. Dis. **9**, 27 (2009)
11. Cameron, A.R., Baldock, F.C.: A new probability formula for surveys to substantiate freedom from disease. Prev. Vet. Med. **34**, 1–17 (1998)
12. Eichner, M., Dietz, K.: Eradication of poliomyelitis: when can one be sure that polio virus transmission has been terminated? Am. J. Epidemiol. **143**, 816–822 (1996)

Statistical Considerations in Infectious Disease Randomized Controlled Trials

Matthew J. Hayat

Abstract Randomized controlled trials (RCT) provide the highest standard of evidence available for assessing treatment efficacy. Causal inferences are enabled and effects may be directly attributed to a treatment. The nature of infectious disease presents challenges to the design, conduct, and analysis of a trial for a new drug or therapy. Many of these challenges are statistical in nature and can be addressed with modern methods for planning and analyzing RCT data. In this chapter, some of these challenges are described and reviewed. Modern statistical modeling methods for analysis of correlated data are covered. Some challenges with sample size determination are outlined and updated methods for data monitoring, interim, and subgroup analyses detailed. Also, discernment is made between multisite and cluster randomized trials. Recommendations for best practices are included.

Keywords Randomized controlled trial · Treatment efficacy · Causal inference · Therapy · Cluster randomized trial

1 Introduction

Many questions abound around the ethicality of conducting a rigorous randomized controlled trial (RCT) to test efficacy of a new therapy in the midst of an infectious disease outbreak. A compelling argument for RCTs was made by [4] and published in *NEJM* at the peak of the 2014 Ebola virus disease epidemic. The authors argued against the exclusion of a concurrent control group, suggesting its necessity in measuring effects of an investigational therapy. In the absence of random allocation, potential imbalances and biases prevent accurate estimation of true treatment effects.

Testing efficacy with an infectious disease RCT necessitates thoughtful statistical thinking and reasoning in the design, conduct, and analysis. The RCT is the scientific gold standard for enabling causal inference and is based on a random allocation of

M.J. Hayat (✉)
School of Public Health, Georgia State University, Atlanta, GA, USA
e-mail: mhayat@gsu.edu

G. Chowell and J.M. Hyman (eds.), *Mathematical and Statistical Modeling for Emerging and Re-emerging Infectious Diseases*,
DOI 10.1007/978-3-319-40413-4_18

treatment. Such randomness of assignment provides a theoretical basis for the control of confounders and a valid inference that any resulting observed efficacy is the result of a preceding treatment cause.

Unique statistical challenges arise with the implementation of an infectious disease RCT. In an acute outbreak, there is often little to no time to properly plan and conduct the traditional phase I and phase II studies that are usually intended to provide the needed information to carefully and thoughtfully plan a phase III RCT. Sample size determination is difficult without a well-informed effect size. Traditional RCTs are known to be tedious and slow, which is ill-aligned with the needs in infectious disease. Fortunately, advances in trial structure and design have attempted to address these modern needs. For example, data monitoring and interim analyses are methodologies that have been developed to reduce the time needed to determine effective treatment, as well as more quickly identify harm and safety concerns [26]. Multilevel studies and cluster randomized trials are designs that offer potential benefit of efficiently handling contamination concerns while addressing multilevel data structures with within-cluster correlation [11].

With the advent of many statistical techniques and paradigms for advancing the science of infectious disease RCTs, inadequacies with the conduct and reporting of new methodologies have unfortunately been problematic [1]. Multiple reviews of studies published in the infectious disease research literature have revealed high quantities of errors in the statistical analysis and/or reporting of results. For example, a review of articles in the journal *Infection and Immunity* found that about half of the reviewed articles had problems with the statistical results presented [20]. A study of the *Journal of Virology* found similar problems [23]. In fact, studies dating back to the 1960's reviewing the health and biomedical literature have attempted to quantify and describe statistical analysis and reporting errors [25]. MacArthur, R.D., and Jackson, G.G. [16] found in their evaluation of the *Journal of Infectious Diseases* that "Almost all of the articles that used statistics contained at least one statistical error."

Renowned statistician Karl Pearson famously said "statistics is the grammar of science" (Pearson 1897). Statistical analysis and reporting provides a framework for using observed study data to best answer the research question of interest. Reporting problems, which may include application of the wrong statistical method, poor or inadequate summary of statistical analyses, or errors in displayed results, give pause to the validity of inferences made and conclusions drawn. Not surprisingly, the scientific community has placed a premium on reporting of RCT results. For example, the Consolidated Standards of Reporting Trials (CONSORT) Group, begun in 1993, was formed [19]. The CONSORT guidelines is a working document with comprehensive recommendations for reporting of clinical trials. The CONSORT team consists of a group of experts in clinical trial methodology, guideline development, biomedical journal editors, and research funders. The effort was created with the intention of addressing the problems resulting from inadequate reporting of RCTs.

The purpose of this chapter is to highlight selected statistical considerations that arise in the design, conduct, and analysis of randomized controlled trials. I focus on considerations that particularly present in the arena of infectious disease trials. This chapter is organized as follows. Four general domains of statistical considerations in the design and analysis of randomized controlled trials are presented and discussed. The first domain pertains to modern approaches appropriate for the statistical analysis of RCT data. Sample size determination and challenges that arise with this important topic are considered in the second domain. The third domain focuses on data monitoring and interim analyses, along with statistical issues with multiple comparisons that arise in these processes. The fourth domain is in the area of multisite and cluster randomized trials.

2 Modern Statistical Analysis of RCT Data

Classical statistical methods, usually the focus in a first or second semester graduate health sciences course in statistics, are inadequate for statistical analysis of clinical trials data. Such conventional statistical methods have been the focus in statistics education for non-statisticians. This means working within the general linear models (GLM) framework. The GLM framework is powerful and very useful in science. Yet, its limitations present challenges for its application in the analysis of clinical trials data since the GLM assumes independent observations. Clinical trials data usually includes 2 or more measurements for each subject, cluster, or unit. Thus, the measurements are correlated and the independence assumption not met.

The nature of study of treatment for infectious disease involves a temporal component. In other words, repeated measurements are taken on each individual at 2 or more distinct time points. Classical statistical methods assume independence between measurements. However, this assumption is violated with repeated measures data. Modern methods for analyzing repeated measures data extends the classical general linear model framework to account for multiple measurements on each participant [10]. This is also known as multilevel data. In particular, the GLM is extended to the general linear *mixed* model (GLMM), which involves the addition of random effects. Mixed refers to the mixing of fixed and random effects. Fixed effects contribute to knowledge about the mean of the dependent variable, whereas random effects add to understanding about its variance. Also commonly known as subject-specific models, GLMM partition the variance of the dependent variable into components to account for the multilevel structure of RCT data.

With the advent and dramatic increase in computing power during the past two decades, procedures to fit the GLMM have been made readily available in modern statistical software packages. This was not always the case. Historically, analyses of experimental studies in the health sciences applied naïve methods of inference [10]. For example, a common practice applied to RCT data with a continuous outcome used to be to calculate pre to post change and apply a classical GLM approach with change as the single outcome measure for each study subject. Another method was to calculate percent change and analyze these percent changes as the dependent variable. These approaches are deeply problematic, as they ignore baseline value and an individual's condition prior to treatment. This can lead to misleading inferences, since change from baseline is usually the effect of interest. Common occurring phenomena with infectious disease outcomes, which limits further the value of only considering change, are floor and ceiling effects with the outcome of interest. In addition, partial data on a subject, a common occurrence in infectious disease trials due to attrition and loss to follow-up, may not be used with these naïve approaches. By contrast, in a GLMM model the baseline and follow-up values(s) are each included together in a dependent variable vector format for each subject. The GLMM uses all available information on each subject, including partial data due to loss to follow-up [5].

Continuous outcome data that can be reasonably assumed to be normally distributed are best modeled with a GLM or GLMM [22]. Other dependent variable types, such as skewed continuous, count, dichotomous, polychotomous, and ordinal, may be handled with a broader framework of linear models referred to as the generalized linear model (GzLM) and generalized linear mixed model (GzLMM). The distribution of the dependent variable can be specified in accompaniment with the link function describing the relationship between the independent and dependent variables.

The GLMM and GzLM are conditional models. They condition on the random effect, thus lending to subject-specific interpretations of slope estimates for fixed effects. This is particularly useful and of interest when it is desirable to make inferences at an individual level by conditioning on covariates for a subject. Marginal models provide an alternative approach to mixed models for analysis of RCT data. Also referred to as population averaged models, slope estimates are averaged over the population, rather than estimated differently for varying subject characteristics. For example, a marginal interpretation may describe the average change each of the treatment and control groups, for a one-unit increase in time or some other covariate. The consensus in the statistics literature is marginal models be used for the analysis of repeated measures binary data, and mixed models otherwise be used with other outcome data types [8, 27]. This is especially useful with respect to infectious disease trials, given the common use of a dichotomous outcome measure (e.g., infected or not, diseased or not, survived or not, protected or not).

3 Sample Size Determination

Sample size is an ethical consideration [17]. An underpowered study lacks sufficient statistical power to detect an effect, resulting in an inability to establish treatment benefit. While an underpowered study is problematic, an overpowered study is also unacceptable since this means exposing more subjects to risk than necessary. There are two approaches for sample size determination deemed acceptable by governmental funding agencies (e.g., NIH, NSF, PCORI). Power analysis is a classical methodology for estimating sample size as a function of the level of significance, statistical power, and effect size, whereas precision estimation inverts a confidence interval and describes the number needed as based on a pre-specified desired level of precision [9].

It is commonplace for researchers to seek a scientifically objective approach to sample size determination. However, power analysis and precision are necessarily applied a priori prior to enrollment. Each approach involves unavoidable subjectivity. For example, the level of significance, statistical power, relevant effect size estimate, between and within subject variability, and/or precision level, need be specified in advance before data are collected. The threshold for allowed Type I error (level of significance) and Type II error (1-statistical power), as well as the pre-defined meaning of efficacy, are subjectively determined by the researcher. There are different schools of thought on deciding effect size [9]. This author suggests effect size specification in an infectious disease trial is best defined with a clinically meaningful change in the primary outcome of interest (Lenth 2001). Effect size can be defined with a defined clinically important change in disease status, or some other primary endpoint. For an alternative approach that attempts an effect size estimate based on observed effects in previous studies is described in [2]. However, the author has encountered significance challenges with this approach. Publications of previously completed clinical trials often present results in the form of summary statistics by treatment arm at each time point. These types of summaries often cannot be properly used in effect size estimation for a future RCT, since the quantity of interest is likely individual change. Summary statistics on change from baseline to follow are needed in order to include a correct variance estimate in the sample size calculation. Further, effect size estimation for binary comparisons may be more arbitrary than for continuous outcomes.

Statistical power is an a priori concept [3]. Study planning should include a rigorous consideration of needed sample size [6]. However, statistical power is not considered in the data analysis. When evaluating analyses on the back end of a clinical trial, statistically significant results means there was sufficient statistical power to find an effect. Lack of statistically significant findings suggests two possibilities: (i) there is really not an effect; or, (ii) the study was underpowered. In fact, there is not a way with classical statistical inference to determine which it is. One approach some researchers try is to perform a *post hoc* power analysis to determine how much statistical power one had with a non-significant finding. This approach is flawed and misleading, as power is a desired and specified (not an observed) quantity, and statistical power has a perfect negative correlation with the p-value [13]. This means that a small p-value equates to high, and a large p-value to low statistical power. Post hoc power analysis is not meaningful and should be avoided [9].

Traditional RCT designs consider a total fixed study sample size to be achieved by completion of data collection, and the sample size is conceptualized as a constant once data collection begins. This is a limitation and presents challenges with the pressing need occurring with infectious disease trials. Methodological developments in the past few decades have included changes to the traditional framework, to allow for sample size as a random variable that may change during the progression of a trial [14]. Termed adaptive designs, these approaches condition on observed data as a study progresses, and allows for change to the sample size as data are accumulated. In order to conduct a power analysis to determine an a priori target sample size, information on effect size and within or between subject variability are needed. This information may not be readily available, or precision in estimates lacking. Commonly termed *sample size re-estimation*, a variety of approaches have been developed in recent years to utilize partial data with pre-planned interim analyses to re-calculate sample size as a trial progresses. For example, [18] describe an approach that begins a trial with a small up-front sample size target. Through interim analyses, efficacy potential is assessed, and if promising results obtained, additional subjects are enrolled and the target sample size increased.

4 Data Monitoring, Interim, and Subgroup Analyses

Data monitoring during data collection is important. Logistical problems may be detected early and considerations of benefit and risk weighed prior to trial completion. Some trials may persist for years in duration. Ethical considerations require that the safety of human subjects be prioritized in the conduct of a clinical trial. This includes closely monitoring safety and efficacy. If a vaccine or treatment for infectious disease can be measured with reasonable certainty to be effective prior to trial end, it may be sensible to make the treatment available to all participants. Conversely, if a vaccine or drug presents undue safety risk, a moral and ethical obligation may be to stop administration of an experimental treatment. An independent committee of clinical and scientific experts make up a trial's data and safety monitoring board/committee (DSMB/DSMC). This group is responsible for data monitoring and closely following the conduct and happenings in a clinical trial with human subjects.

Alpha spending functions were developed to address multiplicity concerns that occur with multiple statistical tests performed on a primary RCT outcome (DeMets and Lan 1995). The traditional RCT prescribes avoidance of data analysis, nor any data looks, prior to total completion of data collection. However, human considerations and ethical concerns quickly arise due to the waiting period needed for RCT completion in the midst of acute outbreak of an infectious disease. Data monitoring is a practice dating back to the 1960's and provided a framework for interim review of accumulated data during the course of a clinical trial. The goal was to provide scientific criteria for early termination of a trial due to (i) unacceptable toxicity, (ii) substantial and persuasive evidence of beneficial effect, or (iii) futility, which results when it is known that continued data collection will not result in a superior treatment. Scientific criteria were developed, and termed *stopping rules*. These describe pre-determined thresholds on which to stop a trial.

Data monitoring and interim data analyses need to be planned, and accompanied by a pre-determined spending allocation plan of the study alpha to the different interim data analyses [15]. Pre-defining the number of interim data looks is essential in order to adequately address the anticipated multiplicity challenges resulting from multiple statistical tests on the same primary endpoint or other measures of interest. Measures of interest in addition to the primary endpoint may also be related to safety [7]. Alpha spending functions are valuable for planning ahead, and many types of functions have been developed to support different analysis strategies.

Three common procedures used are the Pocock, O'Brien-Fleming, and Peto alpha spending functions. The Pocock function assumes a fixed alpha level at each interim look. For instance, for a conventional $\alpha = 0.05$ study wide significance level and planned interim data analyses at 6 and 12 months (with 12 months as the final study endpoint), the Pocock method would assign a testing alpha level of 0.029 at 6 months and 0.029 at 12 months. These values differ from a more simplistic idea of 0.025 at each time point due to the use of a discrete probability distribution for estimated alpha levels. The O'Brien-Fleming spending function protects against easily finding an effect in a trial's early stages. Thus, the alpha level increases with interim looks at the trial progresses. The alpha levels with this method would be 0.005 at 6 months and 0.048 at 12 months. Another useful approach is Peto's function, which is more likely to find an effect at the last time point (end of trial). This method would yield alpha levels of 0.001 at 6 months and 0.05 at 12 months. Alpha spending functions are used to avoid an inflated number of false positives that results with multiple statistical tests.

Henao-Restrepo et al. [12] presented results of an interim analysis for an ongoing Ebola vaccine cluster-randomized trial. Interim results suggested the experimental treatment may be highly efficacious and safe in preventing Ebola virus disease. The authors made use of a conservative O'Brien-Fleming alpha spending function and an independent DSMB reviewed the interim 3 months after trial commencement, with an interim analysis cutoff of $\alpha = 0.0027$. Study results at this interim analysis were based on proportion of clusters with one or more eligible disease cases. Applying Fisher's exact test, the statistical test result was p=0.0036. Since this result failed to reach statistical significance, the trial continued. This study is an exemplar of careful forethought, including an analytic plan with pre-defined interim analyses and established stopping rules with the use of an alpha spending function.

Subgroup analyses is another common practice with analysis of RCT data. Consider a vaccination trial with infection as the primary endpoint. In addition to comparison of treatment and control, consideration of variations in risk for different subgroups is often of interest. For example, risk may differ for men and women, across different age groups, or by a prognostic factor such as a pre-existing condition. It is common for researchers, after conducting a test for efficacy on all subjects, to test for efficacy within a subgroup. This is problematic for two substantial reasons. First, the study was powered on the primary endpoint. As a result, a subgroup analysis will likely suffer from an inadequacy of statistical power. Second, multiple statistical tests on the same measure results in an increased rate of false positives. Deeming a treatment efficacious in absence of a real effect has led some researchers to observe that "subgroups kill people" due to the resulting harm from false positive findings [26].

Heterogeneity of treatment effects often exists with respect to demographics, physiology, pathology, and many other possible characteristics. If a researcher conducting an infectious disease RCT wishes to test for efficacy within subgroups, it is essential for subgroups to be anticipated and predefined. When a substantial subgroup effect is anticipated, a stratified randomization plan by subgroup variables is advisable and preferred. With a stratified randomization, the sample size determination can be approached so that adequate sample sizes for detecting treatment effects are derived for each stratum. While ideal, stratifying by one or more variables multiplicatively increases the sample size needed, which may create an untenable study size due to economic, time, and financial limitations.

In the absence of a possibility of stratification, and a subgroup analysis instead chosen, it is essential it be predefined and planned. In conducting a subgroup analysis, the first analytic step is to test for an interaction (moderation) subgroup-treatment effect. If there is not a significant interaction effect, no further significance tests within subgroups should be performed. In the event of a significant interaction effect, significance tests within subgroups may be done, but should be interpreted with caution. In addition, many statisticians have argued for multiplicity adjustments. [24] suggests the use of an alpha spending function with subgroup analyses to adjust for the multiplicity problems that ensue as a result of multiple statistical tests on the same outcome.

5 Multisite and Cluster Randomized Trials

Classical statistical methods assume independence between observations. Yet, by default, causal inference necessitates a temporal sequence of measurements, in order to establish a preceding cause to a sequential effect. As such, clinical trials usually entail at minimum a baseline and post-treatment measurement for each individual. This lends to a multilevel data structure, since two measurements observed from the same individual possess a within-subject correlation. A traditional RCT with repeated measurements on each subject leads to a 2-level data structure. Further, vaccine and treatment trials for infectious disease are often implemented at more than one site and persons treated at the same site are likely to have commonalities that lend to a within-site correlation. This creates a third level of data.

A clinical trial conducted at multiple sites, with random assignment at the patient level for all subjects at all sites, is a *multisite trial*. The benefits of multisite studies are often seen in the increased access to the number of needed study subjects. However, several challenges may compromise the integrity of a multisite trial. For example, contamination, provider availability, an inability to direct treatment to selected patients, and other practical limitations, may prevent patient randomization. An alternative approach is to randomize at the site level. A *cluster randomized trial* controls for within-cluster correlation by administering the same treatment arm to all individuals within a cluster. The difference between a multisite and cluster randomized trial is with the level of randomization.

Cluster randomized trial data can be analyzed with the use of multilevel statistical models. Variance components of the primary endpoint are partitioned into cluster level and patient level variances. Properly accounting for this multilevel data structure is needed to obtain valid standard error estimates needed for correct inferences. Variance components for each model level are estimated, and conditional on these, mean effects estimated with proper accounting of the within-subject and within-cluster correlations inherent in cluster trials.

6 Discussion

Statistical considerations play an essential role in the design, conduct, and analysis of a clinical trial. Planning and carrying out an infectious disease trial to measure treatment effects presents many challenges. Research on human subjects is complex. Statisticians and methodologists have made valiant efforts to improve statistical approaches, develop new methods, and improve existing ones, to allow for more realistic analysis, understanding, and reporting of clinical trial findings. Researchers apply these methods to attempt to analytically describe the complexities of clinical research, and statistical inference is used to interpret and generalize study results beyond the study sample.

In this chapter I've described modern statistical modeling approaches appropriate for tackling the multilevel data structure inherent in clinical trials data. Sample size determination should be considered in the research planning stages, and meaningful effects of interest carefully defined. Data monitoring is used in infectious disease trials, and managed by the trial's DSMB/DSMC. Interim and subgroup analyses need to be planned before data collection commences, and alpha spending functions used to address the multiplicity problems that ensue with multiple statistical tests on the primary endpoint. Cluster randomized trials present powerful alternatives when patient level randomization is problematic or not possible.

Intensive planning and forethought are needed in the planning of an infectious disease trial. Most of the topics touched on here are considerations to be made before data collection begins. When ready to publish trial findings, the CONSORT report and guidelines provide a cohesive and comprehensive framework for the reporting of clinical trials. Statistical considerations are detailed and clear guidelines given. Structured suggestions and advices are provided in the CONSORT documents for reporting on the different statistical considerations touched on in this chapter.

References

1. Altman, D.G.: The scandal of poor medical research. BMJ **308**, 283–4 (1994)
2. Berben, L., Sereika, S.M., Engberg, S.: Effect size estimation: methods and examples. Int. J. Nurs. Stud. **49**, 1039–1047 (2012)
3. Cox, D.R.: Planning of Experiments. Wiley, New York (1958)
4. Cox, E., Borio, L., Temple, R.: Evaluating Ebola therapies-the case for RCTs. N. Engl. J. Med. **371**(25), 2350 (2014)
5. Diez-Roux, A.: Bringing context back into epidemiology: variables and fallacies in multilevel analysis. Am. J. Publ. Health **88**, 816–822 (1998)
6. Fleiss, J.L.: The Design and Analysis of Clinical Experiments. Wiley, New York (1986)

7. Friedman, L.M., Furberg, C.D., DeMets, D.L.: Fundamentals of Clinical Trials, 4th edn. Springer, New York (2010)
8. Gardiner, J.C., Luo, Z., Roman, L.A.: Fixed effects, random effects and GEE: what are the differences? Stat. Med. **28**, 221Y239 (2009)
9. Hayat, M.J.: Understanding sample size determination in nursing research. West. J. Nurs. Res. **35**(7), 943–956 (2013)
10. Hayat, M.J., Hedlin, H.: Modern statistical modeling approaches for analyzing repeated-measures data. Nurs. Res. **61**(3), 188–194 (2012)
11. Hayes, R.J., Bennett, S.: Simple sample size calculation for cluster-randomized trials. Int. J. Epidemiol. **28**, 319–326 (1999)
12. Henao-Restrepo, A.M., Longini, I.M., Egger, M., Dean, N.E., Edmunds, W.J., Camacho, A., Carroll, M.W., Doumbia, M., Draguez, B., Duraffour, S., Enwere, G., Grais, R., Gunther, S., Hossmann, S., Kondé, M.K., Kone, S., Kuisma, E., Levine, M.M., Mandal, S., Norheim, G., Riveros, X., Soumah, A., Trelle, S., Vicari, A.S., Watson, C.H., Kéïta, S., Kieny, M.P., Røttingen, J.A.: Efficacy and effectiveness of an rvsv-vectored vaccine expressing ebola surface glycoprotein: interim results from the guinea ring vaccination cluster-randomised trial. Lancet **386**(9996), 857–866 (2015)
13. Hoenig, J.M., Heisey, D.M.: The pervasive fallacy of power calculations for data analysis. Am. Stat. **55**, 19–24 (2001)
14. Kairalla, J.A., Coffey, C.S., Thomann, M.A., Muller, K.E.: Adaptive trial designs: a review of barriers and opportunities. Trials **23**(13), 145 (2012)
15. Koch, G.G., Schwartz, T.: An overview of statistical planning to address subgroups in confirmatory clinical trials. J. Biopharm. Stat. 72–93 (2014)
16. MacArthur, R.D., Jackson, G.G.: An evaluation of the use of statistical methodology. J. Infect. Dis. **149**(3), 349–354 (1984)
17. Maxwell, S.E.: Ethics and Sample Size Planning. In: Panter, A.T., Sterba, S.K. (eds.) Handbook of Ethics in Quantitative Methodology, pp. 159–183. Routledge, New York (2011)
18. Mehta, C.R., Pocock, S.J.: Adaptive increase in sample size when interim results are promising: a practical guide with examples. Stat. Med. **30**(28), 3267–3284 (2011)
19. Moher D, Hopewell S, Schulz KF, Montori V, Gøtzsche PC, Devereaux PJ, Elbourne D, Egger M, Altman DG, for the CONSORT Group: CONSORT 2010 Explanation and Elaboration: updated guidelines for reporting parallel group randomised trial. BMJ **340**, c869 (2010)
20. Olsen, C.H.: Review of the use of statistics in Infection and Immunity. Infect. Immun. **71**, 6689–6692 (2003)
21. Pearson, K.: The Grammar of Science. Walter Scott, London (1892)
22. Rabe-Hesketh, S., Skrondal, A.: Multilevel and Longitudinal Modeling Using Stata. Stata Press, College Station (2005)
23. Richardson, B.A., Overbaugh, J.: Basic statistical considerations in virological experiments. J. Virol. **79**(2), 669–676 (2005)
24. Rothwell, P.M.: Treating individuals 2. Subgroup analysis in randomised controlled trials: importance, indications, and interpretation. Lancet **365**(9454), 176–86 (2005)
25. Schor, S., Karten, I.: Statistical evaluation of medical journal manuscripts. JAMA **195**, 1123–8 (1966)
26. Schulz, K.F., Grimes, D.A.: Multiplicity in randomised trials II: subgroup and interim analyses. Lancet **365**(9471), 1657–61 (2005)
27. Twisk, J.W., Smidt, N., de Vente, W.: Applied analysis of recurrent events: a practical overview. J. Epidemiol. Commun. Health **59**, 706Y710 (2005)

Epidemic Models With and Without Mortality: When Does It Matter?

Lisa Sattenspiel, Erin Miller, Jessica Dimka, Carolyn Orbann and Amy Warren

Abstract We use an agent-based computer simulation designed to model the spread of the 1918 influenza pandemic to address the question of whether, and if so, when disease-related mortality should be included in an epidemic model. Simulation outcomes from identical models that differ only in the inclusion or exclusion of disease-related mortality are compared. Results suggest that unless mortality is very high (above a case fatality rate of about 18 % for influenza), mortality has a minimal impact on simulation outcomes. High levels of mortality, however, lower the percentage infected at the epidemic peak and reduce the overall number of cases because epidemic chains are shortened overall, and so a smaller proportion of the population becomes infected. Analyses also indicate that high levels of mortality can increase the chance of oscillations in disease incidence. The decision about whether to include disease-related mortality in a model should, however, take into account the fact that diseases such as influenza, that sicken a high proportion of a population, may nonetheless lead to high numbers of deaths. These deaths can affect a real population's perception of and response to an epidemic, even when objective measures

L. Sattenspiel (✉) · E. Miller · A. Warren
Department of Anthropology, University of Missouri, 112 Swallow Hall, Columbia, MO 65211, USA
e-mail: sattenspiell@missouri.edu

E. Miller
e-mail: elmvw9@mail.missouri.edu

A. Warren
e-mail: alwgyb@mail.missouri.edu

J. Dimka
Department of Epidemiology, School of Public Health, University of Michigan, 1415 Washington Heights, 4667 SPH 1, Ann Arbor, MI 48109-2029, USA
e-mail: jdimka@umich.edu

C. Orbann
Department of Health Sciences, University of Missouri, 501 Clark Hall, Columbia, MO 65211, USA
e-mail: orbannc@health.missouri.edu

G. Chowell and J.M. Hyman (eds.), *Mathematical and Statistical Modeling for Emerging and Re-emerging Infectious Diseases*,
DOI 10.1007/978-3-319-40413-4_19

suggest the impact of mortality on epidemic outcomes is relatively low. Thus, careful attention should be paid to the possibility of such responses when developing epidemic control strategies.

Keywords Agent-based model · Epidemics · Influenza · 1918 influenza pandemic · Epidemic control · Mortality

Infectious diseases have been and continue to be major causes of fear, economic loss, and mortality in human populations worldwide. Many infectious disease models do not include disease-related mortality, however, even when the disease in question can kill large numbers of people. For such diseases, e.g. pandemic influenza or Ebola, the decision to ignore mortality is often questioned, but there are few studies that systematically compare models with and without disease-related mortality to assess whether the added complexity of a model with such mortality is truly necessary. In this paper we explore this issue using agent-based computer simulation, which is well suited to studying these kinds of questions. Unlike most mathematical models, agent-based models can easily incorporate heterogeneity in individual characteristics, such as behaviors that influence the risk of becoming infected or dying, and they can also easily incorporate stochastic factors that are often very important in the spread of real epidemics. Agent-based models possess a higher degree of realism than most mathematical models and can be used to compare scenarios with and without disease-related death while maintaining a constant and significant level of underlying heterogeneity and complexity across models.

We have developed a model to study the spread of the 1918 influenza pandemic in a small fishing community in Newfoundland and Labrador. The choice to model this situation was motivated by several considerations. First, much attention has been directed in recent years to research on the 1918 influenza pandemic (see, for example, the papers in *Vaccine*, Vol. 29, Suppl. 2 (2011)). Many of these studies draw upon the experiences of large and developed cities; studies of smaller populations outside the mainstream of Western Europe and North America are needed to fully understand the impact of this truly global event. Second, from a modeling perspective, an important reason to consider small communities is that the detailed day-to-day activities of community residents can be easily modeled without basing assumptions about individual-level behaviors on idealized understandings of these behaviors. Incorporating realistic activity patterns allows a finer-grained resolution of how individual actions affect epidemic patterns than is possible using either mathematical approaches or larger-scale agent-based models.

Our overall project is also fundamentally multidisciplinary, drawing upon knowledge and methods in mathematics, computer science, anthropology, history, public health, and geography. This multidisciplinary approach combined with the small scale of the study community allows us to firmly ground model structures as well as parameter estimates in historical, ethnographic, and epidemiological data and knowledge. It is important to note, however, that like all models, ours is a simplification of reality, but the assumptions we have made are based on in-depth understanding of how real communities in Newfoundland and elsewhere work.

Because of the nature of this volume and space limitations, this paper focuses on the modeling component of our project, with specific emphasis on the impact of varying levels of mortality on the outcomes of an epidemic model. We first provide a brief description of the essential structure of our model. We then compare results from two versions of the model that are identical in all respects except for the presence of disease-related mortality. We explore the impact of varying levels of mortality alone as well as patterns that are observed when allowing both mortality and one of our other primary model parameters (length of the latent period, length of the infectious period, transmission probability, and population size) to vary simultaneously. We present selected results from extensive sensitivity analyses and conclude the paper by discussing the implications of these results for understanding human experiences with and responses to infectious disease epidemics.

1 An Agent-Based Influenza Model with Mortality

The model used in this project is an agent-based SEIR epidemic model of the spread of influenza in a small human community. The model includes a set of agents (individual entities) placed on a social/geographic space and a suite of rules that govern how each agent behaves during each time step of the model. The model was originally developed using the programming language Java and the Repast Simphony 1.2 simulation libraries and packages [9] and it has also been implemented using NetLogo 5.2 [16].

1.1 Set-up of the Population

The model agents are designed to represent a realistic human population. Agents are assigned an age and sex and are allocated into households based on information in the 1921 census for the community of St. Anthony, Newfoundland and Labrador [8]. This community was chosen because a variety of historical materials are available to provide details about what life was like in the community during the early 20th century. Agents are also assigned a specific dwelling, membership in one of two churches, an occupation, and a disease status. All variables other than disease status are initialized with values that reflect known conditions in the community as represented in the ethnographic and historical literature. At initialization all agents are susceptible; one agent is subsequently given the status of exposed.

Buildings are placed on the model space to facilitate visualization of social activities, but the space is not reflective of true geographical space—it is designed to represent a social space. During a time step agents move directly from one cell on the space to another, dependent on their specific activities for the time step. Social interactions (and opportunities for disease transmission) can only occur between an agent and the four possible von Neumann neighbors surrounding the agent's destination. The agents' instantaneous movement makes the model similar to a traditional network model because it effectively generates links between agents (nodes), but the underlying network changes its character every time step. Agents with similar characteristics are more likely to be linked to one another because they are more likely to move to the same building during a particular time step, but unless they choose a cell adjacent to another agent, they will not have a link to that agent during the time step. Thus, the model's overall social network is fully dynamic and is based only on where agents happen to be at each step of the simulation.

The buildings placed on the model space represent the major types of social activities that would generally occur in a small, early 20th century Newfoundland fishing community. These buildings include 84 houses, an orphanage (known to be present in the study community), a school, a hospital (also known to be present), two churches, and 23 boats. The resulting town map is shown in Fig. 1.

Each day of the simulation is divided into six 4-h time steps. During four of the six steps (6–10 AM, 10 AM–2 PM, 2–6 PM, and 6–10 PM), agents move to new cells in specific buildings corresponding to rules for their behavior based on their assigned occupations (e.g. fisherman, schoolchild, mother with preschool-aged children) and the day of week and time of day the step represents. During the remaining two time steps each day (10 PM–2 AM and 2–6 AM), agents are assumed to be sleeping and no movement occurs. The model is run for a sufficient number of days to allow completion of all or nearly all epidemic simulations; depending on the specific parameter values, true completion is occasionally difficult to achieve. For the simulations described below, all model runs began on a Monday morning at 6 AM.

1.2 Daily Activities Incorporated into the Model

The nature of agents' daily activities was decided using insights drawn from relevant ethnographic and historical materials (e.g., [1, 12]). Mechanistically, the activities involve choosing a destination cell within a specific building in which an agent's assigned activities occur. For example, at the beginning of the Monday–Friday 6–10 AM time step all agents are at home. During that step fishermen move to their assigned boat, school-aged children and teachers move to the school, doctors and nurses move to the hospital, and all other agents (i.e., servants, preschool-aged children, and all adult females who are neither teachers nor nurses) move to a new location within their dwelling.

Illness-related behaviors, such as changes in normal movement patterns, are not included at present, but are planned for the future. All living agents follow their designated movement rules at each time step; only doctors and nurses move to the hospital. Dead agents are moved to a cell at the corner of the space that is designated as the "cemetery", and they no longer participate in the daily activities.

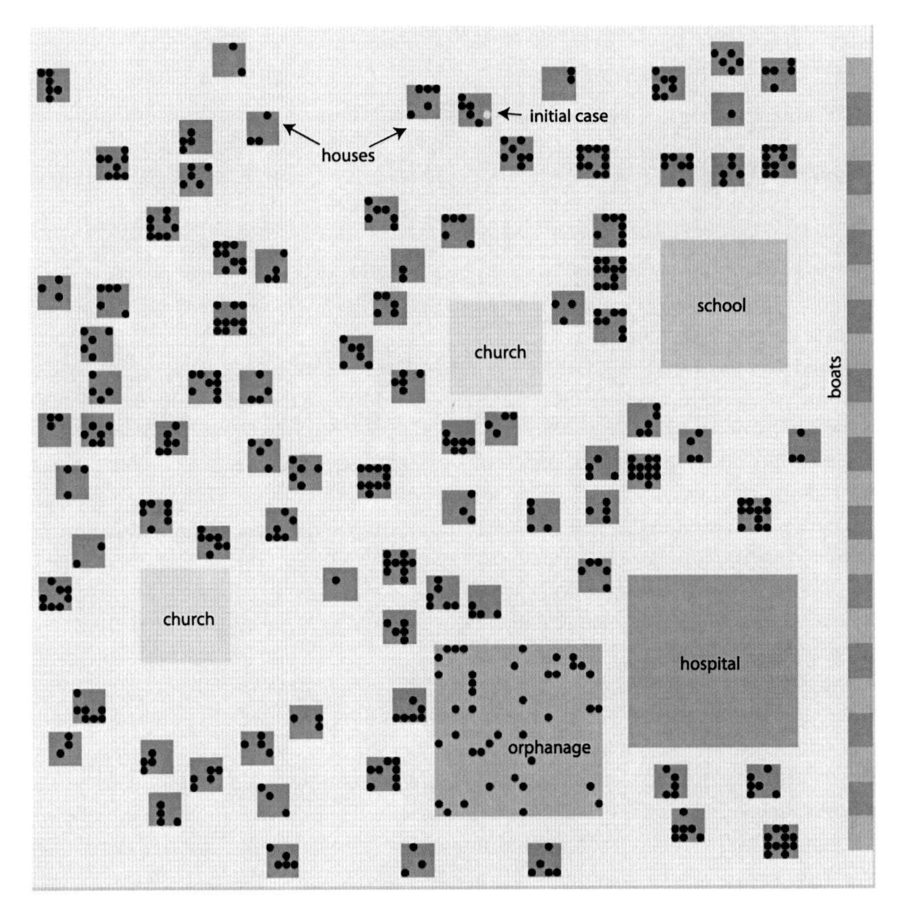

Fig. 1 Idealized representation of the study community, St. Anthony, Newfoundland and Labrador. Boats are represented in two shades only to facilitate visualization; their other characteristics are identical

Sometimes agents have different possibilities for their activities during a time step. In this case the model includes a hierarchical decision-making process to specify which of the possible activities is actually pursued. The suite of activities is similar for all weekdays (M–F); Saturday activities differ slightly from weekday activities since school is not in session. On Sundays every agent (in family groups) goes to church, visits another family, is visited by another family, or remains at home without visitors. A more detailed description of these daily activities can be found in [11].

1.3 The Disease Transmission Process

At the end of each time step, after an agent completes its movement, it determines whether any other agents are situated directly to the north, south, east, or west. Infectious-susceptible pairs of neighbors are identified, and then a random number is drawn to determine whether the pathogen is transmitted to whichever of the two agents is susceptible, an event that happens if the drawn number is below the user-determined and pre-set transmission probability. Because "sleeping" agents may be situated adjacent to other agents within the household, disease transmission is still possible during the night.

An SEIR framework with mortality is used in the model, but because the model is limited to a single, short-lived epidemic, vital statistics are not included (i.e., there are no births or migrations and the only deaths are those due to the pathogen itself). When agents become infected, they enter an exposed (or latent) stage, which lasts a fixed length of time, after which the agent becomes infectious. Transmission of the disease by one agent to another (susceptible) agent can only occur if the transmitting agent is in the infectious stage. Death can occur with a pre-set probability for each 4-h time step included in the infectious period. Agents that survive through the infectious period enter the recovered stage and stay in that state for the remaining steps of the simulation.

Baseline parameter values are designed to represent the conditions present in Newfoundland during the 1918 influenza pandemic. The latent and infectious periods are assumed to be constant, with the latent period set at 1 day (6 time steps) and the infectious period at 3 days (18 time steps). As there is little consensus in the influenza literature about the specific values to use for these parameters, a number of different values were assessed, including published values (e.g., [3, 5–7]) and other approximations within the range of published values. The specific values chosen were the integer values deemed to best represent the information available. The transmission probability was also assumed to be constant at a value of 0.042 per time step throughout the infectious period. This value was chosen so that the average simulation attack rate was approximately 55 %, the midpoint of a range suggested by [5] for the 1918 influenza pandemic. The death data recorded for Newfoundland and Labrador were also used to calculate a growth rate for the epidemic (Chowell, personal communication). This growth rate was then used to derive another estimate of the transmission probability, but the resulting value produced simulated epidemics that did not reflect the overall observed pattern of influenza spread on the island as well as did the value derived using Ferguson et al.'s [5] estimate of the attack rate. The estimate for the probability of death per time step was derived from the known mortality rate (7.5 deaths per thousand population) on the island of Newfoundland [13]. This mortality rate in combination with the estimated 55 % prevalence gave a case fatality rate of 13.6 deaths per thousand cases. Working back from this observed rate, the baseline death probability was estimated at 0.00076 per time step during the infectious period.

At the end of each time step the numbers of agents with each disease status (susceptible, exposed, infectious, removed, and dead) are recorded. Once a simulation has completed its run, data are also collected on the final size and on case-related data such as the ID number and occupation of the first case; time of infection for each infected agent; the ID, occupation, and dwelling of the agent responsible for the infection; and where that infection took place. Data are also collected on when and where agents die.

2 Analysis of the Model

Extensive sensitivity analyses varying the five primary parameters (length of the latent period, length of the infectious period, transmission probability, probability of death, and population size), both singly and in pairs, have been completed. All analyses were performed on sets of 100 runs of the simulation. In the remainder of this paper we discuss some of the results and implications of varying the probability of death.

The model used in analyses with no mortality is an earlier version of the model with mortality; both have the same structure other than the presence/absence of mortality. However, analyses of the earlier model used slightly different parameter values from the baseline values reported above. To ensure that valid comparisons were made between the models with and without mortality, the sensitivity analyses discussed here used the same values as were used in the analyses of the model without mortality. In particular, an infectious period of five days and a transmission probability of 1 were used in the sensitivity analyses when these parameters were held constant. Table 1 provides the specific parameter values used in model analyses. Analyses of simulation data primarily focused on assessing the effects of changes in parameter values on four outcomes: (a) the final numbers of individuals in each disease class, (b) the number or percentage of the population infected at the peak of the epidemic, (c) the timing of the epidemic peak, and (d) the time at which the last infectious agent (last case) is observed. Space does not allow discussion of all the results from these analyses; instead we highlight several insights derived from results of simulations varying the probability of death.

2.1 *General Effects of Adding Mortality to an Epidemic Model*

The effect of including mortality in an epidemic model can be studied by comparing the results of simulations with the probability of death (μ) set at 0 to those with $\mu > 0$. Our model indicates that the overall impact of disease-related mortality is variable and dependent on the specific probability of death being considered. Results demonstrate

Table 1 Parameter values used in model sensitivity analyses

Scenario	Baseline	Default for sensitivity variable analyses[a]	Values in single variable analyses	Values in dual-variable analyses
Latent period	1 day[b]	1 day	1–7 days, 1–day steps	1–7 days, 1–day steps
Infectious period	3 days	5 days	1–10 days, 1–day steps	1–10 days, 1–day steps
Transmission probability	0.042	1	0.01–0.1 in steps of 0.01, plus 0.5 and 1.0	0.01, 0.03, 0.05, 0.1, 0.2, 0.3, 1.0
Population size[c]	503	503	Target of 50–500, increment of 50	Target of 50–500, increment of 50
Probability of death	0.00076	0.00025	0.00005–0.0005 in steps of 0.00005, 0.001, plus 0.01, 0.05, 0.1, 0.4, 0.7, 1.0	0.00005, 0.00025, 0.0005, 0.001, 0.01, 0.05, 0.1, 0.4, 1.0

[a]Default values were used whenever the variable was not being varied. All results discussed in this paper involve varying the probability of death
[b]1 day = 6 time steps (ticks of the model)
[c]In order to retain the realistic household structure designed for the model, values used when varying population size are target numbers ±3 agents. Only the target numbers are used in presenting results

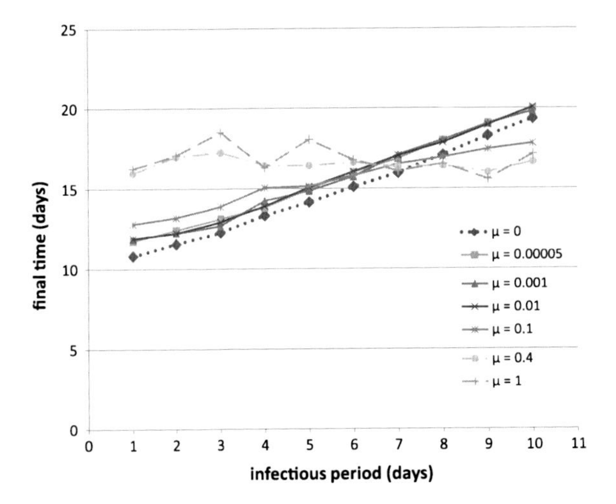

Fig. 2 Change in the time of an epidemic's last case as the infectious period and probability of mortality (μ) vary. Note that curves for $\mu \leq 0.01$ are only slightly different from the curve for $\mu = 0$ and are indistinguishable from each other; the curve for $\mu = 0.1$ varies somewhat more, and the remaining curves are significantly different from the curve for $\mu = 0$. Graphs derived from analyses that varied or co-varied latent period, transmission probability, and population size show even greater similarities between the curves for $\mu \leq 0.01$ and that for $\mu = 0$ and more differences between curves for $\mu \geq 0.1$ and $\mu = 0$

that unless the probability of mortality is high—well above 0.01 per 4-h time step[1]—simulated epidemics with mortality differ only minimally from epidemics generated from an equivalent model without mortality. These results are most easily seen when looking at how different levels of mortality affect patterns observed when varying a second parameter (see Fig. 2, which shows the results for time of the last case). Results also indicate that high levels of mortality ($\mu > 0.01$) substantially lower the percentage of the population infected at an epidemic's peak no matter which other parameter is varied, but the effects on the peak time of an epidemic and the time of the last case are more moderate, with the direction of differences (i.e., delaying or speeding up epidemics) depending on the second parameter.

[1]Note that the fundamental death parameter in the model is the per-tick probability of mortality, μ. This parameter can be converted to a case fatality rate (cfr), but the estimate of the latter is dependent on the value of the infectious period. The cfr can be calculated from the equation $\text{cfr} = 1 - (1 - \mu)^i$, where i is the length of the infectious period; $(1 - \mu)^i$ gives the probability that an individual survives through the entire infectious period assuming a constant probability of death. Thus, one minus this quantity gives the probability of dying while infected. If $\mu = 0.01$ and the infectious period is 18 ticks (3 days), the estimate for the 1918 pandemic influenza, the corresponding cfr is 16.5 %, a value substantially higher than that commonly observed during influenza pandemics. The cfr for $\mu = 0.01$ jumps to 26.0 % if the infectious period is 5 days (as used in the sensitivity analyses).

2.2 *The Effect of Mortality on Ultimate Numbers of Cases and Proportions of a Population Affected by an Epidemic*

It might seem reasonable to assume that the higher the probability of mortality, the more severely an epidemic will affect a population. One unexpected result from our analyses, however, is that this is not necessarily the case. Figure 3 shows the final numbers of cases and dead as the probability of mortality increases under two scenarios: (a) the standard parameter set used in the sensitivity analyses, and (b) the baseline parameter set derived from analysis of epidemiological and historical materials. In both situations, when the probability of mortality is at or below 0.001 per 4-h time step (a case fatality rate (cfr) of about 1.8 % when the infectious period (infper) is 3 days or 3.0 % when infper = 5 days), only a small proportion of those who become infected die. However, above that probability of mortality, the proportion dying increases rapidly, and in both cases when the probability is 0.1 or greater (cfr > 85.0 % for infper = 3, cfr > 95.8 % for infper = 5), almost all cases end in death.

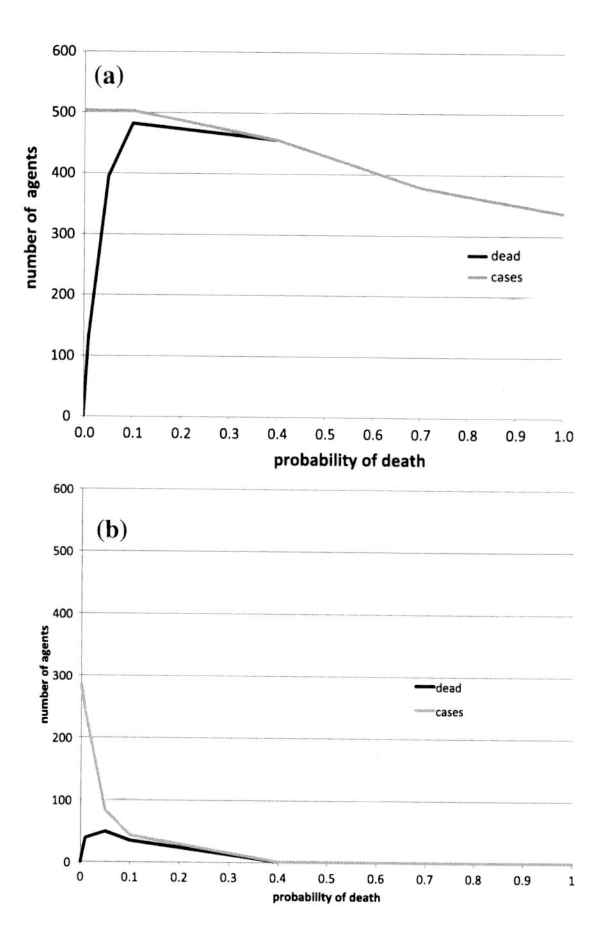

Fig. 3 Change in final epidemic size as the probability of mortality varies. **a** Results from simulations using the parameters chosen for sensitivity analyses (Table 1, Col. 2). **b** Results from simulations using baseline influenza parameters (Table 1, Col. 1)

This is not at all surprising, but what was unforeseen is that the total proportion of the population that gets infected at all is actually lower for very high levels of mortality than it is with moderate levels, and thus the number of deaths is also lower. Thus, in some sense, high mortality provides a type of protective effect for a certain proportion of the population. In fact, a similar *number* of deaths will occur with both low and high mortality rates, although the reasons for these similar values are very different. In the case of low mortality rates, low numbers of deaths occur because the probability of death is low. In the case of very high mortality rates, the relatively low number of deaths occurs because individual chains of infection are severely shortened due to death of infected individuals and so fewer people overall become infected before the epidemic dies out for good. This latter situation is also reflected in the declining number of cases overall as the mortality probability increases.

This counterintuitive behavior under conditions of high mortality makes sense given how diseases and mortality work on populations, but it is important to step back and think about how such a situation would be perceived in a real population. From the perspective of individuals within the population, although the actual numbers of cases may not be as high as with moderate levels of mortality, high levels of mortality will cause the epidemic to be perceived as much worse, because the individuals within a population are much more attuned to the extreme levels of death around them rather than to the fact that a lower proportion may be getting sick at all. This disconnect between the actual impact of an epidemic and the perception of that impact will be discussed further below.

2.3 Models with Mortality and the Development of Oscillations in the Numbers of Infected Individuals over Time

A final aspect of model behavior to be addressed here is the impact of mortality on the overall epidemic patterns across time. Several of the dual variable sensitivity analyses illustrated conditions under which cycling of epidemics may occur. The most marked of these in simulations that vary the probability of death is when that parameter is jointly varied with the length of the latent period. Figure 4 illustrates what happens to epidemic patterns for different lengths of the latent period and a death probability of 0.4 per time step. Cycling is apparent at all values of the latent period and becomes particularly marked at the longest latent periods. In fact, although Fig. 4 indicates dampening fluctuations (as they must since the population size is constant and susceptibles are continuously depleted), simulations with the longest latent periods still had not resulted in extinction of the epidemic when extended to at least 1000 time steps. In these cases, the epidemic appears to die out, but it is actually still in the population—just hidden in exposed individuals. In other words, a sufficient number of cases remain infectious long enough to transmit the epidemic to a few susceptible individuals, but the transmitting cases die before the newly

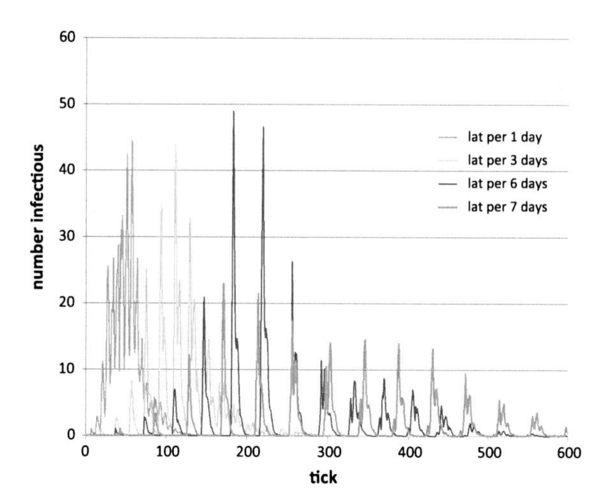

Fig. 4 Averaged epidemic curves of 100 simulations with a probability of death of 0.4 and different values of the latent period. 6 ticks (time steps) = 1 day

exposed individuals become infectious. Under the proper conditions, this behavior can be maintained for extensive periods of time until the last susceptible individual finally becomes infected, although given the stochastic nature of the simulation (and real epidemics as well), die out will likely occur due to chance well before the disease reaches all susceptible individuals.

3 Discussion

Until the development of the model described here, mortality was rarely included in the primary author's influenza models (e.g., [10, 14, 15]), and given that the 1918 influenza pandemic was the epidemic being modeled, numerous comments were received asking why mortality was not being considered. The argument was made that the models were always focused on a single short epidemic and so the effect of mortality was likely negligible. The results presented here provide a more nuanced view of why it may be reasonable to ignore mortality in influenza models. In particular, the case fatality rate for the 1918 influenza pandemic has been estimated to be under 2 %, rates observed for other influenza pandemics of the 19th and 20th centuries were less than 0.1 %, and rates during seasonal outbreaks of influenza are even lower [2]. Even for the 1918 flu, a major pandemic, the case fatality rate is low enough that the results for models with and without mortality are nearly identical. This suggests that for diseases such as influenza, which can result in high *numbers* of deaths because of extreme levels of morbidity, models that ignore mortality may not be far off the mark *as long as the questions of primary interest do not center on deaths during the epidemic.* In other words, the major impact of epidemics of diseases such as influenza relates to the high proportions of the population that become ill and the consequent disruptions in daily life, not to high mortality rates.

Several other infectious diseases common in today's world have low levels of mortality similar to that observed during the 1918 influenza pandemic. Measles case fatality rates in present-day developing countries range from 0.1 to 6 %, although in localities with high levels of malnutrition and other causes of immune suppression, rates can be as high as 30 % [18]. Dengue fever (not including dengue hemorrhagic fever) has a case fatality rate of about 2.5 % [17]; pertussis kills about 3.7 % of unvaccinated infants and 1 % of children aged 1–4 who become infected [4]. Although the specific case fatality rate that results in deviations between models with and without mortality will vary somewhat depending on the particular characteristics of a disease, it is likely that the low case fatality rates observed in all of these diseases would result in the same effects we observed with our influenza model.

One dimension of infectious disease epidemics that researchers often fail to consider is the population's *perception* of the impact of an epidemic. Our model shows clearly that very low levels of mortality do not significantly alter disease dynamics, but real people experiencing an infectious disease epidemic respond to what they see happening in the world around them, not to ideas about how diseases spread in a population. It is important to remember this aspect of the infectious disease experience when evaluating the potential impacts of epidemics, especially when using a model to inform policies about how best to control disease outbreaks. In the case of our Newfoundland study population, a mortality rate of 7.5 per thousand people meant that fewer than four deaths would be expected in the study community of 503 persons, which is not likely to result in high fear levels. But in a population of two million, that same death rate of 7.5 per thousand people would mean that 15,000 people would die. That might not influence overall disease dynamics, but it certainly would affect perceptions about the severity of the epidemic and the willingness of people to comply with different control strategies.

The analyses of the model reported here as well as other, more extensive sensitivity analyses assess the importance of the different base model parameters. One parameter commonly considered in infectious disease models that we have not studied in depth with our model is R_0, the average number of secondary cases generated by a single infectious individual in a totally susceptible population. Although this is an important parameter to consider when designing control strategies for infectious diseases, this is not an explicit parameter in our model; rather, it is probably some complex combination of all of our base model parameters, and its value is not easy to determine when doing sensitivity analyses of the model. Every unique set of parameters in the sensitivity analysis generates a different average curve. These curves and their associated growth rates (which provide insight into the value of R_0) are outcomes of the simulations, not input values that we control. In other words, the curves and their growth rates are emergent properties of the model and not parameters that are manipulated a priori by the modeler. Thus, analyzing the impact of systematic variation in R_0 is not a straightforward process and is beyond the scope of this paper.

The main purpose of the research reported here was to assess whether inclusion of mortality in an influenza model was necessary to accurately represent a real epidemic. To facilitate this goal, the model was parameterized using data related directly to the 1918 pandemic in Newfoundland and Labrador and elsewhere. It is important to remember, however, that our estimate of the value of mortality that is low enough to be negligible depends on the estimate of the length of the infectious period, the assumption that death occurs only during the infectious period, and a further assumption that there is a constant probability of death throughout the entire infectious period. Additional research relaxing these assumptions as well as using models designed for other diseases is needed to assess whether, and if so, to what extent results from our analysis can be generalized to other epidemics, locations, or diseases. Nonetheless, it may well be that putting mortality into models of diseases with low probabilities of death adds unnecessary complexity to a model and should be considered carefully, particularly when dealing with diseases and/or populations for which data are inadequate in quantity or quality.

References

1. Baier, F.: The new orphanage. Among Deep Sea Fish. **22**(2), 54–57 (1924)
2. Brundage, J.F., Shanks, G.D.: Deaths from bacterial pneumonia during 1918–19 influenza pandemic. Emerg. Infect. Dis. **14**(8), 1193–1199 (2008)
3. Cori, A., Valleron, A.J., Carrat, F., Scalia Tomba, G., Thomas, G., Boëlle, P.Y.: Estimating influenza latency and infectious period durations using viral excretion data. Epidemics **4**, 132–138 (2012)
4. Crowcroft, N.S., Stein, C., Duclos, P., Birmingham, M.: How best to estimate the global burden of pertussis? Lancet Infect. Dis. **3**, 413–418 (2003)
5. Ferguson, N.M., Cummings, D.A.T., Cauchemez, S., Fraser, C., Riley, S., Meeyai, A., Iamsirithaworn, S., Burke, D.S.: Strategies for containing an emerging influenza pandemic in Southeast Asia. Nature **437**(7056), 209–214 (2005)
6. Glass, R.J., Glass, L.M., Beyeler, W.E., Min, H.J.: Targeted social distancing design for pandemic influenza. Emerg. Infect. Dis. **12**(11), 1671–1681 (2006)
7. Mills, C.E., Robins, J.M., Lipsitch, M.: Transmissibility of 1918 pandemic influenza. Nature **432**, 904–906 (2004)
8. Newfoundland Colonial Secretary's Department: Census of Newfoundland and Labrador, 1921. Colonial Secretary's Office, St. John's, NF (1923)
9. North, M.J., Collier, N.T., Ozik, J., Tatara, E., Altaweel, M., Macal, C.M., Bragen, M., Sydelko, P.: Complex adaptive systems modeling with repast simphony. Complex Adapt. Syst. Model. **1**, 3. http://www.casmodeling.com/content/1/1/3 (2013). Accessed 4 Aug 2015
10. O'Neil, C.A., Sattenspiel, L.: Agent-based modeling of the spread of the 1918–1919 Spanish flu in three Canadian fur trading communities. Am. J. Hum. Biol. **22**, 757–767 (2010)
11. Orbann, C., Dimka, J., Miller, E., Sattenspiel, L.: Agent-based modeling and the second epidemiologic transition. In: Zuckerman, M.K. (ed.) Modern Environments and Human Health: Revisiting the Second Epidemiologic Transition, pp. 105–122. Wiley-Blackwell, Hoboken (2014)
12. Queen, S.A., Habenstein, R.W.: The Family in Various Cultures, 4th edn. JB Lippincott, Philadelphia (1974)
13. Sattenspiel, L.: Regional patterns of mortality during the 1918 influenza pandemic in Newfoundland. Vaccine **29S**, B33–B37 (2011)
14. Sattenspiel, L., Herring, D.A.: Structured epidemic models and the spread of influenza in the Norway House District of Manitoba, Canada. Hum. Biol. **70**, 91–115 (1998)
15. Sattenspiel, L., Herring, D.A.: Simulating the effect of quarantine on the spread of the 1918–19 flu in central Canada. Bull. Math. Biol. **65**(1), 1–26 (2003)

16. Wilensky, U.: NetLogo. Center for Connected Learning and Computer-Based Modeling, Northwestern University, Evanston, IL. http://ccl.northwestern.edu/netlogo/ (1999). Accessed 4 Aug 2015
17. World Health Organization (WHO): Dengue and severe dengue, Fact sheet No. 117. http://www.who.int/mediacentre/factsheets/fs117/en/ (2015). Accessed 4 Aug 2015
18. Wolfson, L.J., Grais, R.F., Luquero, F.J., Birmingham, M.E., Strebel, P.M.: Estimates of measles case fatality ratios: a comprehensive review of community-based studies. Int. J. Epidemiol. **38**, 192–205 (2009)

Capturing Household Transmission in Compartmental Models of Infectious Disease

Jude Bayham and Eli P. Fenichel

Abstract Social distancing policies may mitigate transmission of infectious disease by shifting individuals time spent in public into household environments. However, the efficacy of such a policy depends on the transmission differential between public and household environments. We extend the standard compartmental model of infectious disease with heterogeneous mixing to explicitly account for the health state of households. Our model highlights the fact that only households with an infectious individual pose a transmission risk to other household members. Moreover, susceptible households become infectious at a rate that depends on household size and the health status of the household members. We demonstrate our model by simulating an epidemic similar to the A/H1N1 2009 outbreak using empirical mixing patterns derived from time-use data in the United States. We find that household transmission accounts for 12–23 % of total cases. These results suggest that while social distancing policies encourage individuals to spend more time at home, the reduction of time in public improves public health outcomes on balance.

Keywords Household transmission · Compartmental model · Epidemics · Infectious disease · Pandemic influenza · Heterogeneous mixing

1 Introduction

Mathematical models of infectious disease are an important tool used to forecast epidemic outcomes and assess public health policy. A useful model is tractable while incorporating relevant features of the real world. Since [18], compartmental models

J. Bayham (✉)
College of Agriculture, California State University, Chico, Chico, CA 95926, USA
e-mail: jbayham@csuchico.edu

E.P. Fenichel
Yale School of Forestry and Environmental Studies, Yale University,
195 Prospect Street, New Haven, CT 06511, USA
e-mail: eli.fenichel@yale.edu

G. Chowell and J.M. Hyman (eds.), *Mathematical and Statistical Modeling for Emerging and Re-emerging Infectious Diseases*,
DOI 10.1007/978-3-319-40413-4_20

have been modified to accommodate realistic contact patterns [1, 12, 23, 26]. The heterogeneous mixing model allows contact rates to vary among different population strata. As researchers operationalize these models by incorporating mixing patterns from observable data [5, 21, 30], new questions arise about how to integrate empirical contact patterns that vary by location into compartmental models.

Incorporating household mixing patterns directly into compartmental models remains a challenge because individual's movements and infectious status are not tracked as in agent-based models, though such agent-based models can rapidly become intractable and over-parameterized. Traditionally, compartmental models were based on static mixing patterns that capture population means across household and public or community locations. However, household mixing patterns are fundamentally different than public contacts because the universe of possible contacts in the household is limited by the number of individuals in the household, contacts are often repeated, of longer in duration, and are likely more intimate than public or community contacts. While household transmission is known to be important, the contribution of household transmission to the total number of cases during an epidemic is still under debate in the literature. Increasingly, infectious disease models use a rule of thumb for household transmission. For example, a commonly cited number is that 30 % of flu transmission is within-household. However, this number is tracked back to an agent-based simulation model calibrated (not estimated) to households in Thailand [14]. We argue that estimates of household transmission can be improved using empirical mixing patterns.

In this chapter, we extend the heterogeneous mixing model to explicitly account for household contact patterns as well as contacts in other locations. Specifically, we separate public from household transmission and provide adjustments for contact patterns based on the composition of the household. The impact of household transmission depends on the concentration of community-acquired infections in households. We illustrate the model using empirical contact matrices derived from time-use data that allow us to distinguish between public and household contacts. We simulate a severe epidemic resulting in approximately twice the number of cases that arose from the 2009 A/H1N1 outbreak to quantify the contribution of household transmission to the total number of cases.

The role of household transmission has received significant attention in the literature. The empirical literature has sought to estimate transmission parameters that may differ across community and household environments using reported and serologic infection data [2, 9, 15, 20]. Theoretical models have been proposed to attempt to capture household transmission dynamics [4]. We bridge these literatures by proposing an extension to the compartmental model with heterogeneous mixing rates, which are based on empirical contact patterns in community and household environments.

Social distancing policies or non-pharmaceutical interventions such as school closure are an important public health policy available to officials during a crisis [6]. Such social distancing policies are designed to mitigate public exposure to disease risk and consequently, increase exposure in the household [11, 17, 22]. Individuals may also engage in voluntary distancing behavior to avoid infection risk

[8, 12, 13, 25]. Regardless of the reason for modifying behavior, the ability to model public and household transmission is critical to forecasting the effect of social distancing policies.

We find that explicitly modeling household transmission heightens the severity of the epidemic at the peak as individuals are more likely to make household contacts with potentially infectious family members. However, household transmission accounts for only 12 % of total cases when new cases concentration into households is density dependent, and 23 % of total cases when new cases are completely dispersed among households.

2 Compartmental Model

The standard compartmental model of infectious disease with heterogeneous mixing is based on mean contact rates between segments of the population [7]. The mean contact rate at the population level is sufficient when all individuals in the population may experience potentially infectious contacts with every other individual in the population. Household mixing patterns differ from public mixing patterns because the universe of potential contacts is limited to the family members that reside in their household.[1] Moreover, a single household can be either safe with no infected individuals or infectious with at least one infected individual. As new individuals become infected, the model must determine the household in which newly infected individuals reside. The population level model is not designed to track the infection status of individuals. We solve this problem by introducing a new set of state variables for the health status of households.

We build on the standard Susceptible-Infectious-Recovered (SIR) model with heterogeneity in mixing rates between subpopulations. The subpopulations are defined by the $K = 35$ combinations of age group and household size {0–4, 5–12, 13–17, 18–24, 25–49, 50–64, 65+} × {1, 2, 3, 4, 5+}. Mixing rates differ between public locations and the household. There are $L = 5$ household sizes $\{1, 2, 3, 4, 5+\}$. A household is considered infected if at least one member of the household is infected. Each individual and each household is susceptible, infected, or recovered for a total of $3(K + L)$ state variables. The transmission dynamics are described by the system of differential equations.

[1] Friends of family members may also be potential contacts but we restrict the household population to family members for simplicity. Moreover, individuals may avoid time with friends during an epidemic in which health status is uncertain.

$$\dot{S} = -\left(S \circ \delta C \left(\frac{I}{N} \right) + ZH_I \circ \left[\frac{S}{N_H} \circ \delta C^h \left(\frac{I}{N} \right) \right] \circ \left[Z \left(1 - \frac{H_I}{H} \right)^{-1} \right] \right);$$
$$\dot{I} = \left(S \circ \delta C \left(\frac{I}{N} \right) + ZH_I \circ \left[\frac{S}{N_H} \circ \delta C^h \left(\frac{I}{N} \right) \right] \circ \left[Z \left(1 - \frac{H_I}{H} \right)^{-1} \right] \right) - \nu I;$$
$$\dot{R} = \nu I \tag{1}$$
$$\dot{H}_S = -\left(Z' \left[S \circ \delta C \left(\frac{I}{N} \right) \right] \circ \frac{H_S}{H} \right);$$
$$\dot{H}_I = -\left(Z' \left[S \circ \delta C \left(\frac{I}{N} \right) \right] \circ \frac{H_S}{H} \right) - \nu H_I;$$
$$\dot{H}_R = \nu I$$

where $\circ$ and / denotes element by element multiplication and division. $\boldsymbol{S}$, $\boldsymbol{I}$, and $\boldsymbol{R}$ are $K \times 1$ vectors of susceptible, infectious, and recovered health classes, $\boldsymbol{H_S}$, $\boldsymbol{H_I}$, and $\boldsymbol{H_R}$ are $L \times 1$ vectors of susceptible, infectious, and recovered household classes, and $\dot{x} = dx/dt$ for $x = \{\boldsymbol{S}, \boldsymbol{I}, \boldsymbol{R}, \boldsymbol{H_S}, \boldsymbol{H_I}, \boldsymbol{H_R}\}$. $\boldsymbol{N}$ is an $K \times 1$ vector of subpopulations in each segment. $\boldsymbol{N_H}$ is a $K \times 1$ vector of the number of households in each subpopulation. $\boldsymbol{H}$ is a $L \times 1$ vector of the number of households in each size class. $\boldsymbol{Z}$ is a $K \times L$ conformability matrix of zeros with ones in each column indicating subpopulations with household size equal to the column number. $\boldsymbol{ZH_I}$ expands the $L \times 1$ vector of the number of households infected by size class into a $K \times 1$ where the size class is repeated for each age group. $\boldsymbol{C}$ and $\boldsymbol{C^h}$ are $K \times K$ public and household probabilistic contact matrices, PCM, [5] that describe the interaction time in minutes between an individual in subpopulation j (rows) and subpopulation k (columns). The PCMs are estimated from time-use data and are described in Sect. 3. δ is the disease-specific infectivity parameter, or conditional probability of transmission per minute of contact between a susceptible and infected individual. $1/\nu$ is the average infectious period constant across classes. We adopt the standard assumption of a constant population, which implies $\boldsymbol{N}(t) = \boldsymbol{S}(t) + \boldsymbol{I}(t) + \boldsymbol{R}(t)$ and $\boldsymbol{H}(t) = \boldsymbol{H_S}(t) + \boldsymbol{H_I}(t) + \boldsymbol{H_R}(t)$ for all t.

Individuals exit the susceptible state and enter the infected state by contracting the infection through public or household contacts [16, 20]. Infections acquired in public locations are governed by the term $\boldsymbol{S} \circ \delta \boldsymbol{C} \left(\frac{\boldsymbol{I}}{\boldsymbol{N}} \right)$. This term is the contact time analog to the standard heterogeneous mixing model. In public locations, susceptible individuals may encounter any infectious individuals in the population. The second transmission term describes transmission in households with at least one infected individual by subpopulation $\boldsymbol{H_I}$; all other households $(\boldsymbol{H} - \boldsymbol{H_I})$ are completely safe because all household members are susceptible or recovered. Household transmission dynamics are similar to those in public, but the set of possible contacts at any moment in time is limited by the number of susceptible individuals in the household ($\boldsymbol{S}/\boldsymbol{N_H}$ in expectation for a randomly chosen household). As the outbreak progresses, the number of susceptible individuals in the household is displaced by recovered individuals.

As the number of new infections rises, multiple infected individuals are likely to be in the same household. The term $Z\left(1-\frac{H_I}{H}\right)^{-1}$ is a contact intensity multiplier that accounts for the relative increase in infection risk in households with a higher concentration of infected individuals relative to the population mean $\left(\frac{I}{N}\right)$.

The second set of state equations determines the health status of households. Susceptible H_S households become infected if at least one member of the household becomes infected. Therefore, the initial infected member(s) of the household must acquire the infection from contacts made in a public location. However, not all new infected individuals are necessarily members of different households. A new infectious individual does not equal a new infectious household. We assume that the rate at which a new infected individual translates into a new infected household is dependent on the density of susceptible households $\left(\frac{H_S}{H}\right)$. Early in the outbreak, most households will be susceptible as each are unlikely to house one of the few infected individuals, which implies that new infected individuals are more likely to be a member of a susceptible household. As the epidemic progresses, the probability that new infections acquired in public reside in already infected households rises, thus increasing the concentration of infected individuals in the infected household. Note the contact intensity term within a household $Z\left(1-\frac{H_I}{H}\right)^{-1}$ is inversely proportional to $\frac{H_S}{H}$. We assume that households recover at the same rate as individuals, which would be true if a household were only infected for a single generation. This recovery rate could vary by household size as larger households may experience several generations.

3 Epidemic Simulation and Probabilistic Contact Matrices

We simulate epidemics under several alternative household infection assumptions to illustrate the role of concentration of infected individuals in households on transmission dynamics. New infections acquired in public may result in a spectrum of infected households ranging from highly concentrated where each new infected individual resides in an already infected household to dispersed where each new infected individual resides in a different household. We simulate epidemics under these two extreme assumptions and compare them to our proposed model with density dependent concentration of new infections.

We calibrate the simulations to an epidemic in the U.S. approximately twice as severe as the 2009 A/H1N1 outbreak. The average infectious period is 2.6 days—chosen to match the 2009 A/H1N1 epidemic [9, 10, 29]. We calibrate the infectivity per minute parameter, δ =0.0016, to produce an epidemic approximately twice as severe as the 2009 A/H1N1 swine flu epidemic, which was estimated to have affected 60.8 [43.3, 89.3] million Americans [24].

The population and mixing patterns data come from the US Census and Bureau of Labor Statistics. The US population, N, in 2011 is approximately 310 million and there are 117 million households, H [28]. The probabilistic contact matrices are estimated from the American Time-Use Survey (ATUS) (2003–2012) [27]. The ATUS is subsampled from the U.S. Current Population Survey—a nationally representative survey that contains detailed demographic and socioeconomic information about respondents older than 15 years old and their family members (including children under 15 years of age). Survey respondents report a 24-h diary of activities, locations, and accompanying persons for every minute of the day. We supplement the ATUS data with time-use data from the National Health and Activity Patterns Survey (NHAPS), a similar time-use survey, that includes children under 15 years old [19]. The combined dataset consists of 146,331 respondents with sample weights that report an average of 16.1 activities per day.

We estimate PCMs, $\boldsymbol{C}$ and $\boldsymbol{C}^h$ for each location or "microenvironment" described in the ATUS by the proportional time mixing (PTM) method [5, 30]. The PTM method assumes that subpopulations (e.g., age 19–24 in two-person households) contact each other in proportion to their share of the population present in a given microenvironment at a given time. Figure 1 illustrates these contact patterns in public and household locations. Details of the PCM calculations are provided in the supplementary information of [5]. Public contacts occur in non-household microenvironments where individuals are likely to experience incidental interactions with non-acquaintances. Household PCMs capture the contact patterns of individuals with

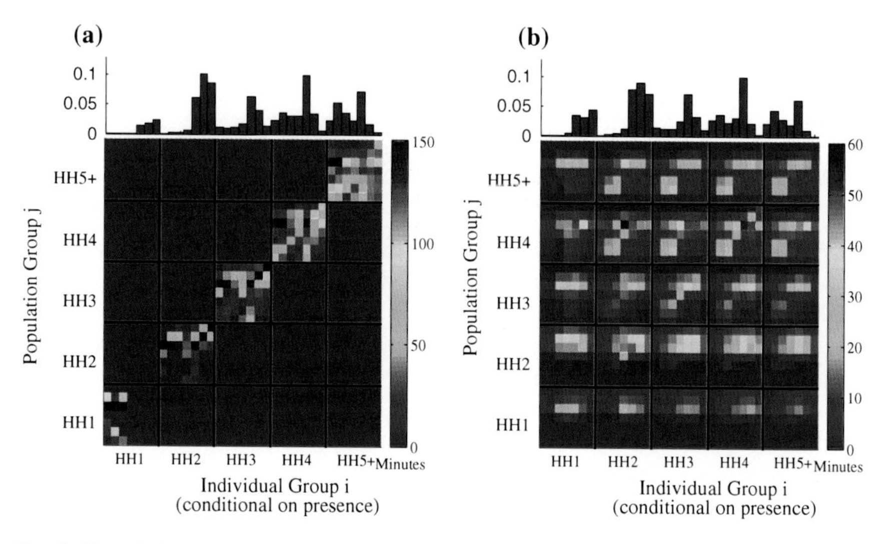

Fig. 1 Household and public PCMs with empirical population distributions above. Dark lines denote the five household size groups. Each household size category consists of the seven age groups for a total of 35 groups ($\{0\text{–}4, 5\text{–}12, 13\text{–}17, 18\text{–}24, 25\text{–}49, 50\text{–}64, 65+\} \times \{1, 2, 3, 4, 5+\}$). Note these bins are not of equal width. A cell represents the number of contact minutes an individual in group i interacts with the population of group j. The vertical sum of cells in a single column is equal to an individual's total contact minutes. The vertical axis of the population distribution (bar chart) is group i percent of the population. Note, these are the transpose of C described in the main text. **a** Household. **b** Public

family members in their home. Each household is treated as a unique microenvironment so that the universe of possible contacts is limited to members of the household. The population-level household PCM is a weighted average of individual household contact patterns resulting in the contact patterns of a representative household with some of each subpopulation. There is no household mixing between household sizes, because every member of the household shares the household size attribute.

4 Results

We compare the epidemic simulation results under a range of assumptions regarding the concentration of new infections in households (Fig. 2). The assumptions form a spectrum where on one end new infected individuals are assumed to be concentrated if they all reside in the same households such that susceptible and infected individuals make no contact in the household (blue solid line in Fig. 2). On the other end of the spectrum, new infected individuals are assumed to fully disperse into susceptible homes maximizing the potentially infectious household contacts (red dashed line in Fig. 2). We also consider a density dependent assumption where new infected individuals are more likely to infect a previously safe household when the proportion of susceptible or safe households is large (yellow dash-dotted line in Fig. 2). The simulation results show that peak prevalence under the density dependent assumption lies between the fully concentrated and fully dispersed assumptions. The attack rate under density dependence is 48 % of the population versus 42 and 55 % under the fully concentrated and fully dispersed assumptions, respectively.

Two opposing forces influence household transmission throughout the epidemic. As individuals become infected, more households necessarily become infected. How-

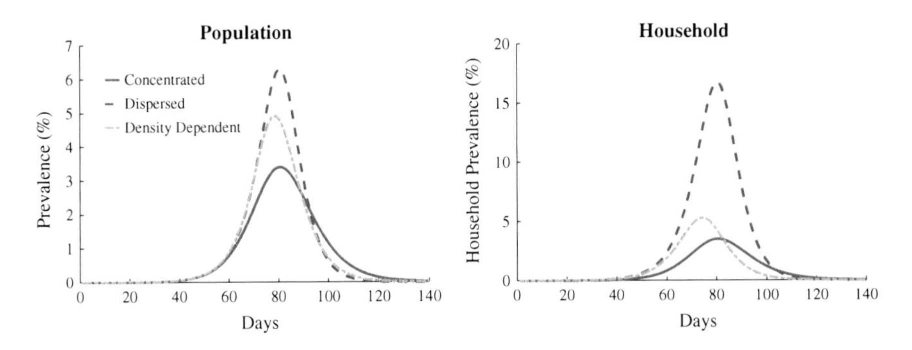

Fig. 2 Aggregate prevalence paths of similar epidemics under alternative household infection assumptions. The Concentrated case assumes that all new infections acquired in public reside in infected households so there is no additional risk to the susceptible population. The Dispersed case assumes that all new infections reside in a different household. The Density Dependent case assumes that new infections are dispersed across susceptible households when few households are infected, and become more concentrated when more households are infected

ever, if those new cases acquired in public return to the same household, the number of newly infected households grows at a slower rate than the number of new infections thus increasing the concentration of infectious people in households. The lower rate of growth in infected households relative to infected individuals (household safety effect) attenuates the impact of household transmission on the overall progress of the epidemic. However, susceptible individuals in households with a higher concentration of infected individuals face increased risk of acquiring the infection (exposure intensity effect). The simulation results suggest that the household safety effect dominates the contact intensity effect since the peak prevalence and overall attack rate are smaller under the density dependent assumption compared to the dispersed assumption.

We find evidence of significant heterogeneity in concentration and exposure intensity between household sizes. Figure 3 depicts the concentration index $\left(1 - \frac{H_S}{N_H}\right)$ by household size throughout the course of the epidemic. The results show that early in the epidemic newly infected individuals are very dispersed across households. As the epidemic gains momentum, the concentration index rises rapidly in each household size. The concentration index reaches 0.57 in households of two and over 0.90 in households of 4 or more. The household size distribution from the United States Census indicates that there are more 2-person households than 4 or more person households (33 % versus 23 % of total households). The high concentration index in larger households is a result of an increased likelihood that at least someone in a household with 4 or more persons becomes infected. However, such statistics are likely to vary greatly across countries. For example, we may expect Thailand to have more 4, 5, or even larger households for cultural, economic, and policy reasons. Figure 4 depicts the exposure intensity $\left(1 - \frac{H_I}{N_H}\right)^{-1}$ by household size over the course of the epidemic. The peak exposure intensity in 2-person households (1.06) is slightly more than half of the exposure intensity in 4 or more person households (1.11).

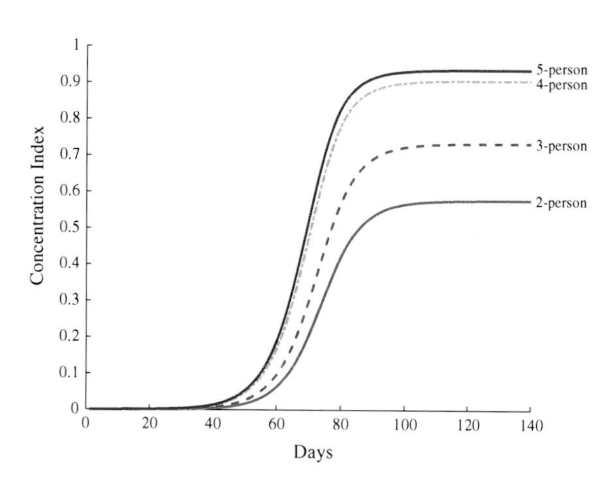

Fig. 3 Concentration index by household size over the course of the epidemic

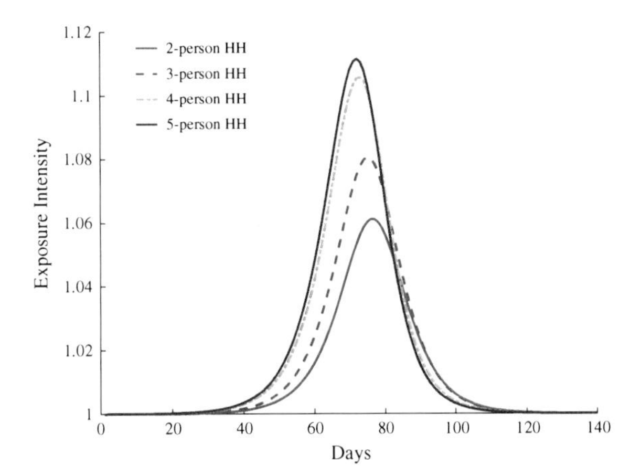

Fig. 4 Exposure intensity by household size over the course of the epidemic

The spectrum of concentration assumptions made for the simulation permits a disentangling of the effects of household versus public or community transmission. The assumption that all new infected individuals concentrate in the same households is equivalent to assuming no household transmission occurs. Therefore, all outcomes under the Concentrated assumption are attributable to public transmission. Given the simulation under the Density Dependent and Dispersed assumptions are conducted under identical epidemic conditions, we can infer that any additional cases resulting from these assumptions are attributable to household transmission. We find that household transmission accounts for 12 % of total transmission under the Density Dependent assumption and 23 % of total transmission under the Dispersed assumption. Thus, the [14] estimate of nearly a third of transmission resulting within households may be reasonable for societies with large household sizes (though this would also depend on contact patterns), but is likely to high for western societies with smaller household sizes.

5 Discussion

Household transmission has received significant attention in the empirical epidemiology literature. However, many studies focus on secondary infections once an index case has been introduced [9]. Our results suggest that household transmission, while important, especially to those susceptible individuals in infected households, is likely small relative to public or community transmission. The relative magnitude of public transmission also supports voluntary or mandatory social distancing that leads people to spend more time at home [5].

We assume that a higher concentration of infected individuals in a household increases the risk of infection to the susceptible individuals in the same household. This intuition is consistent with the Reed–Frost model in which contacts are considered independent events and cumulatively increase infection risk as contacts increase [3, 15]. Alternatively, the impact of additional infectious individuals beyond one may not significantly impact infection risk because the pathogen is already in the environment. Indeed, [9] find that larger households exhibit lower secondary attack rates than smaller households. Our exposure intensity measure may be exaggerating the infection risk in larger households.

Despite our efforts to incorporate realistic features of household transmission, the compartmental model is a population level model. Consequently, households are not distinct units. The mechanics of the model effectively allow individuals within a household size to instantaneously move among like households. While this is not strictly accurate, accounting for the concentration of new infected individuals into households can help mitigate the overestimation of transmission.

6 Conclusion

We extend the SIR compartmental model of infectious disease with heterogeneous mixing to include household transmission. We introduce new household health compartments to track the health status of households over the course of the epidemic. Explicitly modeling household compartments permits a calculation of the concentration of newly infected individuals. We parameterize density dependent concentration of newly infected individuals, which captures the likely early dispersal of new infections into susceptible households and the increased concentration as few susceptible households remain by the end of the epidemic. The model highlights the countervailing forces of more safe households as concentration rises with the higher exposure intensity of those susceptible individuals in infected households. Finally, we quantify the relative contribution of household transmission to public or community transmission and find that it ranges from 12 to 23 % in the United States depending on the concentration assumption.

References

1. Anderson, R.M., May, R.M.: Age-related changes in the rate of disease transmission: implications for the design of vaccination programmes. J. Hyg. **94**(3), 365–436 (1985)
2. Ball, F., Neal, P.: A general model for stochastic SIR epidemics with two levels of mixing. Math. Biosci. **180**(1–2), 73–102 (2002). doi:10.1016/S0025-5564(02)00125-6
3. Ball, F., Mollison, D., Scalia-Tomba, G.: Epidemics with two levels of mixing. Ann. Appl. Probab. **7**(1), 46–89 (1997)
4. Ball, F., Sirl, D., Trapman, P.: Analysis of a Stochastic SIR Epidemic on a Random Network Incorporating Household Structure. Math. Biosci. **224**(2), 53–73 (2010). doi:10.1016/j.mbs.2009.12.003
5. Bayham, J., Kuminoff, N.V., Gunn, Q., Fenichel, E.P.: Measured voluntary avoidance behaviour during the 2009 A/H1N1 epidemic. Proc. R. Soc. B **282**(1818), 20150814 (2015). doi:10.1098/rspb.2015.0814

6. Bell, D., Nicoll, A., Fukuda, K., Horby, P., Monto, A.: Nonpharmaceutical interventions for pandemic influenza, national and community measures. Emerg. Infect. Dis. **12**(1), 88–94 (2006). doi:10.3201/eid1201.051371
7. Brauer, F., Castillo-Chávez, C.: Mathematical Models for Communicable Diseases. Society for Industrial and Applied Mathematics, Philadelphia (2013)
8. Caley, P., Philips, D.J., McCracken, K.: Quantifying social distancing arising from pandemic influenza. J. R. Soc. Interface **5**(23), 631–639 (2008). doi:10.1098/rsif.2007.1197
9. Cauchemez, S., Donnelly, C.A., Reed, C., Ghani, A.C., Fraser, C., Kent, C.K., Finelli, L., Ferguson, N.M.: Household transmission of 2009 pandemic influenza A (H1N1) virus in the United States. N. Engl. J. Med. **361**(27), 2619–2627 (2009). doi:10.1056/NEJMoa0905498
10. Chowell, G., Echevarría-Zuno, S., Viboud, C., Simonsen, L., Tamerius, J., Miller, M.A., Borja-Aburto, V.H.: Characterizing the epidemiology of the 2009 influenza A/H1N1 pandemic in Mexico. PLoS Med. **8**(5), e1000436 (2011). doi:10.1371/journal.pmed.1000436
11. Eames, K.T., Tilston, N.L., White, P.J., Adams, E., Edmunds, W.J.: The impact of illness and the impact of school closure on social contact patterns. Health Technol. Assess. **14**(34), 267–312 (2010)
12. Fenichel, E.P., Castillo-Chavez, C., Ceddia, M.G., Chowell, G., Parra, P.A., Hickling, G.J., Holloway, G., et al.: Adaptive human behavior in epidemiological models. Proc. Natl. Acad. Sci. **108**(15), 6306–6311 (2011). doi:10.1073/pnas.1011250108
13. Fenichel, E.P., Kuminoff, N.V., Chowell, G.: Skip the trip: air travelers' behavioral responses to pandemic influenza. PLoS ONE **8**(3), e58249 (2013). doi:10.1371/journal.pone.0058249
14. Ferguson, N.M., Cummings, D.A.T., Cauchemez, S., Fraser, C., Riley, S., Meeyai, A., Iamsirithaworn, S., Burke, D.S.: Strategies for containing an emerging influenza pandemic in Southeast Asia. Nature **437**(7056), 209–214 (2005). doi:10.1038/nature04017
15. Fraser, C., Cummings, D.A.T., Klinkenberg, D., Burke, D.S., Ferguson, N.M.: Influenza transmission in households during the 1918 pandemic. Am. J. Epidemiol. **174**(5), 505–514 (2011). doi:10.1093/aje/kwr122
16. House, T., Keeling, M.J.: Household structure and infectious disease transmission. Epidemiol. Infect. **137**(05), 654–661 (2009). doi:10.1017/S0950268808001416
17. Kelso, J.K., Milne, G.J., Kelly, H.: Simulation suggests that rapid activation of social distancing can arrest epidemic development due to a novel strain of influenza. BMC Public Health **9**(1), 117 (2009). doi:10.1186/1471-2458-9-117
18. Kermack, W.O., McKendrick, A.G.: Contributions to the mathematical theory of epidemics, Part 1. Proc. R. Soc., Lond. Ser. A **115**, 700–721 (1929)
19. Klepeis, N.E., Nelson, W.C., Ott, W.R., Robinson, J.P., Tsang, A.M., Switzer, P., Behar, J.V., Hern, S.C., Engelmann, W.H.: The national human activity pattern survey (NHAPS): a resource for assessing exposure to environmental pollutants. J. Expo. Anal. Environ. Epidemiol. **11**(3), 231–252 (2001)
20. Longini, I.M., Koopman, J.S., Monto, A.S., Fox, J.P.: Estimating household and community transmission parameters for influenza. Am. J. Epidemiol. **115**(5), 736–751 (1982)
21. Machens, A., Gesualdo, F., Rizzo, C., Tozzi, A.E., Barrat, A., Cattuto, C.: An infectious disease model on empirical networks of human contact: bridging the gap between dynamic network data and contact matrices. BMC Infect. Dis. **13**(April), 185 (2013). doi:10.1186/1471-2334-13-185
22. Maharaj, S., Kleczkowski, A.: Controlling epidemic spread by social distancing: do it well or not at all. BMC Public Health **12**(1), 679 (2012). doi:10.1186/1471-2458-12-679
23. Morin, B.R., Fenichel, E.P., Castillo-Chavez, C.: Sir dynamics with economically driven contact rates. Nat. Resour. Model. **26**(4), 505–525 (2013). doi:10.1111/nrm.12011
24. Shrestha, S.S., Swerdlow, D.L., Borse, R.H., Prabhu, V.S., Finelli, L., Atkins, C.Y., Owusu-Edusei, K., et al.: Estimating the burden of 2009 pandemic influenza A (H1N1) in the United States (April 2009–2010). Clin. Infect. Dis. **52**(suppl 1), S75–82 (2011). doi:10.1093/cid/ciq012
25. Springborn, M., Chowell, G., MacLachlan, M., Fenichel, E.P.: Accounting for behavioral responses during a flu epidemic using home television viewing. BMC Infect. Dis. **15**(1), 1–14 (2015). doi:10.1186/s12879-014-0691-0

26. Towers, S., Chowell, G.: Impact of weekday social contact patterns on the modeling of influenza transmission, and determination of the influenza latent period. J. Theor. Biol. **312**(November), 87–95 (2012). doi:10.1016/j.jtbi.2012.07.023
27. United States Department of Labor. Bureau of Labor Statistics. "American Time Use Survey." (2012)
28. US Census Bureau. "Summary File 1, Tables H4, H16, and H17." (2010)
29. Yang, Y., Sugimoto, J.D., Elizabeth Halloran, M., Basta, N.E., Chao, D.L., Matrajt, L., Potter, G., Kenah, E., Longini, I.M.: The transmissibility and control of pandemic influenza A (H1N1) virus. Science **326**(5953), 729–733 (2009). doi:10.1126/science.1177373
30. Zagheni, E., Billari, F.C., Manfredi, P., Melegaro, A., Mossong, J., John Edmunds, W.: Using time-use data to parameterize models for the spread of close-contact infectious diseases. Am. J. Epidemiol. **168**(9), 1082–1090 (2008). doi:10.1093/aje/kwn220

Bistable Endemic States in a Susceptible-Infectious-Susceptible Model with Behavior-Dependent Vaccination

Alberto d'Onofrio and Piero Manfredi

Abstract Several new vaccines have the characteristic of being "imperfect" that is their protection wanes over time and supplies only partial protection from infection. On the other hand recent research has shown that the agents' behavioral responses have the potential to dramatically affect the dynamics and control of infections. In this paper we investigate, for a simple susceptible-infective-susceptible (SIS) infection, the dynamic interplay between human behavior, in the form of an increasing prevalence-dependent vaccine uptake function, and vaccine imperfections. The mathematical analysis of the ensuing SISV model shows a complexly articulated bifurcation structure. First, the inclusion of the simplest possible hypothesis about vaccination behavior is capable to trigger, in appropriate windows of the key parameters, phenomena of multistability of endemic states. Second, as far as the stability of the disease-free equilibrium is concerned, the model preserves the backward bifurcation which is characteristic of SIS-type infections controlled by imperfect vaccines.

Keywords Vaccination · Behavior · Multistability · Epidemic models · Transmission dynamics · Backward bifurcation

1 Introduction

Multistability, i.e. the presence of multiple co-existing locally stable equilibria, is a critical concept in nonlinear dynamics, which has numberless and deep implications in biology and medicine. Two fields of biomedicine where this concept is increasingly

---

A. d'Onofrio (✉)
International Prevention Research Institute, 95 Cours Lafayette, 69006 Lyon, France
e-mail: alberto.donofrio@i-pri.org

P. Manfredi
Department of Economics and Management, University of Pisa,
Via Ridolfi 10, 56124 Pisa, Italy
e-mail: piero.manfredi@unipi.it

G. Chowell and J.M. Hyman (eds.), *Mathematical and Statistical Modeling for Emerging and Re-emerging Infectious Diseases*,
DOI 10.1007/978-3-319-40413-4_21

gaining prominent are immunology and molecular biology. In the latter, in particular, the word bistability has became of quite common use also among experimental scientists.

For several decades the vast majority of mathematical epidemiology research has focused on monostable systems, and on their well-known paradigm that can be summarized as follows: *there is an appropriate threshold parameter, often termed the reproduction number (RN) of the model, such that if the RN is smaller than one then the disease-free equilibrium (DFE) is unique and globally attractive, whereas if the RN it is larger than one then the DFE is unstable and a unique endemic equilibrium (EE) appears. Most often the EE is also globally attractive, in other cases, though far less frequently, it is surrounded by self-sustained oscillations* [18].

In last twenty years, however, it has been shown that certain feedback loops, such as those stemming from vaccine imperfection or waning, may complicate this scenario since they may induce the onset of bistability through so called "backward bifurcations" (BB). This type of bifurcation is typically characterized as follows: there is a value $b \in (0, 1)$ such that, although the DFE is locally asymptotically stable (unstable) for $RN < 1$ ($RN > 1$), nevertheless for values of the RN in the interval $(b, 1)$ there are two endemic equilibria: one unstable and the other one locally stable. Therefore, for $b < BRN < 1$ bistability occurs, with the birth at $RN = b$ of an endemic equilibrium that co-exists with the stable DFE. Note that for $RN > 1$ the DFE still exists but becomes unstable. This makes the BB deeply different from the more known hysteresis bifurcation, where there never is the coexistence of an even number of equilibria. Backward bifurcations have been found initially in a number of simple epidemic models [8, 16, 22, 23], in particular in models for infections without immunity, as the susceptible-infective-susceptible (SIS) model, when the vaccine is imperfect [23]. There is evidence that the phenomenon is also frequent in more realistic models, so that BB are also becoming important, due to their negative implications for infection elimination, from the public health viewpoint [20].

Classical epidemiological models are built upon some founding principles, namely the law of mass action of statistical mechanics, which is used to model at once social contacts between individuals and infection transmission. Though critical in promoting the take off of mathematical epidemiology as a discipline, the law of mass action is a gross simplification or reality whereby individuals entering into social contacts are represented as "collisions" between the particles of a perfect gas. This in turn implies that social contacts and transmission parameters are dealt with as "universal constants" which are therefore unaffected by e.g. the states of the infection and the disease. Said otherwise, individuals would continue to come into contact at the same rate, irrespective of how low or high is the risk of acquiring the infection, or of dying from it, that they might perceive from the available information on current and past infection prevalence and seriousness. The idea that human behavior is static is far distant from the reality and constitutes one of the strongest limitation of traditional epidemiological models. By their intimate nature, human beings are neither static nor passive. Changes in humans' behavior in response to infection threats are indeed well documented already in outbreaks in historical epochs (where however they mostly occurred in the form of community-enforced measures), but seem to be a rule ([15]

and references therein) in current societies, possibly stemming from the continued progress of scientific knowledge on diseases and communications technologies [6]. Modern individuals can therefore spontaneously change in a complicate manner their social behavior in response to a pandemic threat, as well documented for the 2009 H1N1 pandemics [15], or can shift their sexual activity towards partners that are perceived as being as less-at-risk in response to news about a threatening STI [21]. But they might also decide not to vaccinate their children after having compared perceived costs and benefits of a vaccination program, or to stop vaccinating after a rumour, thereby threatening the success of the program, as it has been the case for the pertussis whole-cell vaccine scare, and the persistent decline in MMR vaccine coverage in the UK due to the alert for the suspected relation between MMR and autism ([6] and references therein). From the latter standpoint human behavior is representing an increasing challenge not only for modelers but also for public health policies. Indeed, depending on not-easy-to-predict circumstances, the effects of human behavior on infection dynamics can range—and switch—from policy-enforcing to policy-threatening [7].

The importance of human behavior for the understanding of infection dynamics and for the development of resilient policy interventions has led in the last fifteen years to the take-off of the new branch that we termed the *behavioral epidemiology* (BE) of infectious diseases [6]. A major area of current behavioral epidemiology of infections deals with immunization choices, particularly in relation to childhood vaccine preventable infections. This interest in motivated not only by the aforementioned vaccine crises related to the big "vaccine scares" but also by the dramatically changed context of mass immunization in modern societies. This epochal change is the consequence of decades of successful mass immunization against traditionally threatening infections, within the overall changed landscape of infectious diseases in industrialized countries, due to the continued success of man in controlling diseases threats thanks to medical progress [6]. A major implication of these successes is for example the full overturning of perceived risks [28], with the perceived risk of vaccine adverse events becoming the major determinant of vaccination [12].

After a few forerunners [6, 17, 19], the last epoch has seen an explosion of studies of the interplay between the diffusion of information about perceived risks due to the infection on the one hand, and risks of vaccine adverse events on the other hand, and the infection dynamics and control. These investigations have resorted to a variety of different approaches, either "behavior implicit" or "behavior explicit" based e.g. on game-theoretic or other representations of behavior, to unfold the complicate relationship between human choices and infection control (e.g. [3–5, 10–14, 24–27, 29, 30] and references therein).

However, in this fast growing literature on the behavioral epidemiology of vaccination no studies have investigated, to the best of our knowledge, the dynamic implications of vaccinating behavior within the framework of models for imperfect vaccines showing backward bifurcations. Given the peculiar role played by vaccine characteristics in promoting or not BBs, it is of interest to investigate whether the interplay between vaccinating behavior and imperfect vaccines might trigger further interesting dynamic phenomena.

In this paper we study a model including a simple behavioral assumption about vaccination within one of the simplest framework capable to yield a backward bifurcation, namely the SIS model with imperfect vaccination (SISV) by Kribs-Zaleta and Velasco-Hernandez [23]. In particular vaccinating behavior is incorporated following the "behavior implicit" [6], phenomenologically-based, formulation proposed in [10] where the vaccine uptake at birth is specified as an increasing function of current infection prevalence.

2 The SISV Model with Prevalence-Dependent Vaccine Uptake and Its Disease-Free Equilibrium

The modelling framework considered is that of a stationary and homogeneously mixing population where an infection without immunity can be controlled by immunization at birth (instead than [23] who considered vaccination at constant rate). The vaccine is assumed to be "imperfect" i.e. protection wanes over time and moreover vaccinated subjects can acquire infection, though at a reduced rate compared to fully susceptible individuals. Vaccination is assumed to be voluntary according to a prevalence-dependent schedule $p(I) \in [0, 1]$, where I denotes the relative infection prevalence and p an increasing function with $p(0) \geq 0$. This formulation [10] amounts to assume that parents decide to vaccinate or not their children depending on the perceived risk of infection, possibly measured by the publicly available current information on infection prevalence. Though oversimplified, because behavior-implicit, this model can be shown to be consistent with more refined behavioral schemes, for example with a prevalence-dependent behavior-explicit vaccination schedule based on an imitation process [4], provided the social spread of behavior is fast compared to other processes [13]. These hypotheses yield the following SISV model:

$$\begin{aligned} S' &= \mu(1 - p(I)) - \mu S - \beta I S + \gamma I + \theta V, \\ I' &= I\left(\beta(S + \sigma V) - (\mu + \gamma)\right), \\ V' &= \mu p(I) - \sigma\beta I V - (\mu + \theta)V \end{aligned} \tag{1}$$

where: $S, I, V, S + I + V = 1$, respectively denote the fractions of susceptible, infective, and vaccinated individuals, μ denotes both the death and birth rates (taken equal to ensure that the population remains stationary over time), β the transmission rate for naive susceptibles, $\sigma\beta$ $(0 < \sigma < 1)$ the reduced transmission rate for vaccinated subjects, γ the rate of recovery from infection, θ the vaccine waning rate. By the equality $S + I + V = 1$ one of the model equations can be eliminated yielding a 2-dimensional system. Using $S = 1 - (I + V)$ we get:

$$I' = \beta I\left(p_{cr} - I - (1 - \sigma)V\right), \tag{2}$$

$$V' = \mu p(I) - (\mu + \theta + \sigma\beta I)V \tag{3}$$

In (2) the constant p_{cr} is the critical immunization threshold [1] for infection elimination by a (hypothetical) perfect vaccine, in absence of behavioral effects:

$$p_{cr} = 1 - \frac{1}{R_0}$$

where $R_0 = \beta/(\mu + \gamma)$ denotes the basic reproduction number of the infection, representing the number of secondary infections caused by a single infective case in a wholly susceptible population (therefore in the absence of any immunization).

As a preliminary step, note that from the differential inequality

$$I' \leq \beta I (p_{cr} - I)$$

it is trivial to show that it asymptotically holds:

$$0 < I(t) < p_{cr}.$$

Thus in the following we shall study system (2) and (3) in the set

$$A = \{(I, V) | I \in [0, p_{cr}] \; AND (V, I) \geq (0, 0) \; AND \; I + V \leq 1\}$$

System (2) and (3) always admits the following disease free equilibrium (DFE):

$$DFE = \left(0, \frac{\mu}{\mu + \theta} p(0)\right).$$

A linearization of system (2) and (3) straightforwardly yields that the local asymptotic stability (LAS) of the DFE is governed by the equation:

$$i' = \beta i \left(p_{cr} - (1 - \sigma) \frac{\mu}{\mu + \theta} p(0)\right).$$

This means that the DFE will be LAS if the following condition holds:

$$p(0) > p_{cr} \frac{1}{1 - \sigma} \left(1 + \frac{\theta}{\mu}\right), \tag{4}$$

which can also be reformulated as $R_V < 1$ where R_V is the vaccine reproduction number:

$$R_V = R_0 \frac{\theta + \mu(1 - p(0)) + \sigma \mu p(0)}{\theta + \mu}, \tag{5}$$

Condition (4) states that the local stability of the DFE requires that the "zero-prevalence" vaccine uptake, i.e. the vaccine uptake that spontaneously arises under conditions of minimal perceived risk of infection, must exceed the critical elimination threshold p_{cr} by a factor $(1-\sigma)^{-1}(1+\theta/\mu)$. Note that this factor is increasing in both parameters (σ and θ) tuning the degree of "imperfection" of the vaccine. Suppose now that the average length of vaccine-induced immunity (θ^{-1}) is significantly smaller than the average lifespan μ^{-1}. In such a case, condition (4) might be fulfilled only for diseases that in the same time: (i) are characterized by a low critical threshold; (ii) can induce, also when their prevalence is low, a large perceived risk. This condition extends to the present SISV model the result that in our past work on behavior-implicit SIRV models we termed "elimination: mission impossible" [13].

In order to proceed further, let us rewrite system (2) and (3) in the following equivalent form that we will adopt in the next sections:

$$I' = \beta(1-\sigma)I\left(L(I)-V\right), \tag{6}$$
$$V' = (\mu+\theta+\sigma\beta I)\left(\Psi(I)-V\right) \tag{7}$$

where:

$$L(I) = \frac{p_{cr}-I}{(1-\sigma)}$$

is the nullcline $I'=0$; and:

$$\Psi(I) = \frac{\mu p(I)}{(\mu+\theta+\sigma\beta I)}$$

is the nullcline $V'=0$.
Endemic equilibria of (6) and (7) are the non-trivial intersections of the two nullclines.

3 Instability of the Disease-Free State: Mono Versus Multistability

In this section we shall assume that the baseline vaccination rate $\mu p(0)$ is not sufficient to guarantee the elimination of the infection, i.e. we shall assume that

$$0 < p(0) < p_{cr}\frac{1}{1-\sigma}\left(1+\frac{\theta}{\mu}\right). \tag{8}$$

Note preliminarily that in the case of prevalence-independent vaccine uptake the following result holds:

Lemma *If $p(I)$ is constant and (8) holds then (6) and (7) admit a unique endemic equilibrium point.*

We now show that if Ψ is non-monotonic then there may be either a single or multiple equilibrium points.

As a first step, note that the local stability properties of all endemic equilibria of (6) and (7) depend on the following characteristic polynomial

$$\lambda^2 + (\mu + \theta + (1+\sigma)\beta I_e)\lambda + \beta I_e(\mu + \theta + \sigma\beta I_e)\left(1 + (1-\sigma)\Psi'(I_e)\right), \quad (9)$$

The condition for the local stability of endemic states therefore reads as follows:

$$\Psi'(I_e) > -\frac{1}{1-\sigma}. \quad (10)$$

i.e.

$$\Psi'(I_e) > L'(I_e). \quad (11)$$

The interpretation of condition (10) is immediate: if the linearized nullcline $V' = 0$ at a generic endemic equilibrium (EE) of (6) and (7) is steeper than the linearized nullcline $I' = 0$ at EE, then that particular endemic state EE is LAS, otherwise it is unstable.

As far as the V-nullcline $\Psi(I)$ is concerned, it is worth to note that:

Lemma *Under condition (8), if $\Psi(I)$ is monotone, i.e. if*

$$\mu p'(I) > \sigma\beta\Psi(I) \; OR \; \mu p'(I) < \sigma\beta\Psi(I),$$

or constant then system (6) and (7) has a unique equilibrium point.

Note, however, that uniqueness of the endemic state can also occur for some non-monotone $\Psi(I)$.

If there is a unique endemic equilibrium point, the following proposition holds:

Proposition *If system (6) and (7) has a unique equilibrium point EE_u then it is globally stable in A.*

Proof First, it is straightforward to verify that EE_u cannot be unstable, otherwise it could not be the unique endemic equilibrium. Then, denoting as F the bi-dimensional vector field associated to system (6) and (7) and applying the Dulac–Bendixon theorem with weigth function $1/I$ one gets:

$$div\left(\frac{1}{I}F\right) = -\beta - \sigma\beta - \frac{\mu+\theta}{I} < 0.$$

□

A necessary condition for the presence of multiple co-existing endemic equilibrium points, i.e. for endemic multistability, is that the V-nullcline $\Psi(I)$ is non-monotone. Depending on the parameters of the system, for example σ or c, which are embedded in the functions $L(I)$ and $\Psi(I)$ these equilibria can vary, thus determining hysteresis or pitchfork bifurcations (see next subsection for a noteworthy example).

Note that the type of bifurcation described here differs from the backward bifurcation phenomenon well known in mathematical epidemiology. Indeed the backward bifurcation describes the onset of bistability where one of the two co-existing locally stable equilibria is the disease-free equilibrium. Here, instead all the coexisting LAS equilibria are endemic equilibria. In the next subsection we will develop the relevant bifurcation analysis based on a particular form of the vaccine uptake function $p(I)$.

3.1 Bistable Endemicity Induced by a Linear-Saturated Vaccine Uptake $p(I)$

Let us consider the following linear-saturating vaccination rate:

$$p(I) = min(p(0) + cI, 1) \tag{12}$$

which increases for

$$0 < I < I_*(c) = \frac{1 - p(0)}{c}$$

and is constant thereafter.

It follows that for $I > I_*(c)$ the function $\Psi(I)$ is a decreasing hyperbolic function:

$$\Psi(I) = \frac{\mu}{\mu + \theta + \sigma\beta I} \tag{13}$$

which *does not depend on* c. The latter fact is of relevance when considering c as the bifurcation parameter. Instead, for $0 < I < I_*(c)$ the function $\Psi(I)$ depends on c as follows:

$$\Psi(I) = \frac{\mu(p(0) + cI)}{\mu + \theta + \sigma\beta I} \tag{14}$$

This implies that the condition for Ψ to be increasing in $0 < I < I_*(c)$ is

$$c > \sigma\beta\frac{p(0)}{\mu + \theta}.$$

Finally, if $\Psi(I)$ is increasing in $0 < I < I_*(c)$ then the condition for bistability is that the two solutions of the following equation

$$\frac{\mu}{\mu + \theta + \sigma\beta I} = \frac{p_{cr} - I}{1 - \sigma} \tag{15}$$

are both larger than $I_*(c)$.

Taking c as the bifurcation parameter, makes it the analysis of the system quite simple. Note preliminarly that if the Eq. (15) has no real positive solutions (i.e. if the hyperbolic function (13) does not intersect the nullcline $L(I)$) then there is only a unique endemic equilibrium. The other case is that the hyperbolic function (13) intersect the linear nullcline $L(I)$ in two points of positive abscissae I_l and $I_h > I_l$. If

$$I^*(c) \in (I_l, I_h)$$

then there is again a unique endemic equilibrium with

$$I_e = I_h,$$

i.e. independent of c. On the contrary if

$$I^*(c) < I_l$$

i.e. if

$$c > c_l = \frac{1 - p_0}{I_l} \tag{16}$$

then there is multistability with three co-existing endemic equilibria: (i) I_h which is LAS and constant, thus independent of c; (ii) I_l which is unstable and again constant, thus independent of c; (iii) a third equilibrium point $I_{small}(c)$ that is LAS and decreasing function of c, with

$$I_{small}(c_l) = I_l.$$

Finally, note that condition (16) for multistability is equivalent to state that

$$\Psi(I^*(c)) > L(I^*(c)). \tag{17}$$

In order to consider the role of σ as bifurcation parameter, it is useful to define the following functions

$$(\Psi_1(I;\sigma), L_1(I)) = (1-\sigma)(\Psi(I), L(I))$$

which have the following properties: $L_1(I)$ does not depend any more on σ, whereas $\Psi_1(I;\sigma)$ is a strictly decreasing function of σ.

As a consequence, let us consider a pair (c_0, σ_0) where $c_0 < c_l(\sigma_0)$. In such a case we have the above mentioned three equilibria, which also depend on σ. If one increases σ then the function $\Psi_1(I;\sigma)$ is pushed downward, the equilibrium $I_h(\sigma)$ increases whereas the other two initially get closer and then both disappear. In other words we are describing a scenario of a classical hysteresis bifurcation (Figs. 1 and 2).

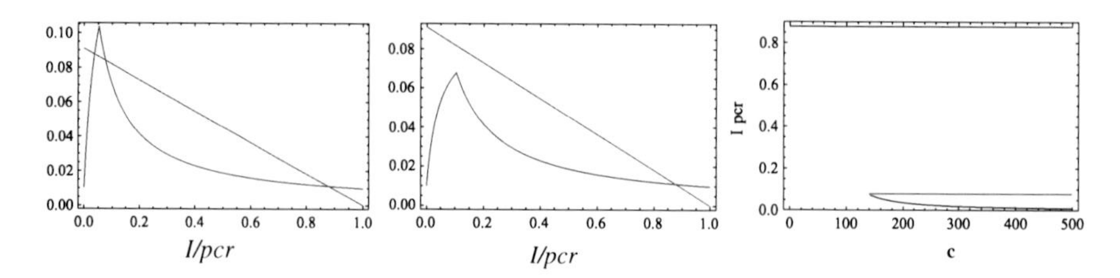

Fig. 1 Impact of the behavior-related parameter c on the number and location of endemic equilibria. In all panels $\sigma = 0.333$. *Left panel* for $c = 200$ the system exhibits three co-existing equilibria, as resulting from the intersection for the curves $\Psi_I(I)$ and $L_I(I)$; *Central panel* for $c = 10$ the central and the left endemic equilibria disappeared, whereas the right equilibrium was not affected at all by the change in the value of c; *Right panel* the full bifurcation diagram. Note that not only the largest equilibrium is constant, but also the central one (when it exists, i.e. for $c > c_I$)

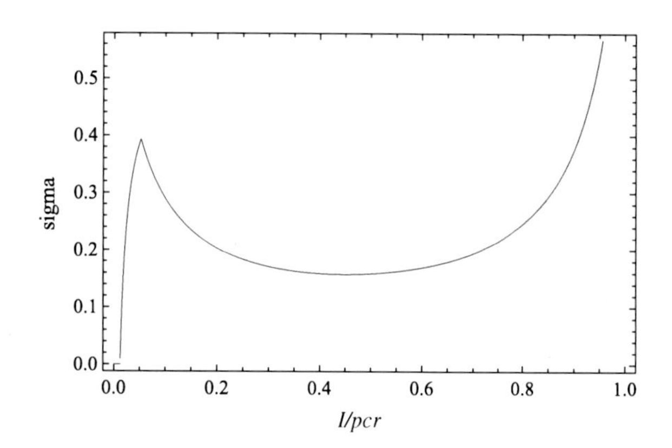

Fig. 2 Impact of the parameter σ on the number and location of endemic states: bifurcation diagram in the form I_e vs σ, under $c = 200$

4 Local Stability of the Disease-Free: Global Stability Versus Backward Bifurcations

In this section, for the sake of mathematical completeness, we shortly consider the issue of backward bifurcations, which is expected to occur in our model due to its SISV structure. We therefore focus on the case where the disease-free state is locally stable, i.e. the case where:

$$p(0) > p_{cr}\frac{1}{1-\sigma}\left(1 + \frac{\theta}{\mu}\right),$$

or equivalently

$$\Psi(0) > L(0). \tag{18}$$

First let us consider the case where the DFE is the unique equilibrium. Not surprisingly, the following proposition holds:

Proposition *If $\Psi(I) \geq L(I)$, i.e. if DFE is the unique equilibrium, then DFE is also Globally Asymptotically Stable (GAS) in A.*

Proof Let us define the following set:

$$B = \{(I, V) \in A | V \geq L(I)\} .$$

It is straightforward to show that if

$$\Psi(I) \geq L(I),$$

then B is a positively invariant set. The GAS of DFE in B then immediately follows by the following LaSalle–Liapunov function:

$$\mathcal{L}(I) = I.$$

□

Remark The above GAS condition yields:

$$p(I) > \frac{(p_c r - I)(\mu + \theta + \sigma\beta I)}{\mu(1 - \sigma)},$$

i.e. if the vaccination behavioral response function is greater than the LHS function, then the global eradication is reachable.

Note however that, still under (18), if the two nullclines intersect then (excluding the trivial case of tangency) there must be an even number of intersections, as it follows by applying elementary analysis to the function

$$D(I) = \Psi(I) - L(I).$$

Thus we are dealing again with a multistable case where however one of the LAS equilibrium states involved is represented by the disease-free equilibrium. Therefore, the related bifurcation which appears when, due to appropriately varying the model parameters, the system makes a transition from the situation where the DFE is the unique and globally asymptotically stable equilibrium to such type of multistability is exactly a "backward bifurcation" of the type described for SISV systems in [23].

5 Concluding Remarks

In relation to the current epoch of development of behavioral epidemiology [25], a large part of the modeling investigations of the potential effects of immunizations choices on the dynamics and control of infectious diseases have focused on the case of vaccine preventable infections, such as measles, which confers permanent immunity. Consequently most efforts in the literature have concentrated on susceptible-infective-removed (SIR) frameworks [3–5, 9–14, 24–26, 29, 30], see also the review in [6] about the historical development of the subject, and references therein. In relation to this, much of the emphasis has concentrated, though not exclusively, on the issue of the difficulty to eliminate the infection, and possible ways to prevent this drawback, and on the complicate dynamic patterns (e.g. oscillations) that can be triggered by more appropriate, both behavior-implicit and explicit, modeling of individual behavioral responses. This emphasis on traditional vaccine preventable SIR-type infections by no means exhausts the range of infections for which complicate behavioral responses by agents might be triggered by the introduction of a vaccine. Many other important infections conform instead to the SISV-type framework that has been considered in this paper. Among the many instances in relation to this there are for example bacterial infections, such as Meningococcal Meningitis. Though characterised by a complex epidemiology, Meningococcal Meningitis does not impart immunity and both vaccines that have been introduced to protect against the two Meningococci types widely circulating in Europe, namely groups C and B, are "imperfect". Another critical example, though based on a more complicate model structure, is tuberculosis [20]. As demonstrated in this paper the introduction of even the simplest possible hypothesis about human behavior, namely that of a behavior-implicit, prevalence-dependent vaccine uptake function, is capable to enrich the spectrum of possible dynamical behaviors of SISV-type models, by adding to the possibility of multi-stability on the sub-threshold side, the further possibility of multistability on the above-threshold side. The practical meaning of this finding is that the presence of agents' behavioral responses to the introduction of the vaccine might cause the appearance and coexistence of a number of stable (over appropriate basins) endemic states. This was to our knowledge the first theoretical investigation in this direction, based on a very simple, almost trivial, hypothesis on the agents' behavioral response. The follow-up of this first effort should therefore acknowledge a number of realistic features that just for the sake of simplicity had been neglected here. First of all one should, still within the boundary of behavior implicit models, consider the effects of time-delays, both in information supply and agents response, as opposed to the instantaneous adaptation of behavior postulated in this paper. These time-delays can generate complicate dynamical patterns even under simpler modeling frameworks, as the SIR model with information-dependent delay [10]. Even more interesting would be the inclusion of more structured, namely behavior explicit, behavioral responses, through e.g. imitation processes or their extensions [4, 5, 13, 14], or game-theoretic frameworks [2, 3, 27, 29, 30].

Acknowledgments The authors want to thank the anonymous referees for their important suggestions (e.g. the remark in Sect. 4), and the editors of this book, G. Chowell-Puente and J. (Mac) Hyman, for their kind assistance and remarkable patience....

References

1. Anderson, R.M., May, R.M.: Infectious Diseases in Humans: Dynamics and Control. Oxford University Press, Oxford (1991)
2. Bauch, C.T., Galvani, A.P., Earn, D.J.D.: Group interest versus self-interest in smallpox vaccination policy. Proc. Natl. Acad. Sci. USA **100**, 10564–10567 (2003)
3. Bauch, C.T., Earn, D.J.D.: Vaccination and the theory of games. Proc. Natl. Acad. Sci. USA **101**, 13391–13394 (2004)
4. Bauch, C.T.: Imitation dynamics predict vaccinating behavior. Proc. R. Soc. Lond. B **272**, 1669–1675 (2005)
5. Bauch, C.T., Bhattacharyya, S.: Evolutionary game theory and social learning can determine how vaccine scares unfold. PLoS Comp. Biol. **8**(4), e1002452 (2012)
6. Bauch, C.T., d'Onofrio, A., Manfredi, P.: Behavioral epidemiology of infectious diseases: an overview. In: Manfredi, P., d'Onofrio, A. (eds.) Modeling the Interplay Between Human Behavior and the Spread of Infectious Diseases, pp. 1–19. Springer, Heideberg (2013)
7. Bhattacharyya, S., Bauch, C.T.: Emergent dynamical features in behaviour-incidence models of vaccinating decisions. In: Manfredi, P., d'Onofrio, A. (eds.) Modeling the Interplay Between Human Behavior and the Spread of Infectious Diseases, pp. 243–254. Springer, Heideberg (2010)
8. Brauer, F.: Backward bifurcations in simple vaccination models. J. Math. Anal. Appl. **298**(2004), 418–431 (2004)
9. Buonomo, B., d'Onofrio, A., Lacitignola, D.: Global stability of an SIR epidemic model with-information dependent vaccination. Math. Biosci. **216**, 9–16 (2008)
10. d'Onofrio, A., Manfredi, P., Salinelli, E.: Vaccinating behaviour, information, and the dynamics of SIR vaccine preventable diseases. Theor. Popul. Biol. **71**, 301–317 (2007)
11. d'Onofrio, A., Manfredi, P., Salinelli, E.: Fatal SIR diseases and rational exemption to vaccination. Math. Med. Biol. **25**, 337–357 (2008)
12. d'Onofrio, A., Manfredi, P.: Vaccine demand driven by vaccine side effects: dynamic implications for SIR diseases. J. Theor. Biol. **264**, 237–252 (2010)
13. d'Onofrio, A., Manfredi, P., Poletti, P.: The impact of vaccine side effects on the natural history of immunization programmes: an imitation-game approach. J. Theor. Biol. **273**, 63–71 (2011)
14. d'Onofrio, A., Manfredi, P., Poletti, P.: The interplay of public intervention and private choices in determining the outcome of vaccination programmes. PLoS ONE **7**(10), e45653 (2012)
15. d'Onofrio, A., Manfredi, P.: Impact of human behavior on the spread of infectious diseases: a review of evidences and models, under review at Ecological Complexity (2015)
16. Dushoff, J., Huang, W., Castillo-Chavez, C.: Backwards bifurcations and catastrophe in simple models of fatal diseases. J. Math. Biol. **36**, 227–248 (1998)
17. Fine, P.E.M., Clarkson, J.A.: Individual versus public priorities in the determination of optimal vaccination policies. Am. J. Epidemiol. **124**, 1012–1020 (1986)
18. Gao, L., Mena Lorca, J., Hethcote, H.W.: Four SEI endemic models with periodicity and separatrices. Math. Biosci. **128**, 157–184 (1995)
19. Geoffard, P.Y., Philipson, T.: Disease eradication: private versus public vaccination. Am. Econ. Rev. **87**, 222–230 (1997)
20. Gerberry, D.J.: Practical aspects of backward bifurcation in a mathematical model for tuberculosis. J. Theor. Biol. **S0022–5193**(15), 00496–00498 (2015)
21. Gregson, S., Garnett, G.P., Nyamukapa, C.A., Hallett, T.B., Lewis, J.J.C., et al.: HIV decline associated with behavior change in Eastern Zimbabwe. Science **311**, 664–666 (2006)
22. Hadeler, K.P., van den Driessche, P.: Backward bifurcation in epidemic control. Math. Biosci. **146**, 15–35 (1997)
23. Kribs-Zaleta, C.M., Velasco-Hernanndez, J.X.: A simple vaccination model with multiple endemic states. Math. Biosci. **164**, 183–201 (2000)
24. Manfredi, P., della Posta, P., d'Onofrio, A., Salinelli, E., Centrone, F., Meo, C., Poletti, P.: Optimal vaccination choice, vaccination games, and rational exemption: an appraisal. Vaccine **28**, 98–109 (2009)

25. Manfredi, P., d'Onofrio, A. (eds.): Modeling the Interplay Between Human Behavior and the Spread of Infectious Diseases. Springer, New York (2013)
26. Reluga, T.C., Bauch, C.T., Galvani, A.P.: Evolving public perceptions and stability uptake. Math. Biosci. **204**, 185–198 (2006)
27. Reluga, T.C., Galvani, A.P.: A general approach for population games with application to vaccination. Math. Biosci. **230**(2), 67–78 (2011)
28. Salmon, D.A., Teret, S.P., MacIntyre, C.R., Salisbury, D., Burgess, M.A., Halsey, N.A.: Compulsory vaccination and conscientious or philosophical exemptions: past, present and future. Lancet **367**, 436–442 (2006)
29. Shim, E., Kochin, B., Galvani, A.P.: Insights from epidemiological game theory into gender-specific vaccination against rubella. Math. Biosci. Eng. **6**(4), 839–854 (2009)
30. Shim, E., Grefenstette, J.J., Albert, S.M., Cakouros, B.E., Burke, D.S.: A game dynamic model for vaccine skeptics and vaccine believers: measles as an example. J. Theor. Biol. **295**(2012), 194–203 (2012)

Index

G. Chowell and J.M. Hyman (eds.), *Mathematical and Statistical Modeling for Emerging and Re-emerging Infectious Diseases*,
DOI 10.1007/978-3-319-40413-4